CLINICAL
NEUROPHYSIOLOGY

To my wife

CONTENTS

ACKNOWLEDGEMENTS

In writing this book I have received much help from friends and colleagues. In particular I should like to thank Professor A. E. Ritchie for reading the whole text and for many helpful comments. Dr A. M. Fleming and Mr I. Jacobson also read portions of the manuscript and Dr Fleming helped to select some of the illustrative material. The line drawings were prepared by Miss M. Benstead, medical artist Dundee University, and the manuscript was typed by Mrs Norma Spain. It is a pleasure to acknowledge the courtesy and generosity of authors and publishers who have granted permission to reproduce previously published illustrations. The source of each illustration has in each case been acknowledged in the caption. Lastly I am indebted to Mr Per Saugman, Mr Nigel Palmer and the staff of Blackwell for their help, patience and cooperation.

PREFACE

The purpose of this book is to give an account of those aspects of the physiology of the nervous system which have a particular bearing on clinical neurology. It is written primarily for clinicians with an interest in neurology or psychiatry who wish to appreciate the physiological background to neurological disease. As such it is hoped that it may prove useful to postgraduate students in the neurological sciences and also perhaps to undergraduates who have completed introductory courses in anatomy and physiology and are about to embark on clinical studies.

Although neurophysiology has developed as a laboratory discipline, the clinical study of the patient has contributed much to basic knowledge. At the same time physiological techniques have been applied increasingly to clinical investigations. The field of investigation is now very large and includes not only the methods of bedside examination, which depend on the application of physiological principles but also a wide range of specialized diagnostic techniques. These include such diverse applications as electroencephalography, electromyography, tests of auditory and vestibular function, the cystometrogram, the measurement of cerebral blood flow and a wide range of methods used by the clinical psychologist. Likewise, much of the treatment of neurological disease, medical or surgical, depends on the application of physiological principles. The present discussion is primarily concerned with the basic concepts and experimental techniques of neurophysiology and their application to the understanding of clinical problems, but particular emphasis has been placed on the application and interpretation of physiological investigations. In so wide a field the treatment must inevitably be selective and so far as possible, material has been included which seems to be of current clinical interest. No attempt has been made to be exhaustive but it is hoped that sufficient references have been included in each chapter to enable the reader to go back to original sources.

CHAPTER 1

The Cerebrospinal Fluid

The brain and spinal cord are surrounded by a fluid which is formed in the cerebral ventricles and passes out of these to surround the brain and spinal cord in the subarachnoid space. It is reabsorbed into the blood stream by passing through the arachnoid villi into the dural venous sinuses. Since the membranes which surround the brain and spinal cord extend for some distance beyond the termination of the cord at the level of the first lumbar vertebra a needle inserted through one of the lumbar intervertebral spaces can readily and safely enter the subarachnoid space and remove cerebrospinal fluid (CSF). When this procedure of lumbar puncture is carried out with the subject lying horizontal the pressure recorded by a manometer attached to the lumbar puncture needle is between 100 and 150 mm of CSF. The total volume of cerebrospinal fluid is approximately 120 ml and it is formed at a rate of probably more than 500 ml/day.

The cerebrospinal fluid has an important protective function in that it provides a fluid support for the delicate tissues of the central nervous system. Since the brain is in effect floating it is protected from direct physical contact with the walls of the cranium and movement of the brain relative to the skull when the head moves is reduced. In addition it has the important function of providing a medium for the passage of substances between the blood and the extracellular fluid of the brain. Obstruction or disturbance to the free flow of the cerebrospinal fluid will cause serious alterations in the pressure relationships within the skull, and in disease of the nervous system the composition of the cerebrospinal fluid may be altered. The whole subject has been extensively reviewed by Davson (1967).

ANATOMY OF THE SUBARACHNOID SPACE AND VENTRICULAR SYSTEM

The ventricles are what remain of the cavity of the primitive neural tube from which the brain is developed. They consist of two lateral ventricles situated in

1

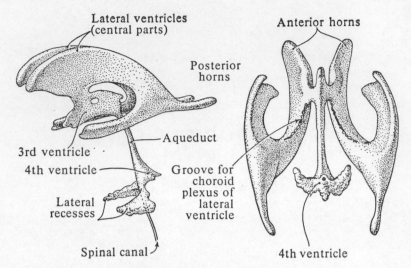

FIG. 1.1. Morphology of ventricular system.

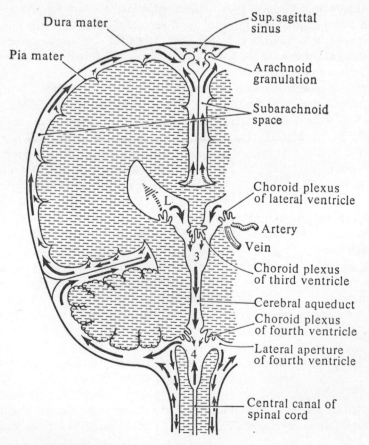

FIG. 1.2. (a) Circulation of cerebrospinal fluid.

the cerebral hemispheres which connect with the third ventricle in the midline by the foramina of Munro. The third ventricle is joined caudally to the fourth ventricle by the aquaduct of Sylvius and the fourth ventricle opens into the sub-arachnoid space through the single median foramen of Magendie and the two foramina of Luschka. (Fig. 1.1).

The ventricles contain a vascular structure known as the choroid plexus and there is convincing evidence that the cerebrospinal fluid is formed in the choroid

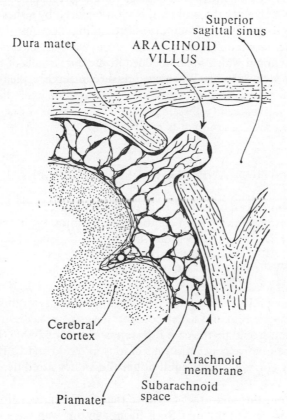

FIG. 1.2. (b) Structure of arachnoid villus.

plexus. Thus if one foramen of Munro is blocked in the dog the lateral ventricle on the side of the blocked foramen increases in size; on the other hand if the choroid plexus has previously been removed no dilatation occurs and instead the ventricle collapses (Dandy, 1919).

The subarachnoid space lies between the arachnoid mater which separates it from the dura and the pia mater which covers the surface of the brain and spinal cord. The major cerebral and spinal arteries run on the surface of the pia mater and bleeding from one of these arteries will give rise to blood in the subarachnoid space. Since the pia is closely applied to the surface of the brain and the arachnoid to the dura, subarachnoid spaces develop in the region of the sulci between the pia and arachnoid and these are particularly large over the base of the brain. The larger of these spaces are known as cisterns and the cisterna magna receives cerebrospinal fluid from the fourth ventricle through the foramen of Magendie.

The pia mater is separated from the substance of the brain by a layer of glial cells. A small cuff of pia-arachnoid extends for a short distance along the larger blood vessels which enter the brain but is soon replaced by a sheath of neuroglia which separates the artery from the surrounding nervous tissue. The subarachnoid space communicates with the dural venous sinuses through outgrowths of arachnoid which are embedded in the dural walls of the sinuses and are known as arachnoid villi. When the pressure in cerebrospinal fluid is higher than the venous pressure in the sinus, as is normally the case, fluid passes from the subarachnoid space into the sinus. The villus acts as a one-way valve and collapses if the pressure gradient is reversed (Fig. 1.2).

COMPOSITION AND FLOW OF CEREBROSPINAL FLUID

The composition of cerebrospinal fluid is very similar to that of a protein free dialysate of plasma (Table 1.1). Thus the concentration of protein in CSF is of the order of 30 mg/100 ml compared with about 7·0 g/100 ml in plasma but all substances in CSF have a concentration of the same order of magnitude as in plasma. However if the CSF is dialyzed against plasma the concentration of a number of substances in the CSF alters which it would not do if it were a simple filtrate of plasma. In particular CSF has higher concentrations of sodium, chloride and magnesium and lower concentrations of potassium, calcium, urea and glucose than would be the case if it were a simple dialysate (Davson, 1958). Moreover if the relative concentrations of ions in blood and CSF are calculated according to a Gibbs-Donnan equilibrium the values are different from those observed.

It is clear from this and other evidence that CSF is a secretion produced by the choroid plexuses but not all CSF is formed in this way since some is formed by filtering directly into the wall of the ventricles. In this way substances may also pass from cerebral capillaries into the brain and thence into the CSF. Similarly it is likely that the arachnoid villi do not account entirely for the absorption of CSF and that a proportion may be absorbed into the spinal veins or into the brain substance. The passive escape of CSF which takes place largely through the arachnoid villi has been given the name of bulk flow. The main driving force for this process is the hydrostatic pressure of the CSF which is greater than that of the venous blood within the dural sinuses. The difference in colloid osmotic pressure between the CSF with its low protein content and the plasma is probably not an important factor since the pores in the villi are large enough to allow the escape of red blood cells and changing the osmotic pressure of an artificial CSF perfused into the ventricles has no proportionate effect on flow (Davson *et al.*, 1970). Certain substances, one example is creatinine, enter the CSF relatively slowly but pass out unimpeded through the arachnoid villi so that the concentration in CSF is consistently lower than in blood. Another mechanism which applies only to particular substances in appropriate concentrations is reabsorption by active transport, a process which seems to be confined to the choroid plexus within the fourth ventricle. This mechanism may account for the failure of penicillin given by intramuscular injection to penetrate the CSF in significant concentration (Pappenheimer *et al.*, 1961).

Various methods have been adopted to measure the rate of formation of CSF in man; for example, flow rates have been recorded during lumbar or ventricular drainage and the time taken for the pressure to be restored after removal of fluid

TABLE 1.1. Chemical composition of cerebro-spinal fluid in comparison with blood plasma.

Constituent		CSF	Blood plasma
Protein		15–40	6000–8000
Glucose	mg/100 ml	50–75	70–100
Urea		15–35	10–40
pH		7·33	7·4
Na$^+$		146	136–145
Cl$^-$	mEq/l	125	100–106
K$^+$	mEq/l	3·0	3·5–5·0
HCO$_3^-$		23·6	24·9

from the lumbar theca has been measured, but these have given conflicting results. The most reliable method has been to perfuse an artificial CSF through the ventricles containing a substance such as dextran which does not pass into the adjacent tissues and calculate the rate of CSF formation from the rate at which the test substances undergoes dilution. This method has been extensively applied to animals (Pappenheimer *et al.*, 1962) and recently has been applied to human subjects in whom ventriculolumbar perfusions with chemotherapeutic agents has been combined with perfusion with a test substance such as albumen labelled with an isotope. This method gives a rate of formation of between 3·0 and 4·0 ml/min or about 500 ml/day (Cutler *et al.*, 1968). Both animal experiments and human studies have shown that the rate of secretion is reduced by the carbonic anhydrase inhibitor, acetazolamide.

It is evident from the fact that CSF is formed in the ventricles and reabsorbed from the subarachnoid space that an outward flow takes place from the ventricles to the cisterns and over the convexity of the hemisphere. How far there is a circulation up and down the spinal subarachnoid space is uncertain. The concentration of protein in the CSF is higher in fluid obtained from the spinal theca than in ventricular or cisternal fluid which would be consistent with re-absorption of fluid taking place during the course of circulation.

THE BLOOD–BRAIN BARRIER

Early observations with dye stuffs, in particular with acid dyes such as trypan blue, showed that if these were injected intravenously they stained the tissues but not the brain. They would however enter the brain if injected into the CSF. The explanation for this was that in plasma these dyes become associated with protein molecules which are too large to enter either the CSF or the brain. On the other hand in the CSF there is not enough protein for binding to occur. This illustrates one aspect of the blood–brain barrier, namely that certain substances cannot pass from the blood either to the CSF or to the brain because their molecules are too large or because they are firmly bound to large protein molecules. Generally, ionisable substances will pass freely and so also will other substances provided they are soluble in lipids. The barrier between blood and brain is not identical with the barrier between blood and CSF because in general substances pass more freely from blood to brain than from blood to CSF. However, the transfer between CSF and brain is considerably freer than that between blood and CSF. The ready passage of substances from the brain to the CSF and the rapid escape of substances from CSF to blood by bulk flow and in some cases active reabsorption through the choroid plexus has a valuable protective function towards nervous tissue. If a substance which is toxic to nervous tissue is absorbed into the brain this 'sink' action of the cerebrospinal fluid enables it to be rapidly cleared from the brain. This is particularly effective if it cannot readily enter the CSF from the blood. The reverse effect takes place with certain substances which may be important for cerebral metabolism. Thus glucose and certain amino acids pass from blood and CSF to brain so readily that it is likely that this takes place through some process of active transport. How this takes place is not known but it is possible that the foot processes of the astroglia which invest the intracerebral capillaries may have an active secretory function both in secreting the extracellular fluid of the brain and promoting active transport of substance between the blood and CSF and the extracellular fluid.

There has been some uncertainty concerning the nature and extent of the extracellular space in the central nervous system. Electron micrographs have shown the brain to be so tightly packed with cells that there is scarcely room for an extracellular space of 3–4 per cent. However, calculation of the extracellular space by diffusion methods gives substantially higher values suggesting that the electron microscope appearances may be modified by other factors such as post-mortem swelling. If the ventriculoatrial system of a live dog is perfused with an artificial CSF containing inulin or dextran diffusion into the cerebral substance occurs in concentrations which would be consistent with an extracellular space of between 7 and 14 per cent (Rall *et al.*, 1962).

EXAMINATION OF THE CEREBROSPINAL FLUID

The CSF can be readily examined by withdrawing a sample from the lumbar subarachnoid space with a lumbar puncture needle inserted between the second and third or the third and fourth lumbar vertebrae. The CSF pressure may be measured with a manometer attached to the needle and if the patient is horizontal it is between 100 and 150 mm of CSF. When the manometer is in place the pressure is seen to show small fluctuations corresponding to respirations. If the jugular vein on one side is compressed, the rise in venous pressure leads to a rise in intracranial pressure which is transmitted to the manometer, unless there is a block in the spinal theca as may be caused for example by a tumour compressing the cord. Pressure on the abdomen will cause a rise in pressure in the spinal theca which will affect the manometer even in the presence of a spinal block. Where a spinal block is suspected and there is impaired conduction following jugular compression abdominal compression is a useful method of confirming that the needle is patent. In the presence of a long standing spinal block the protein content of the CSF obtained at lumbar puncture may be markedly elevated and the normally clear colourless fluid may be yellow in colour. CSF may also be obtained by the procedure of cisternal punture in which case a needle is inserted between the occipital bone and the atlas vertebra into the cisterna magna.

Insertion into the subarachnoid space of contrast media permits radiographic demonstration of abnormalities in the system. Thus if myodil is inserted through a lumbar puncture needle into the lumbar sac, tilting of the patient in front of a fluoroscopic screen may reveal a block or indentation in the spinal theca. Partial replacement of CSF by air through a lumbar puncture (lumbar air encephalography) makes it possible to outline the ventricular system radiologically and this can also be carried out by passing a cannula into a ventricle through a burr hole in the skull and inserting air or myodil (ventriculography).

Analysis of the CSF may be helpful in reaching a clinical diagnosis. Thus in infections of the central nervous system there may be a marked increase in the cell count and in bacterial infections there is frequently a fall in the sugar content. If there has been haemorrhage into the subarachnoid space as may occur after rupture of an intracranial aneurysm the CSF is found to be uniformly mixed with blood. After a single haemorrhage red cells may remain in the CSF for a week or a little longer. In the course of the first 24 hours after the bleeding the CSF takes on a yellow colour (xanthochromia) which may persist for up to about 10 days. Tumours of the brain or spinal cord, particularly neurofibromata, may be associated with an increase in the protein content of the fluid and this is also sometimes raised in demyelinating disease, neurosyphilis and peripheral neuropathy. In demyelinating disease and neurosyphilis there may be an increase in the proportion of γ-globulin in the total protein.

THE CONTINUOUS RECORDING OF INTRACRANIAL PRESSURE

Provided there is no obstruction to the circulation of CSF the measurement of CSF pressure by means of a manometer attached to a needle in the lumbar theca gives a reasonable measure of the intracranial pressure. However, there are advantages in recording directly the intracranial pressure and this can be done either by means of a catheter inserted into the ventricular system through a burr hole and connected to a pressure transducer or by means of a transducer which is inserted directly through a burr hole into the epidural space. With either method it is possible to monitor the intracranial pressure continuously and this has given valuable information regarding pressure changes which occur under general anaesthesia and in neurosurgical operations. In this application it is useful to record the pressure in mm of mercury so that it can easily be related to intravascular pressures. In the normal subject the ventricular fluid pressure lies within the range of 1–10 mmHg. If the ventricular fluid pressure is monitored in patients with a moderate elevation in intracranial pressure periodic elevations of pressure to levels exceeding 60 mmHg may be seen to occur. These elevations of pressure may last for as long as 20 min and have been described as plateau waves (Lundberg, 1972).

HYDROCEPHALUS

Interference with the circulation of cerebrospinal fluid can lead to excessive fluid accumulating in the ventricular system which becomes enlarged, a condition which is spoken of as hydrocephalus. Hydrocephalus can be due to a block within the ventricular system when it is known as non-communicating or obstructive hydrocephalus. If there is communication between the ventricles and the subarachnoid space the condition is known as communicating hydrocephalus. In this the commonest cause is obstruction in the region of the basal cisterns so that CSF cannot pass into the subarachnoid space overlying the convexity to reach the dural venous sinuses where absorption takes place. Another possible mechanism is failure to absorb CSF due to occlusion of a venous sinus but the clinical occurrence of this mechanism is doubtful. Overproduction of CSF is probably a rare mechanism which can occur if there is a papilloma of the choroid plexus. The early experiments of Dandy (1919) threw considerable light on the possible mechanisms of hydrocephalus. He showed that non-communicating hydrocephalus could readily be produced in dogs by obstructing the foramina of Munro or the aqueduct and he produced communicating hydrocephalus by wrapping gauze soaked in an irritant around the midbrain where the resulting adhesions prevented fluid from reaching the cerebral subarachnoid space where it is absorbed. He showed also that if a dye such as phenolsulphonphthalein is injected into a lateral ventricle it will appear promptly in the lumbar CSF in communicating hydrocephalus but not at all in obstructive hydrocephalus.

Non-communicating hydrocephalus can develop at any time of life as the result of intracranial tumour and communicating hydrocephalus as a result of basal adhesions following meningitis or subarachnoid bleeding. In infancy congenital abnormalities can obstruct the outflow of CSF from the ventricles and again meningitis may be a cause of basal adhesions.

The surgical treatment of hydrocephalus was developed very largely by Dandy, who devised the operation of third ventriculostomy for obstructive hydrocephalus and surgical destruction of the choroid plexus for communicating hydrocephalus. These operations have largely been superceded by shunting procedures which enable the CSF to bypass the obstruction to its circulation. In Torkildsen's operation, which is particularly useful where there is stenosis of the aqueduct, a tube is inserted between the lateral ventricle and the cisterna magna. The development of unidirectional valves has made it possible to pass a tube between the lateral ventricle and the superior vena cava, and this method which allows CSF to pass directly from the ventricle to the blood stream can be used for both obstructive and non-communicating hydrocephalus.

There is accumulating evidence that abnormalities in spinal fluid dynamics may also affect the spinal cord. Gardner has suggested that in syringomyelia the fluid containing cavity in the cervical cord results from a congenital anomoly in which outflow of CSF from the fourth ventricle is obstructed and the fluid is driven into the central canal of the spinal cord giving rise to a diverticulum which forms the syrinx (Gardner, 1965; Appleby *et al.*, 1968).

An important effect of hydrocephalus is that the intracranial pressure rises, which may produce symptoms in form of headache, drowsiness and eventually coma and death due to shift and distortion of the brain causing damage to vital centres. Since the optic nerve is part of the brain and invested with a subarachnoid space an increase in intracranial pressure will be transmitted to this space and compress the central retinal vein which leads to oedema of the optic nerve and gives rise to the characteristic ophthalmoscopic appearances of papilloedema. If the intracranial pressure rises sufficiently it may reduce the arterial blood flow to the brain which may cause anoxia to the medulla and cause reflex changes in blood pressure (Cushing, 1902; see Chapter 2). Temporary relief from the the effects of raised intracranial pressure may be obtained by the intravenous infusion of hypertonic solutions, such as mannitol, which lead to the passage of fluid along an osmotic gradient between the brain and the blood stream. Cerebral oedema may be likewise reduced by the administration of glucocorticoids such as dexamethasone.

Even in the absence of raised intracranial pressure, abnormal dilatation of a ventricle as a result of progressive hydrocephalus may produce severe but often reversible damage to the surrounding cerebral tissue. This so-called normal pressure hydrocephalus syndrome is most commonly due to communicating hydrocephalus developing in adult life, sometimes as a sequal to subarachnoid haemorrhage (Adams *et al.*, 1965). In this condition if radioiodinated serum albumen (RISA) is injected into the lumbar theca it fails to pass over the surface of the cerebral hemisphere; instead it enters the ventricular system where it may still be detected 48 hours after the injection (Bannister *et al.*, 1967; Bannister, 1970).

REFERENCES

ADAMS, R. D., FISHER, C. M., HANKIN, S., OJEMANN, R. G. and SWEET, W. H. (1965). Symptomatic occult hydrocephalus with 'normal' cerebrospinal-fluid pressure: a treatable syndrome. *New Engl. J. Med.*, **273**, 117–126.

APPLEBY, A., FOSTER, J. B., HANKINSON, J. and HUDGSON, P. (1968). The diagnosis and management of the Chiari anomalies in adult life. *Brain*, **91**, 131–140.

BANNISTER, R. GILFORD, E. and KOCEN, R. (1967). Isotope encephalography in the diagnosis of dementia due to communicating hydrocephalus. *Lancet*, ii, 1014–1017.

BANNISTER, R. (1970). The place of isotope encephalography by the lumbar route in neurological diagnosis. *Proc. roy. Soc. Med.* **63**, 921–925.

CUSHING, H. (1902). Some experimental and clinical observations concerning states of increased intracranial tension. *Amer. J. Med. Sci.* n.s. **124**, 375–400.

CUTLER, R. W. P., PAGE, L., GALICICH, J. and WATTERS, G. V. (1968). Formation and absorption of cerebrospinal fluid in man. *Brain* **91**, 707–720.

DANDY, W. E. (1919). Experimental hydrocephalus. *Ann. Surg.*, **70**, 129–142.

DAVSON, H. (1967). *The Physiology of the Cerebrospinal Fluid.* London: Churchill.

DAVSON, H. (1958). Some aspects of the relationship between the cerebrospinal fluid and the central nervous system. In: *Ciba Foundation Symposium on the Cerebrospinal Fluid.* Ed. Wolstenholme, G. E. W. and O'Connor, Cecilia M. London: Churchill. 189–203.

DAVSON, H., HOLLINGSWORTH, G. and SEGAL, M. B. (1970). The mechanism of drainage of the cerebrospinal fluid. *Brain*, **93**, 665–678.

GARDNER, W. J. (1965). Hydrodynamic mechanism of syringomyelia: its relationship to hydrocele. *J. Neurol. Neurosurg. Psychiat.*, **28**, 247–259.

LUNDBERG, N. (1972). Monitoring of the intracranial pressure, in *Scientific Foundations of Neurology*, Ed. Critchley, M., O'Leary, J. L. and Jennett, B. London: Heinemann.

PAPPENHEIMER, J. R., HEISEY, S. R., JORDAN, E. F. and DOWNER, J. DE C. (1962). Perfusion of the cerebral ventricular system in unanesthetized goats. *Amer. J. Physiol.*, **203**, 763–774.

RALL, D. P., OPPELT, W. W. and PATLAK, C. S. (1962). Extracellular space of brain as determined by diffusion of inulin from the ventricular system. *Life Sciences*, **1**, 43–48.

CHAPTER 2

The Cerebral Circulation

Although the nerve cells in the brain constitute less than 0·10 per cent of the total body weight the oxygen consumption of the brain is about 18 per cent of that of the whole body. Arrest of the cerebral circulation is followed almost immediately by loss of consciousness and only a few minutes of impaired circulation will cause irreversible damage to the brain. Under normal circumstances the blood flow through the brain and the supply of oxygen to the neurones is maintained remarkably constant even when considerable changes take place in the circulation to other parts of the body. At the present time disease of the cerebral vessels is a major cause of disability and mortality, and the physiology of the cerebral circulation is of particular clinical importance.

ANATOMICAL BASIS

The brain receives its blood from four main arteries, viz., the two internal carotid arteries and the two vertebral arteries. The venous drainage is through cerebral veins which drain into the large intracranial venous sinuses from which blood flows into the internal jugular veins. The four major arteries are joined by an anastomotic connection at the base of the brain which is known as the circle of Willis (Fig. 2.1). Under normal circumstances blood from either internal carotid or vertebral artery passes to the brain on the same side, but crossed circulation through the circle of Willis can occur to compensate if the blood flow to one hemisphere is inadequate. The effectiveness of this crossed circulation varies in different individuals because the circle of Willis is subject to considerable anatomical variation so that in many instances the anastomosis is incomplete. In addition to the circle of Willis there is also an external anastomosis which can enable blood to flow between the branches of the external and the internal carotid. The main arteries give off perforating branches which penetrate the cerebral substance and the main pial branches which supply the greater part of

11

the cortex and the underlying white matter. Some anastomosis takes place between the pial branches and also between their terminal capillary networks but this anastomosis is seldom adequate to compensate fully for occlusion of a major vessel.

In disease of the cerebral circulation these anastomotic connections are of great importance. Many people remain well after occlusion of one internal carotid artery, or after the artery has been surgically ligated, in which case the affected hemisphere derives its blood supply from anastomotic connection with healthy vessels. Such a situation may be precarious, however, if the circle of Willis is defective or if the total cerebral blood flow is reduced as a result of external stress, such as a fall in blood pressure. Cerebral vascular insufficiency arising in this manner is one aspect of the complex pathogenesis of cerebral infarction.

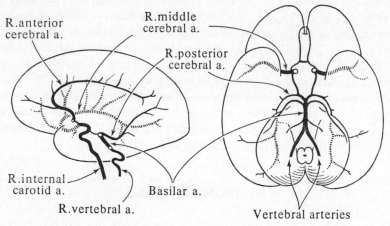

FIG. 2.1. Arterial supply to the brain.

METHODS OF STUDYING CEREBRAL BLOOD FLOW

The complex anatomical arrangements of the arteries and veins to the brain make it difficult to measure cerebral blood flow quantitatively by anything but an indirect method. In experimental animals much useful information has been obtained by direct observation of the pial vessels through a transparent window in the skull (Forbes, 1928; Fog, 1934; Byrom, 1954). By this means it has been possible to study the effect of changes in blood pressure, of nerve stimulation and the action of drugs on the calibre of the vessels. In the monkey, blood flow has been measured directly by use of a flowmeter in both common carotid arteries after ligation of the external carotid and basilar arteries (Schmidt *et al.*,

1945). Indirect methods in which the clearance of an indicator is determined according to the Fick principle correlate well with the direct technique and are suitable for use in man (Kety and Schmidt, 1945).

In the study of the human cerebral circulation clearance methods using diffusable indicators have been of particular value in obtaining quantitative measurements of blood flow through the brain. Other methods using non-diffusable indicators have been of clinical value but have provided largely qualitative information. This applies particularly to the techniques of angiography, in which X-ray photographs are taken after injection of a radio-opaque substance into the carotid or vertebral arteries. The blood flow in individual arteries has been studied by means of electromagnetic flow meters. In this section a few of the methods which have provided quantitative information in man will be considered (see also reviews by Schmidt, 1950; Lassen, 1959; Harper, 1967 and 1969).

The Nitrous Oxide Method

This method was introduced by Kety and Schmidt in 1945 and is an indirect method depending on an application of the Fick principle. According to this the blood flow to any organ of the body can be expressed as the ratio between the uptake of an inert gas per unit time and the arteriovenous inert gas difference across the organ. In measuring the cardiac output this principle can be applied exactly because it is possible to measure the difference in oxygen concentration between arterial and venous blood while the up ake of oxygen through the lungs is measured independently. In measuring cerebral blood flow the use of an inert gas depends on the fact that although the brain does not selectively remove foreign substances from the blood it is able to absorb an inert gas such as nitrous oxide into physical solution. If nitrous oxide in low concentration is inhaled over ten minutes the concentrations in arterial blood, brain tissue and the cerebral venous blood are in equilibrium. The cerebral venous concentration thus provides a measure from which the quantity of gas taken up by the brain can be derived. The arteriovenous difference is more difficult to obtain because it has been changing continuously throughout the 10-min period, and it is necessary to calculate an integrated value.

The practical procedure is to breathe a mixture containing 15 per cent nitrous oxide and 21 per cent oxygen over about 10 min during which period simultaneous samples of arterial blood and blood from the right internal jugular vein are withdrawn at intervals and analysed for nitrous oxide content. A refinement is to have continuous withdrawal of blood samples so that an integrated value for the arteriovenous difference can be obtained. If an isotope such as krypton-85 is used instead of nitrous oxide, the concentration of gas can be determined by measuring the radioactivity of the blood samples with a Geiger counter. At the end of the experiment the amount of nitrous oxide lost per 100 ml of blood passing through the brain and the total amount of nitrous oxide taken up by the brain can be calculated and hence the blood flow per 100 g of brain. Such experiments show that blood flow is normally about 54 ml/100 g/min. If the arteriovenous difference is also determined for oxygen the rate of oxygen consumption can be calculated and is found to be about 3·3 ml/100 g/min. For a 1360 g brain flow is thus about 740 ml/min and oxygen usage about 45 ml/min. This method has many advantages and much of the fundamental work on cerebral blood flow and metabolism has been carried out by means of it. It has the disadvantage that it does not give a direct measure of total cerebral blood flow, and it gives no information about differences of flow in particular regions of the brain.

Measurement of Total Cerebral Blood Flow

This was first done by Gibbs, Maxwell and Gibbs in 1947 using a dye dilution technique. A known amount of Evans blue was injected into one internal carotid artery and the dilution of the indicator followed by taking samples from one or both internal jugular veins. If the total quantity of indicator injected is known the total blood flow per minute can be derived from the dye dilution curves.

Diffusable indicators can also be used to measure total cerebral blood flow. This method consists in using a radioactive substance which is either inhaled (Krypton-79) or given by intravenous injection (Iodine-131-labelled antipyrine). The cerebral radioactivity is measured with scintillation counters and the arteriovenous difference is determined from serial arterial and jugular venous samples. The ratio of the changing brain content of isotope to the arteriovenous difference enables the total cerebral blood flow to be calculated.

Each of these methods has advantages but all are limited by technical complexity which restricts their clinical application.

Measurement of Regional Blood Flow

The dye dilution method has been developed by Nylin *et al.* (1960) to measure the total cerebral flow and also to compare the flow in the two hemispheres. This method uses radioactive-labelled red cells as indicator and these are injected into both carotids while blood is sampled from each internal jugular vein. Computer analysis is necessary and the method is unsuited for regular clinical use.

An important advance in the diffusable indicator methods is the use of radioactive krypton-85 or xenon-133, both of which are much more soluble in air than in blood. The result of this is that when they are given by intra-arterial injection they are excreted as soon as they reach the lungs so that no recirculation occurs. If the γ emissions are recorded by means of scintillation counters, the clearance of gas can be calculated without the necessity for taking samples of venous blood (Lassen and Ingvar, 1961; Glass and Harper, 1963). If multiple scintillation counters are used estimates of regional blood flow can be made. If the clearance curves are plotted on semi-log paper two components can be recognized (Fig. 2.2). Interpretation of these clearance curves in terms of regional blood flow is difficult because γ radiations are highly penetrating and can be recorded from a considerable distance. Studies on the exposed cortex of the monkey, however, have given more accurate regional information since β radiation, which is much less penetrating, can be monitored on the exposed cortex, and this gives reliable information concerning local cortical blood flow. It is found that cortical blood flow as determined from β counting correlates closely with the fast component of the γ clearance curve. On the basis of this

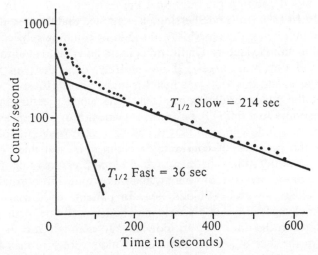

FIG. 2.2. Clearance curve for Xenon-133, plotted on semi-logarithmic paper to show two exponential components which have been extracted from the primary curve. The fast component may be related mainly to blood flow through grey matter, the slow to flow through white matter. T- refers to time taken for radioactivity to reach half its initial value. Harper, A. M. (1967). *Scot. med. J.*, **12**, 349–360.

method of compartmental analysis, it has been assumed that the slow component of the clearance curves represents blood flow in the white matter and the fast component blood flow in the grey matter (Harper and Jennett, 1968).

The above method has been widely applied and despite its complexity has provided information of great clinical interest. It suffers from the disadvantage that the isotope is administered by injection into the internal carotid artery. The attempt has therefore been made to avoid the necessity for arterial puncture by developing a method whereby a mixture of xenon-133 in air is inhaled for 5 min, and clearance curves are obtained from scintillation counters applied to the skull (Veall and Mallett, 1966). This method is subject to the difficulty that during inhalation the whole body takes up isotope so there is contamination of the clearance curves by recirculating isotope, and there is also further contamination from isotope which is circulating in the tissues of the scalp. To overcome these difficulties very complex computer analysis is necessary, but the complete safety of the method makes it attractive for clinical application.

CONTROL OF CEREBRAL BLOOD FLOW

The rate of cerebral blood flow depends on the balance between the head of pressure of blood entering the brain and the resistance offered by the cerebral blood vessels. In 1890 Roy and Sherrington suggested that the vascular resistance of the brain, and hence the blood flow through it, could be subject to modification by local metabolic factors. On the other hand Hill (1896) maintained that the cerebral blood flow was largely, if not entirely, dependent on the systemic arterial pressure, and this view was held for many years. However, in 1934 Fog showed that the pial arterioles contracted if the blood pressure increased and dilated in response to a fall in pressure. It is evident also from measurements of total cerebral blood flow in man that the blood flow through the brain remains constant in the presence of considerable changes in systemic arterial blood pressure. In a healthy subject neither a fall in blood pressure of up to 50 per cent nor a rise in blood pressure of comparable magnitude will normally have any measurable effect on cerebral blood flow. In patients with arteriosclerosis or hypertension changes in blood pressure may be less well tolerated and in malignant hypertension the ability of an individual to maintain a constant cerebral blood flow in the face of a changing level of blood pressure may be restricted (Finnerty *et al.*, 1954).

Effect of Carbon Dioxide and Oxygen

Drugs in general have little effect on cerebral blood flow, and the most important substances which influence it are carbon dioxide and oxygen. In man inhalation of 5 per cent carbon dioxide will result in a 50 per cent increase in cerebral blood flow, and breathing a gaseous mixture containing 8–10 per cent oxygen at atmospheric pressure will likewise bring about a 40 per cent increase in blood flow. On the other hand breathing pure oxygen at 1 atmosphere pressure will cause a reduction of blood flow of about 12 per cent (Lassen, 1959).

How carbon dioxide tension and oxygen lack exert their effect in increasing cerebral blood flow is unknown, but evidence has accumulated for the hypothesis that the effect is brought about by a direct relaxing action on the smooth muscle of the arteriolar walls. It has been postulated that the common factor is a change in pH of the extracellular fluid in relation to the arteriolar smooth muscle. Carbon dioxide may thus exert its effect by diffusion into the extracellular fluid;

oxygen lack on the other hand renders the tissue fluid acid by allowing the accumulation of acid metabolites (Severinghaus, 1968). At present the evidence that pH is the determining factor is not conclusive and the subject has been reviewed in detail by Harper (1969).

Nervous Control of Blood Flow

Anatomical studies have shown that nerve fibres accompany cerebral vessels both in man and animals. These include adrenergic vasoconstrictor fibres derived from the sympathetic and in addition cholinergic axons have also been demonstrated which probably represent vasodilator fibres. The nerve supply is most profuse in the larger vessels but although the innervation of the pial vessels is clearly established there is much less certainty regarding the extent of the nerve supply to the intracerebral vessels.

In 1928 Forbes and Wolff, using the skull window technique, showed that stimulation of the cervical sympathetic would cause some constriction of the pial arteries. It has been generally held, however, that this is a relatively feeble effect of little importance in the regulation of cerebral blood flow, and this is supported by the failure to demonstrate significant clinical response to cervical sympathectomy in patients with cerebral vascular disease. It has, however, been found that the response to CO_2 stimulation in experimental baboons is enhanced after sympathectomy when the cerebral blood flow also becomes more dependent on changes in blood pressure. Similar effects are observed after vagotomy when the dependence of cerebral blood flow upon blood pressure becomes particularly marked (James *et al.*, 1969). Harper *et al* (1972) have suggested that there may be a dual control of the cerebral circulation, the arteries outside the brain parenchyma being predominantly under the influence of the sympathetic whereas in the intracerebral vessels chemical control through the action of tissue metabolites is correspondingly important. The evidence regarding the possible importance of nervous factors in the control of cerebral blood flow has been extensively reviewed by Purves (1972).

Autoregulation

The process whereby the cerebral circulation is maintained relatively constant in the presence of marked changes in blood pressure is known as autoregulation and the mechanisms for this are not wholly understood. In 1902 Bayliss showed that the muscular coat of arteries, like smooth muscle elsewhere in the body, reacts to a stretching force by contracting so that a natural response of the arteries to distending pressure could be contraction with relaxation and dilatation when the pressure falls. On the other hand the muscular coat of the cerebral arteries is less well developed than in comparable vessels elsewhere in the body, and it is possible that intrinsic vascular tone is less important in the cerebral circulation than in tissues such as the muscles and kidneys where autoregulation is also important. Another possible explanation is that a rise in blood pressure causes an increase in tissue pressure so that the vessels become compressed. This certainly occurs in the presence of high arterial pressures but is of more doubtful significance with moderate changes in pressure. A third possible mechanism is a metabolic one on the basis that a rise in blood pressure by increasing local blood flow could wash out carbon dioxide from the tissue fluid and by making it more alkaline lead to vasoconstriction. If the hydrogen ion concentration of the extracellular fluid is a major factor determining cerebral vascular tone this becomes an attractive hypothesis (Zwetnow, 1968). The possible importance of the nervous control of blood flow in autoregulation has been referred to above.

CLINICAL ASPECTS OF CEREBRAL BLOOD FLOW AND OXYGEN

Physical and intellectual effort appear to have little effect on total cerebral blood flow or oxygen consumption but when regional blood flow is measured using 133 Xenon changes in cortical blood flow have been recorded during mental activity (Ingvar and Risberg, 1967). Local changes in blood flow have also been recorded over the dominant hemisphere during speech and reading (Ingvar, 1973). In sleep there may be a small increase in blood flow (Mangold *et al.*, 1955) but in anaesthesia and certain varieties of coma oxygen consumption may fall from the normal level of $3 \cdot 4$ ml/100 g/min to less than 2 ml/100 g/min (Kety, 1949). It is of interest that although barbiturate anaesthesia is associated with a fall in oxygen consumption and in cerebral blood flow, certain volatile anaesthetics such as halothane and trichlorethylene, although they decrease cerebral oxygen uptake, have a vasodilator action which results in an increase in cerebral blood flow. This increase in blood flow may be associated with a rise in intracranial pressure which may be important if these agents are used in connection with intracranial surgery (McDowall, 1972). In dementia where there is likely to be marked loss of cerebral substance there may be correspondingly low levels of oxygen consumption.

Blood Flow During Convulsions

If convulsions are induced in monkeys by the administration of metrazol or picrotoxin there is a marked increase both in cerebral blood flow and in oxygen consumption (Schmidt *et al.*, 1945). Information about blood flow during seizures in man is scanty but McCall and Taylor (1952) found a marked increase in oxygen consumption in a single patient with toxaemia during an eclamptic seizure. This increase in oxygen consumption during seizures is of interest since it is evident that a marked increase in cerebral blood flow is necessary to compensate if the blood during a seizure is unsaturated on account of inadequate air entry.

Intracranial Pressure

If there is a rise in intracranial pressure, compression of the cerebral vessels may impede the cerebral blood flow. Cushing (1902) observed that in dogs with raised intracranial pressure there was a marked increase in systemic arterial blood pressure, and he suggested that this was due to a compensatory reflex in the brain stem which led to generalized vasoconstriction and hence to an increase in blood pressure, which in turn could augment the cerebral blood flow. The rise in blood pressure may however occur in the absence of a marked rise in intracranial pressure, and it is likely that in many instances the operant factor is ischaemic damage to the brain stem resulting from cerebral trauma or shift of intracranial structures.

Hypertension

The vasoconstriction of the cerebral arterioles which occurs in response to moderate rises in blood pressure as part of the normal process of autoregulation becomes particularly important in hypertension. As early as 1876 Gowers commented on the narrowing of the retinal vessels which could be seen in patients with Bright's disease in the presence of high blood pressure. In 1948 Kety *et al.* showed that hypertension in man is accompanied by a marked rise in the vascular resistance of the cerebral circulation. In 1954 Byrom described observations on the pial vessels through a transparent window on the skull on rats which had been made hypertensive by clamping the renal artery. In mild hypertension the only change observed was some constriction of the terminal vessels. With extremely high pressures there was slight dilatation of the larger vessels with tight constriction of the terminal vessels. Although some vessels show segments of dilatation and also of constriction the overall appearance is one of intense vascular narrowing. Lowering the blood pressure produced rapid reversal of these changes (Byrom, 1968).

In a careful study in primates Meyer *et al.* (1960) have tried to distinguish between the effects of a simple rise in blood pressure and the possible action of a vasoconstrictor substance such as might be found in chronic hypertension. Hypertension was produced mechanically by clamping the thoracic aorta distal to the origin of the cerebral vessels. This led to constriction of the small cerebral arteries which was less marked than that which occurs in renal hypertension. If occlusion was maintained swelling of the brain took place possibly as a result of increased filtration pressure in the smaller vessels. This swelling led to compression of the vessels with further narrowing. If renal hypertension was produced in the animals by clamping the renal arteries a much more profound cerebral vasoconstriction occurred suggesting that a vasoconstrictor substance was also important. It is of interest that in these cases also, lowering the blood pressure produced a rapid reversal of the effect.

Skinhøj and Strandgaard (1973) have suggested that an important factor in the development of hypertensive encephalopathy may be a breakdown in auto-regulation which takes place when the perfusion pressure reaches a certain critical level. They measured cerebral blood flow during controlled hypertension and found that the blood flow remained constant as the blood pressure increased until a certain level of pressure was reached when the cerebral blood flow might increase by as much as 100 per cent. The level of pressure at which this occurred varied in different subjects and appeared to be related to the CO_2 tension of the blood. Failure of autoregulation brought about in this way might precipitate symptoms through hyperperfusion of the brain giving rise to cerebral oedema.

Effect of Local Anoxia on Blood Flow

In the presence of cerebral anoxia there may be a breakdown in the mechanism of autoregulation which normally regulates cerebral flow. This can be seen in deep anaesthesia, following strokes, in the presence of brain tumours and also following direct trauma to the brain or neurosurgical operative procedures. Lassen (1966) has suggested that the mechanism for this may be a local metabolic acidosis which can readily occur in conditions of anoxia. The effect of this is that the vessels in the affected area become dilated and lose their response both to changes in intravascular pressure and to carbon dioxide tension. There is localized hyperaemia with poor extraction of oxygen so that the cerebral venous blood becomes abnormally red. This has been termed the 'luxury-perfusion syndrome'. Its clinical importance lies in the fact that in the anoxic brain the blood flow may become solely dependent on the perfusing pressure and measures such as carbon dioxide inhalation may not only be ineffective in increasing blood flow to the ischaemic area but may actually divert blood to other regions of the brain (Lassen, 1969). Fazekas (1968) has shown that in a proportion of patients with chronic cerebral arteriosclerosis, cerebral blood flow is unresponsive to changes in carbon dioxide tension possibly because the vessels are already maximally dilated in response to chronic vascular insufficiency.

REFERENCES

BAYLISS, W. M. (1902). On the local of the arterial wall to changes of internal pressure. *J. Physiol. (Lond.)*, **28**, 220–231.

BYROM, F. B. (1954). The pathogenesis of hypertensive encephalopathy and its relation to the malignant phase of hypertension. *Lancet*, **ii**, 201–211.

BYROM, F. B. (1968). The calibre of the cerebral arteries in experimental hypertension. *Proc. roy. Soc. Med.*, **61**, 605–606.

CUSHING, H. (1902). Some experimental and clinical observations concerning states of increased intracranial tension. *Am. J. med. Sci.*, **124**, 375–400.

FAZEKAS, J. F. (1968). Maximal dilation of cerebral vessels. *Arch. Neurol. (Chic.)*, **11**, 303–309.

FINNERTY, F. A. Jr., WITKIN, L. and FAZEKAS, J. F. (1954). Cerebral haemodynamics during cerebral ischaemia induced by acute hypotension. *J. clin. Invest.*, **33**, 1227–1232.

FOG, M. (1934). Om pia arteriernes vasomotoriske seaktioner, Copenhagen, Munksguard. Cited by Lassen, N. A., 1959. *Physiol. Rev.*, **39**, 183–238.

FOG, M. (1938). The relationship between the blood pressure and the tonic regulation of the pial arteries. *J. Neurol. Psychiat.*, **1**, 187–197.

FORBES, H. S. (1928). The cerebral circulation. I: Observation and measurements of pial vessels. *Arch. Neurol. Psychiat. (Chic.)*, **19**, 751–761.

FORBES, H. S. and WOLFF, H. G. (1928). Cerebral circulation. III. The vasomotor control of cerebral vessels. *Arch. Neurol. Psychiat. (Chic.)*, **19**, 1057–1086.

GIBBS, F. A., MAXWELL, H. and GIBBS, E. L. (1947). Volume flow of blood through human brain. *Arch. Neurol. Psychiat. (Chic.)*, **57**, 137–144.

GLASS, H. I. and HARPER, A. M. (1963). Measurement of regional blood flow in cerebral cortex of man through intact skull. *Brit. med. J.*, **i**, 593.

HARPER, A. M. (1967). Measurement of cerebral blood flow in man. *Scot. med. J.*, **12**, 349–360.

HARPER, A. M. (1969). Regulation of the cerebral circulation. *The Scientific Basis of Medicine*. Annual Reviews 1969. London: Athlone Press, 60–81.

HARPER, A. M., DESHMUKH, V. D., ROWAN, J. O. and JENNETT, W. B. (1972). The influence of sympathetic nervous activity on cerebral blood flow. *Arch. Neurol. (Chic.)*, **27**, 1–6.

HARPER, A. M. and JENNETT, W. B. (1968). In: *Blood Flow Through Organs and Tissues*. Ed. Brain W. and Harper A. M., Edinburgh.

HILL, L. (1896). An Experimental Research. In: *The Physiology and Pathology of the Cerebral Circulation*. London: Churchill

INGVAR, D. H. and RISBERG, J. (1967). Increase of regional cerebral blood flow during mental effort in normals and patients with focal brain disorders. *Expl. Brain Res.*, **3**, 195–211.

INGVAR, D. H. (1973). Speech functions of the dominant hemisphere studied by regional cerebral blood flow measurements. X International Congress of Neurology. *Excerpta Medica*, **296**, 158.

JAMES, I. M., MILLAR, R. A. and PURVES, M. J. (1969). Observations on the extrinsic neural control of cerebral blood flow in the baboon. *Circulation Research*, **25**, 77–93.

KETY, S. S. (1949). Physiology of the human cerebral circulation. *Anaesthesiology*, **10**, 610–614.

KETY, S. S. and SCHMIDT, C. F. (1945). The determination of cerebral blood flow in man by the use of nitrous oxide in low concentrations. *Amer. J. Physiol.*, **143**, 53–66.

KETY, S. S., SHENKIN, H. A. and SCHMIDT, C. F. J. (1948). The effects of increased intracranial pressure on cerebral circulatory effects in man. *J. clin. Invest.*, **27**, 493–499.

LASSEN, N. A. (1959). Cerebral blood flow and oxygen consumption in man. *Physiol. Rev.*, **39**, 183–238.

LASSEN, N. A. (1966). The luxury-perfusion syndrome and its possible relation to acute metabolic acidosis localised within the brain. *Lancet*, **ii**, 1113–1115.

LASSEN, N. A. (1969). Cerebral circulation in cerebrovascular diseases. II. Abolition of the normal regulation of cerebral blood flow after anoxia and trauma ('luxury perfusion syndrome'). *Proc. 4th Int. Congress of Neurological Surgery and 9th Int. Congress of Neurology*. Ed. Drake C. G. and Duvoisin. R. Amsterdam: Excerpta Medica Foundation.

MANGOLD, R., SOKOLOFF, L., THERMAN, P. O., CONNOR, E. H., KLEINERMAN, J. I. and KETY, S. S. (1955). The effects of sleep and lack of sleep on the cerebral circulation and metabolism of normal young man. *J. clin. Invest.*, **34**, 1092–1100.

McCALL, M. L. and TAYLOR, H. W. (1952). Effects of barbiturate sedation on brain in toxaemia of pregnancy. *J. Am. med. Ass.*, **149**, 51–54.

McDOWALL, D. G. (1972). *Anaesthesia for Neurosurgery. Scientific Foundations of Neurology*. Ed. Critchley, M., O'Leary, J. L. and Jennett, B. London: Heinemann.

MEYER, J. S., WALTZ, A. G. and GOTOH, F. (1960). Pathogenesis of cerebral vasospasm in hypertensive encephalopathy. I and II. Neurology (Minneap.), **10**, 735–744; 859–867.

NYLIN, G., SILVERSKIOLD, B. P. LOFTSTEDT, S., REGNSTROM, O. and HEDLUND, S. (1960). Studies on cerebral blood flow in man, using radioactive-labelled erythrocytes. *Brain*, **83**, 293–335.

PURVES, M. J. (1972). The Physiology of the Cerebral Circulation. *Monographs of the Physiological Society No. 28*. London: Cambridge University Press.

ROY, C. S. and SHERRINGTON, C. S. (1890). On the regulation of the blood-supply of the brain. *J. Physiol. (Lond.)*, **11**, 85–108.

SCHMIDT, C. F. (1950). The Cerebral Circulation. In: *Health and Disease*. Springfield, Illinois: Thomas.

SCHMIDT, C. F. KETY, S. S. and PENNES, H. H. (1945). The gaseous metabolism of the brain of the monkey. *Amer. J. Physiol.*, **143**, 33–52.

SEVERINGHAUS, J. W. (1968). Outline of H^+-blood flow relationships in brain. *Scand. J. clin. Lab. Invest.*, *suppl.*, 102, VIII: K.

SKINHØJ, E. and STRANDGAARD, S. (1973). Pathogenesis of hypertensive encephalopathy. *Lancet* I, 461–462.

VEALL, N. and MALLETT, B. L. (1966). Regional cerebral blood flow determination by ^{133}Xe inhalation and extracranial recording: the effect of arterial recirculation. *Clin. Sci.*, **30**, 353–369.

ZWETNOW, N. (1968). Effects of intracranial hypertension: acid-base changes and lactate changes in CSF and brain tissue. *Scand. J. clin. Lab. Invest.*, *suppl.*, 102, III: D.

CHAPTER 3

The Neurone and Transmission of the Nerve Impulse

NERVE CELLS AND GLIA

The cells of the nervous system are derived from the germinal cells which line the neural tube of the embryo. These give rise to three varieties of primitive cell, viz., the neuroblasts, the spongioblasts and the ependymoblasts. The neuroblasts are the precursors of nerve cells, the spongioblasts give rise to the neuroglia or supporting tissue of the nervous system and the ependymoblasts to the ependymal cells which line the ventricles. The neuroglia consists of astrocytes and oligodendrocytes, which are derived from spongioblasts, and traditionally it has been regarded as comprising also the microglia. The microglial cells, however, are of mesodermal origin and pass into the nervous system from the meninges at a relatively late stage of embryonic development. The microglial cells are actively phagocytic and are found in profusion in areas of brain where there is inflammation or injury.

The neurone or nerve cell, with its fibre, is the structure which is responsible for the conduction of nerve impulses. Histologically it has a cell body with a nucleus, and it gives off many small branches or dendrites and a long single branch, known as the axon which constitutes the nerve fibre (Fig. 3.1). According to the neurone theory each neurone is a separate entity, the axon of which makes contact by means of nerve endings with the surface of an effector cell such as muscle or with the cell body or dendrites of another neurone. Division of nerve cells does not occur after early infancy and nerve cells cannot be replaced if destroyed. It has been estimated that in the human brain the cerebral cortex contains in excess of the order of $2 \cdot 6 \times 10^9$ nerve cells (Pakkenberg, 1966).

If neurones are examined under the light microscope they are seen to contain a densely staining nucleus surrounded by cytoplasm which contains material known as Nissl particles which stain deep blue. These may be present both in the cell body and in the dendrites but are not seen in the axon or the axon hillock where the axon joins the cell body. Examined under the electron microscope the

Nissl particles are seen to consist of small bodies that contain ribonucleic acid (RNA) and which are known as ribosomes and which are closely related to a fine tubular structure known as endoplasmic reticulum. The nucleus is composed of chromatin material that contains desoxyribonucleic acid (DNA) which is the genetic material of the cells. The nucleolus is a dense structure within the nucleus

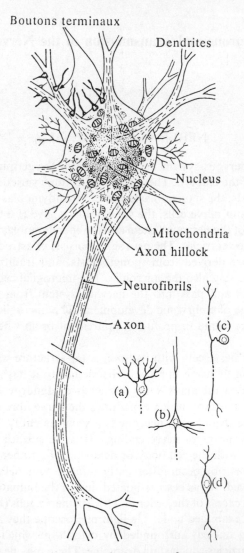

FIG. 3.1. Diagram to illustrate general structure of neurone and morphology of examples of particular varieties: (a) multipolar, (b) pyramidal, (c) pseudounipolar, and (d) bipolar.

which contains RNA and is the site of ribosome formation. Protein synthesis takes place in the ribosomes and the amino acid sequence in synthesized protein depends on the sequence of nucleotides in the genetic material. In the nucleus this sequence is transcribed from DNA to messenger RNA which passes to the cytoplasm where a further process, which involves ribosomal RNA and transfer RNA, establishes the amino acid sequence in the protein molecules. The neurones also contain particles known as mitochondria which contain the enzymes necessary for oxidative phosphorylation. Mitochondria are present in all parts of the cytoplasm including the axon and cell body and they may be profuse in the dendrites.

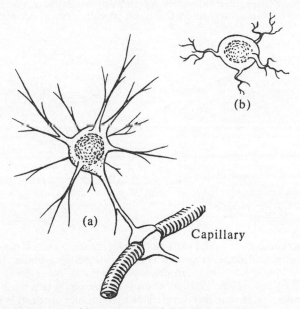

Fɪɢ. 3.2. Neuroglial cells: (a) astrocyte and (b) oligodendrocyte.

The neuroglial cells (Fig. 3.2) in the human cortex are more numerous than neurones but much about their function remains unknown. The astrocytes are particularly important in maintaining the stability of the neuronal environment. They are found throughout the nervous system, their processes ramifying along the surface of the neurones. They invest the walls of the intracerebral capillaries and have an important function in the formation of the extracellular fluid of the brain and in the transport of substances across the blood–brain barrier. The oligodendroglia exist as perineural satellites in the grey matter of the brain and as interfascicular glia in the white matter, where they lie between the myelinated fibres and have the function of forming, and possibly maintaining, the myelin sheaths of the myelinated fibres (see review by Bunge, 1968).

In vertebrates all but the smallest nerve fibres outside the autonomic system are surrounded by a myelin sheath (Fig. 3.3). This myelin sheath forms an insulating layer surrounding the nerve, and it is interrupted at regular intervals along its course by gaps, known as nodes of Ranvier, where the axis cylinder comes into direct contact with the tissue fluid outside the nerve. The number of nodes is constant in a given nerve throughout life so that as the nerve grows the internodal distance increases, and in the adult nerve may be of the order of 1 mm. Myelin is composed of lipid material, and it is this which contributes the white colour to peripheral nerve and the white matter of the central nervous system.

In peripheral nerve the myelin sheath is formed by the Schwann cells which are found along the course of the nerves. Electron microscopy has shown that the Schwann cell cytoplasm surrounds the axon in the form of an outer and inner

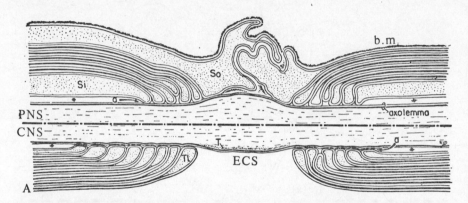

FIG. 3.3. Diagram to show nodal region of myelin sheath in central nervous system (CNS) and peripheral nervous system (PNS). In PNS in addition to the inner collar (Si) provided by the Schwann cell there is also an outer collar (So) which extends into the nodal region and the whole is covered by a basement membrane. At the CNS nodes there may be considerable extracellular space. It is now known that the special areas of density between the axolemma and the Schwann cell loops which are shown in the CNS node are also present in the PNS nodes. They may be concerned with restricting diffusion out of the periaxonal space (a). Bunge, R. P. (1968), *Physiol. Rev.*, **48**, 197–251.

collar on either side of the myelin sheath (Fig. 3.4). The nucleus of the Schwann cell lies outside the myelin sheath at about the mid-point of the internodal segment. The myelin is laid down by the Schwann cell as it spirals round the axon, the lipid layers each being separated by a film of protein. A single Schwann cell thus gives rise to an internodal myelin segment. At the nodes the Schwann cells on either side remain separate but send out processes which cover the greater part of the nerve. The basement membrane of the Schwann cells is continuous and covers the nodal regions. It is now clear that the sheath of Schwann or neurolemma, which surrounds the axon, is a cellular structure composed of

Schwann cells and their basement membrane. Schwann cells also are found in association with unmyelinated fibres indicating that they must have other important functions with regard to the nerve fibre apart from the laying down of myelin. With these fibres the axons are invaginated into a Schwann cell, and it is commonly found that a single Schwann cell will have several non-myelinated fibres invaginated within it.

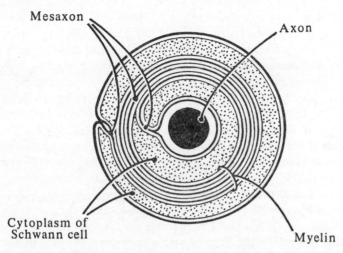

FIG. 3.4. Diagram to show cross-section of peripheral nerve axon surrounded by Schwann cell cytoplasm.

In the central nervous system Schwann cells are not found, but electron microscope studies have shown that here also myelin is laid down in a spiral around the nerve fibres with a collar of cytoplasm both deep and superficial to it. This cytoplasm is connected, sometimes by long processes to oligodendrocytes in the vicinity of the nerve fibre. The node of Ranvier in the central nervous system differs morphologically in a number of respects from that of peripheral nerve; for example, it is not surrounded by interdigitating processes comparable to those derived from the Schwann cell, and there is no basement membrane which crosses the node. An important functional difference between nerves in the brain ands pinal cord and peripheral nerve is that after nerve injury peripheral nerve will regenerate but regeneration does not take place in the central nervous system. The myelin sheath with its interrupted course along the nerve fibre has important effects on the conduction of the nerve impulse and nerve conduction is faster along myelinated than along unmyelinated nerve fibres. In both the central nervous system and peripheral nerve the myelin sheaths are vulnerable to disease and injury, and demyelination in either situation may readily give rise to neurological disability.

THE NERVE IMPULSE

Passage of Nerve Impulse in Non-conducting Medium

A convenient way to study the conduction of the nerve impulse is to stimulate a nerve with a negative electrical pulse with electrodes placed over the nerve at a distance from the stimulating electrode so that the electrical disturbance associated with the impulse can be recorded on a galvanometer or oscilloscope. If this is done with the nerve in an electrolyte medium, such as Ringer's solution, or left in the body in contact with the tissue fluid, the character of the evoked potential will be modified by the characteristics of the conducting medium which is known as a volume conductor. The analysis is much simpler if the nerve is excised and placed in a moist chamber where it is connected to the stimulating and recording electrodes and surrounded only by a thin film of Ringer solution. Alternatively in the intact animal the nerve can be separated from the surrounding tissues by an insulating medium such as mineral oil. With either of these arrangements if the nerve is stimulated a wave of surface negativity will travel along the nerve fibre which will make the first recording electrode negative with respect to the second. By convention the input leads to the recording apparatus are so arranged that this negative potential will be represented by an upward deflection on the oscilloscope. As the disturbance passes further along the nerve it comes in contact with a second electrode so that the first electrode is now positive with respect to the second and a deflection appears in the opposite direction.

In studying the properties of nerve fibres there are disadvantages in studying the diphasic potential evoked in this manner. A monophasic action potential can be obtained if the nerve fibre underlying the second electrode is permanently depolarized and therefore unaffected by the wave of negativity. This state of affairs can be achieved by crushing the nerve under the second electrode or by the local application of potassium salts.

The All-or-Nothing Principle

If a portion of a nerve is blocked by a narcotic, the strength of stimulus necessary to effect conduction through the blocked area remains constant until conduction fails completely. Sometimes a small increase in the threshold stimulus occurs shortly before conduction fails and this is due to conduction failing initially in a few of the most excitable fibres. These observations suggest that conduction in a nerve fibre does not depend on the strength of the stimulus provided the stimulus is adequate (Adrian, 1914). This is known as the all-or-nothing law which is further illustrated by studying the effects of altering stimulus intensity on the size of action potentials in nerve. If a weak stimulus is applied to a nerve trunk a small action potential will be evoked and this will increase in size as the stimulus is increased until a certain level is reached. When a further increase in stimulus strength has no effect on action potential magnitude the nerve is said to be excited supramaximally. The effect of a supramaximal stimulus is to excite all the component fibres of the nerve trunk.

Studies on single nerve fibres have shown that if a stimulus is strong enough to excite a nerve fibre any further increase in the strength of the stimulus will have no effect on the size of the action potential. This all-or-nothing relationship applies to all propagated responses in nerve or muscle fibres. Non-propagated responses, such as postsynaptic potentials in neurones, end-plate potentials in muscle and generator potentials in sense organs may on the other hand be graded in character.

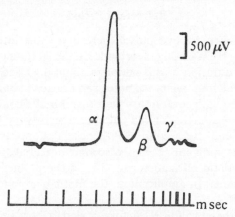

FIG. 3.5. The complex of compound action potential obtained from stimulating frog's sciatic nerve. After J. Erlanger and H. S. Gasser (1937). *Electrical Signs of Nervous Activity*. University of Pennsylvania Press.

The Compound Action Potential

If a nerve is excited with the recording arrangements adjusted so as to give a monophasic deflection, it will be seen that the compound action potential of the nerve trunk contains several components which become more widely separated the further apart the stimulating and recording electrodes are placed (Fig. 3.5). The later components of the potential may only appear as the strength of the stimulus is increased. These observations indicate that the nerve contains fibres which conduct impulses at different velocities and that the more rapidly conducting fibres are the more easily excited. On this basis it has been possible to separate the different fibre types in a nerve trunk in terms of their excitability and conduction velocity, a classification which correlates reasonably well with one based on histological measurement of fibre diameter (see below).

If the time course of the compound action potential is followed for $\frac{1}{2}$ sec after the main deflection, it will sometimes be seen that changes in potential occur which are associated with changes in the excitability of the nerve during the recovery phase after the nerve impulse. The first is a small negative deflection which occurs at the termination of the spike potential, which may last about 10 msec and which is known as the negative after-potential. This is followed by a small positive deflection which may last for longer than 50 msec and is known as the positive after-potential. The duration of these after-potentials is longer in smaller nerve fibres of slower conduction velocity. The negative after-potential corresponds with a period when the nerve is hyperexcitable and the positive after-potential with a period of reduced excitability. These two phases are known as the super-normal and sub-normal periods.

Refractory Period

If a nerve is stimulated by two pulses there is a short interval after the first stimulus when the nerve is wholly inexcitable. In the larger more rapidly conducting nerve fibres the duration of this period is about 0.5 msec. It is followed by a longer period of a few msec when the nerve can be excited but only by a stronger stimulus. This is the relative refractory period and in the compound nerve trunk it can be measured by applying paired pulses and increasing the interval between them progressively until the second evoked potential appears. If supramaximal stimuli are used the moment when the second potential first appears corresponds with the absolute refractory period, and the moment when the second potential becomes equal in amplitude to the first corresponds with the relative refractory period.

The duration of the absolute refractory period is very similar to that of the action potential of the single nerve fibre, and it corresponds to the recovery period of the nerve fibre after excitation which is dependent on the distribution and movement of ions across the nerve fibre membrane (see p. 36). The duration of the refractory period is dependent on changes of temperature and is of longer duration at low temperatures. It tends to be of longer duration in smaller nerve fibres of relatively slow nerve conduction velocity. During the relative refractory period the velocity of nerve conduction is slowed. An important consequence of the refractory period of nerve fibres is that it limits the frequency at which a nerve can be excited and conduct impulses.

Intensity-duration Curve

Since the strength of stimulus required to excite a nerve depends on the length of time it continues, the excitability of the nerve can be expressed in the form of a curve in which the intensity required for excitation is plotted against the duration of the exciting stimulus. Certain points in the intensity or strength-duration curve are of interest. The smallest or threshold stimulus that will excite the nerve if allowed to continue indefinitely is known as the rheobase, and the duration of an effective stimulus of twice the rheobase strength is known as chronaxie. The strength-duration curve is of clinical significance because its time course and the values of rheobase and chronaxie between nerve and muscle. Since innervated muscle is normally excited through its motor nerve the characteristic intenstity-duration curve for muscle will only be obtained when the muscle is isolated from its motor nerve and in clinical practice this may provide reliable evidence of denervation (see chapter 5).

Accommodation

The most effective stimulus to a nerve is a square wave which reaches its maximum intensity in the shortest possible space of time. A slowly rising current may be ineffective so that the nerve becomes refractory without giving rise to an action potential. There is considerable difference between nerves in respect of the property of accommodation which moreover is more marked in nerve than in muscle (see chapter 5).

Nerve Fibre Size and Conduction Velocity

Analysis of the compound action potential of nerve has shown that nerve fibres can be divided into three important categories. Electrophysiological and histological studies of single nerve fibres have provided detailed information regarding the properties of these groups and shown also that the main groups can be divided into subgroups. The three principal categories are as follows.

A Fibres

These are large myelinated fibres of somatic nerves with a diameter varying from 1–20 μm and having a conduction velocity ranging from 5–150 metres/sec. They include both motor and sensory fibres and have been divided into α, β, γ and δ groups in order of decreasing diameter and conduction velocity.

B Fibres

These are small thinly myelinated fibres with a diameter of less than 3 μm and a conduction velocity of less than 15 metres/sec. They include preganglionic autonomic fibres.

C Fibres

These are unmyelinated and do not exceed 1 μm in diameter and conduct at less than 2 metres/sec. They include both sensory and autonomic fibres.

In considering sensory nerves a numerical classification which is based on fibre size has been found useful. In this classification groups I, II and III have an approximate correspondence with different sizes of A fibres and group IV corresponds with C fibres. Group Ia fibres include afferent fibres from muscle spindles and group Ib afferents from Golgi tendon organs. Group II and III fibres are found in both muscle and cutaneous nerves (Lloyd, 1943; Hunt, 1954).

The conduction velocity of nerve fibres is dependent on fibre diameter and is more rapid in the larger nerve fibres. Myelinated fibres conduct more rapidly than unmyelinated nerves, and the myelin sheath has been of great importance in the evolution of the nervous system since it has made possible the development of rapidly conducting nerve fibres of relatively small size so that the complex nervous system of higher vertebrates can accommodate large numbers of fibres within a relatively small space. The relationship between nerve fibre diameter and conduction velocity is complex and differs in the two types of fibre; in the larger myelinated fibres the approximate relationship between fibre diameter and conduction velocity is a linear one, whereas in unmyelinated fibres conduction velocity is proportional to the square root of fibre diameter.

THE PROPAGATION OF THE NERVE IMPULSE

The Injury Potential

It has been known for more than a century that if a nerve or muscle fibre is injured, the injured end becomes electrically negative if its potential is compared with that of an electrode placed at a distance from it on the surface of the fibre. This demarcation potential or injury potential may exceed 50 mV in amplitude and is accounted for by the fact that there is a potential difference across the nerve fibre membrane the outside positive with respect to the inside.

The Membrane Theory

Bernstein in 1902 put forward the hypothesis that the passage of the nerve impulse with its accompanying action potential is due to depolarization of the membrane which spreads along the length of the fibre. He argued that in the resting state the membrane was permeable to potassium only, but that during excitation it became permeable to other ions such as chloride and sodium and that the free passage of these ions through the membrane abolished the potential difference across it. It is now clear that during excitation the nerve fibre is not merely depolarized, but the polarity is reversed so that the inside of the fibre becomes positive with respect to the outside (Hodgkin and Huxley, 1939).

Our present understanding of these events is the result of observations which have been made by passing microelectrodes through the external membrane of nerve and muscle so that the potential difference across it can be measured. The study of nerve in this way became possible when it was found that the squid has a giant unmyelinated nerve fibre with a diameter of 0.5–1.0 mm which may survive for as long as 24 hours after removal from the animal (Young, 1936). It was found by Hodgkin and Huxley that if a glass capillary electrode were passed into the axon a potential difference of between 50 and 70 mV was recorded between the internal electrode and the fluid outside the nerve, the outside of the membrane positive to the inside. It was found also that if the nerve was excited, this potential difference was reversed so that the inside of the membrane became 40–50 mV positive with respect to the outside, giving rise to an action potential having a total amplitude of greater than 100 mV (Fig. 3.6). These observations, and the detailed analyses which have followed, have provided the experimental background for the membrane theory of nerve conduction (see reviews by Hodgkin, 1964, and Katz, 1966).

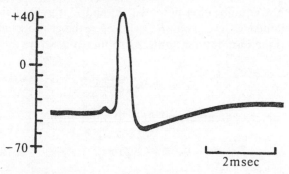

FIG. 3.6. Action potential recorded from axon of squid by means of internal electrode. Zero represents potential of surrounding sea water. After A. L. Hodgkin and A. F. Huxley (1939). *Nature*, **144**, 710–711.

The Resting Membrane Potential

The resting potential of nerve and muscle is particularly important since it is concerned with their excitability and ability to propagate an impulse. It is, however, a general property of cells and depends on the selective permeability of membranes to particular ions. In the squid axon the concentration of potassium is approximately 20 times as great as that in the extracellular fluid. On the other hand the concentration of sodium is about 9 times as great outside the fibre as within it. Chloride ions are about 14 times as concentrated in the extracellular fluid as in the nerve. The anions within the nerve fibre are for the most part organic acids with large molecules which cannot pass through the cell membrane. The osmotic pressures exerted by the extracellular and intracellular fluids are the same and in the resting state the only ion to which the membrane is permeable is the potassium ion. Under these circumstances potassium ions will tend to diffuse along the concentration gradient from within the cell to the extracellular fluid. Since, however, they are not accompanied by the negatively charged anions, which cannot pass through the membrane, further passage of potassium ions across the membrane will be opposed by the attraction of the negative ions which have remained within the fibre. A potential difference will now exist across the fibre membrane, which has been charged like a capacitor, and this potential difference constitutes the resting membrane potential. If the membrane potential were determined entirely by the permeability of the membrane to potassium and the concentration gradient of potassium across it, it would correspond to the value determined by the Nernst equation for the potassium equilibration potential:

$$E_k = \frac{RT}{F} \log_e \frac{(K_o)}{(K_i)}$$

(where E_k is the K equilibration potential, K_i and K_o the potassium concentrations inside and outside the cell and R, T and F are the gas constant, the absolute temperature and the Faraday constant). At room temperature this can be simplified to:

$$E_k = 57 \log_{10} \frac{(K_o)}{(K_i)}$$

If K_i is approximately 400 mmol and K_o is 20 mmol then

$$E_k = 57 \log_{10} \frac{1}{20}$$

$$= 57 \times 2.699$$

$$= -74 \text{ mV}$$

This corresponds with the resting potential which has been recorded in intact squid axons.

Further experimental support for the dependence of the membrane potential on the potassium concentrations inside and outside the cell has been gained from studies in which the fibre has been immersed in fluid containing differing concentrations of potassium and sodium, and by experiments in which the axoplasm has been squeezed out of the fibre and replaced by a fluid in which the ionic concentrations can be altered (Baker, Hodgkin and Shaw, 1961).

The Excitation of Nerve

Excitation in the nerve comes about when there is a change in the fibre so that it becomes permeable to sodium ions. This occurs when the resting potential falls to what is known as the threshold level. In the squid axon this is about 15 mV below the resting potential. When the membrane is depolarized to the threshold level the permeability to sodium increases in an explosive manner so that sodium flows into the fibre transferring a positive charge from the outside to the interior. This leads to a further reduction in membrane potential and a further increase in permeability to sodium. It is of interest that this explosive entry of sodium is different from the effect of a condenser discharge where according to Ohm's law the rate of flow of current falls as the potential difference decreases. At the peak of the action potential the inside of the membrane is perhaps 40 mV positive with respect to the outside and the membrane is now selectively permeable to sodium (Fig. 3.6). At this stage the membrane potential corresponds to the sodium equilibration potential:

$$E_k = \frac{RT}{F} \log_e \frac{(Na_o)}{(Na_i)}$$

The high permeability or conductance to sodium persists for 1–2 msec and then terminates, and it is followed by an enhanced conductance to potassium which is of relatively long duration and leads to an outflow of potassium so that the resting condition is re-established as the action potential subsides (see review by Hodgkin, 1951; Hodgkin and Huxley, 1952 and 1953). At the end of the action potential a gradual process of recovery takes place in which the membrane conductances return to their normal value. The last process to occur is to return the sodium that has entered the fibre during excitation to the extra-cellular fluid. This must take place against the concentration gradient and the process of active transfer by which this takes place has been given the name of the sodium pump.

The process of excitation which has been described is a similar process to that of amplification, in that a small change in membrane potential to the threshold level initiates a change in potential which develops rapidly and greatly exceeds the original change. The essential factor in this process is that the conductance of the membrane to sodium is dependent on the resting potential so that the conductance increases as the potential falls allowing sodium to enter the fibre at an increasing rate along the concentration gradient. How the membrane potential controls the permeability of the membrane to sodium and also to potassium is unknown. The effect of the reversal in membrane potential which accompanies excitation is to set up a difference in potential between the affected part of the fibre and the portion immediately adjacent. As a result of this a current will flow through the surrounding tissue fluid between the depolarized part of the nerve and the next part of the fibre to lower the resting potential. If this is lowered to the threshold level the process of explosive depolarization will again occur and in this way the disturbance is propagated along the nerve fibre. This passive spread of an electrical change from one part of a fibre to another is sometimes referred to as an electrotonic current. It has a particularly important function in transmission along myelinated nerves (fig. 3.7).

This explanation of the nerve impulses has been supported by a number of experimental observations. In the first place the use of radioactive tracers has shown that there is an uptake of sodium and loss of potassium with each nerve impulse which is sufficient to account for the electrical changes which occur with the nerve impulse (Keynes, 1951). Further evidence has been obtained by what is known as the voltage clamp technique.

The voltage clamp is an arrangement whereby an electrode on either side of the membrane is connected to a voltage source so that the membrane potential can be shifted to any desired level. As the membrane potential is adjusted there is a flow of current through the membrane which can be measured. If the ionic concentrations in the bathing fluid are measured during current flow, it is possible to construct curves relating current flow to time in association with the concentrations of ions in the extracellular fluid and so measure the ionic flow accompanying the passage of current. It is also possible to calculate the conductance of the membrane to sodium and potassium ions at particular levels of membrane potential. If the membrane is suddenly depolarized a rapid inward flow of current is first recorded which corresponds to the explosive entry of sodium ions into the cell. After about a msec the inflow of sodium is replaced by an outward current corresponding to the outward flow of potassium ions from the nerve fibre.

During the phase of potassium outflow the membrane becomes impermeable to sodium and remains in this state until the membrane potential has returned to normal at the end of the action potential. This reduction in sodium conductance is not a simple reversal of the increase in permeability which has been brought about by depolarization but is a separate process known as inactivation which is also initiated by depolarization but develops more slowly. Depolarization thus has three effects on membrane permeability which may all depend on separate alterations in the molecular configuration of the surface of the membrane, viz., increased sodium conductance, inactivation of sodium conductance and increased potassium conductance. The first effect develops rapidly, the other two develop more slowly.

During the phase of inactivation of sodium conductance the nerve cannot be excited and it is during this period of time that the nerve is refractory. Since the process of inactivation has come to an end at about the time the action potential terminated, the duration of the refractory period corresponds approximately to that of the action potential. The slow development of inactivation of sodium permeability may also explain accommodation. If a rapidly rising current is used to produce depolarization to the threshold level, the explosive entry of sodium ions will take place before inactivation of sodium conductance has had time to develop. On the other hand if the exciting stimulus is a slowly rising one the sodium permeability may be inactivated before the threshold level is reached and the action potential will fail to develop (Hodgkin and Huxley, 1952; see also reviews by Hodgkin 1951 and 1964).

The Sodium Pump

Since each nerve impulse is accompanied by entry of sodium and loss of potassium from the nerve fibre, repeated activation would lead to the fibre becoming loaded with sodium and depleted of potassium if there were not some mechanism for restoring the original ionic concentrations. To do this sodium and potassium must move against a concentration gradient so that it is necessary to postulate some system of active transport. In theory an active transport system comprising a carrier pathway for pumping sodium out of the cell would be sufficient also to restore the concentrations of potassium since the passage of sodium out of the cell would give rise to a negative potential within the cell which would attract potassium. The evidence, however, suggests that the active transport mechanism is not confined to pumping sodium out of the nerve but also is concerned with the inward movement of potassium (Hodgkin and Keynes, 1955). Little is known about the nature of the sodium pump but it is likely that, at least in nerve, its energy is derived from oxidative metabolism since it can be blocked by substances such as dinitrophenol and cyanide which interfere with oxidative metabolism. Although these substances will block the outward flow of sodium during the stage of recovery, they have no effect on the propagation of action potentials so it would seem that the processes involved in the recovery processes of the membrane are distinct and separate from those regulating the changes in permeability which occur at the time of the action potential. The energy for the sodium transport mechanism is probably derived in the first instance from the breakdown of ATP, but it is likely that other sources of high energy phosphate such as arginine phosphate, or in vertebrates creatine phosphate, may also be necessary. The process has been studied in isolated nerve using radioactive tracers to measure the outflow of sodium to the surrounding fluid, and it has been found that if sodium transport is blocked by poisoning with cyanide, the movement of sodium can be restored by the injection of ATP or arginine phosphate into the axon (Caldwell *et al.*, 1960).

Saltatory Conduction

Conduction of the nerve impulse as it occurs in non-myelinated nerve fibres by propagation along the membrane is a comparatively slow process. In myelinated nerve the inward flow of sodium and the outward flow of potassium occurs only at the nodes of Ranvier. The myelin sheath which surrounds the internodes is of high resistance and is an effective insulator so that an action potential at a nodal area gives rise to depolarization at the next node by passive spread of current outside the myelinated internodal segment. This conduction of the nerve impulse through the action of local circuits between the nodes of Ranvier is very much more rapid than the direct conduction of an impulse along the membrane of an unmyelinated fibre (Fig. 3.7).

Much evidence has accumulated to support the theory of saltatory conduction. For example, the threshold for stimulation in myelinated nerve is lower at the nodes of Ranvier than it is in the region between the nodes. Secondly, substances which block the transmission of the impulse, such as cocaine, are effective at the nodes and ineffective at the internodes. If action potentials are recorded along different points of the internodal segments of an isolated nerve, it is found that in each segment they occur synchronously but measurably later than in the preceding segment; this stepwise increase in conduction latency at the nodes is consistant with the active process being largely confined to the nodal areas. (Fig.

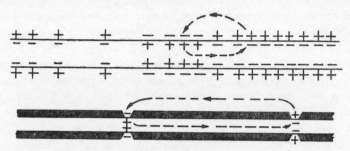

FIG. 3.7. Diagram to illustrate local circuit theory in unmyelinated (upper sketch) and myelinated nerve fibre (lower sketch). Hodgkin, A. L. (1964). *The Conduction of the Nerve Impulse.* Liverpool: University Press.

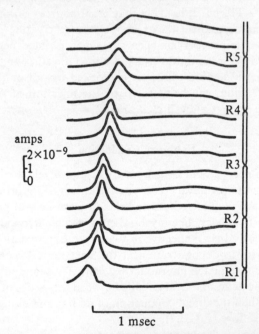

FIG. 3.8. Action potentials recorded at successive points along single fibre of frog's sciatic nerve using capillary partition. Records from any one internode are practically synchronous and conduction latency increases stepwise from node to node. Huxley, A. F. and Stampfli, R. (1949). *J. Physiol. (Lond.),* **108,** 315–339.

3.8) Further evidence has been provided by an experiment in which an isolated nerve fibre is extended between two microscope slides with each end in a pool of saline and at least one node of Ranvier in the gap; in this arrangement the nerve will only conduct if a thread soaked in Ringer solution is placed between the pools of saline to establish electrical continuity (Huxley and Stämpfli, 1949; Tasaki, 1953).

In both myelinated and non-myelinated nerve fibres the speed of conduction is dependent on the nerve fibre diameter. In myelinated nerve fibres, however, fibres of relatively small diameter can conduct impulses at a rapid rate, so that in the more complex forms of life enormous numbers of rapidly conducting fibres can be included in a nerve trunk which remains relatively small in size. When nerve injury occurs it is significant that loss of the myelin sheath results in a marked slowing of nerve conduction velocity.

NERVE INJURY

Wallerian Degeneration and Demyelination

Disease or injury to a nerve fibre can affect the whole nerve including axon and myelin sheath, or can give rise to selective loss of myelin with preservation of the axon. If a nerve is sectioned or crushed the process which occurs in the distal segment is known as Wallerian degeneration. In the first 12–24 hours changes take place in the axons, starting in the distal portions, the fibre first shrinking and then breaking into fragments so that continuity is lost within 4–5 days. Degeneration of the myelin sheath takes place at the same time. The earliest change is that the myelin shrinks and retracts at the nodes of Ranvier exposing a length of unmyelinated nerve at the nodal area. Within 48 hours much of the myelin is broken up into globules and in the course of the next month the debris of myelin and axis cylinders disappears. The above description applies particularly to peripheral nerve fibres. In the central nervous system the changes of Wallerian degeneration are broadly similar, but the changes take place more slowly, little change being evident in the smaller fibres before the end of the first 10 days. In peripheral nerve, regeneration is possible because the basement membrane of the Schwann cell survives and forms a continuous tube along which the regenerating axon can grow. After peripheral nerve section sprouts can be seen emerging from the proximal end of the nerve within about 12 hours and after a few days new axons can be recognized growing down the neurolemma. As regeneration proceeds the new nerve may grow down the neural tube at a rate approaching 3.0 mm/day. As the axons grow they become invaginated into the Schwann cells so that a spiral of myelin forms round them and nodes of Ranvier reform.

Degenerative changes affecting both myelin sheath and axis cylinder occur also if a nerve fibre is damaged by ischaemia or affected by certain toxins of which tri-ortho-cresyl phosphate is an example which has been carefully studied

(Cavenagh, 1964). It may also occur in disease which affects the anterior horn cells such as poliomyelitis and motor neurone disease. On the other hand loss of the myelin sheath with little change in the axis cylinder may occur in a number of other conditions affecting the peripheral nerves, notably diphtheritic and diabetic neuropathy, experimental allergic neuritis and sometimes following local pressure on a nerve. This demyelination starts in the paranodal region and spreads to involve whole internodal segments. Frequently the nerve is affected in a patchy manner so that while some internodal segments are affected others are preserved. Characteristically there is little change in the axon although peripheral neuropathies occur in which there is a combination of both nerve fibre degeneration and segmental or paranodal demyelination. In the central nervous system a similar distinction applies between disorders in which the pathological change applies to both axon and myelin sheath and those in which it is largely confined to the myelin. The first group includes conditions where there is direct damage to nervous tissue through trauma, pressure and anoxia, in which Wallerian degeneration occurs and the system degenerations where a similar but slower process follows atrophy of nerve cells. The second includes the demyelinating disorders, such as multiple sclerosis, acute disseminated encephalomyelitis and the leucodystrophies where the process affects the myelin sheaths, often with preservation of the axons.

Nerve Conduction Velocity Measurement

In the study of disorders of peripheral nerve in man the measurement of nerve conduction velocity has proved a valuable method. This can readily be carried out by stimulating a peripheral nerve at two points along its course and recording evoked potentials from the muscle which it supplies (Piper, 1908). Sensory conduction can be recorded by st mulating digital nerves and recording evoked potentials from proximal portions of the nerve (Dawson, 1956) (Fig. 3.9).

Following nerve section, conduction ceases in the distal segment in about 4 days and during that period the action potential decreases in size but there is little change in conduction velocity (Landau, 1953; Gilliatt and Taylor, 1959). During recovery although action potent als have been recorded in recovering nerve about 3 weeks after the injury in nerve which has been experimentally sectioned and resutured (Berry *et al.*, 1944), nerve conduction velocity cannot normally be measured in the human subject until re-innervation has occurred in the muscle supplied by the nerve. Conduction velocity is slow for long periods after clinical recovery has occurred and in many cases never returns to normal (Hodes *et al.*, 1948; Cragg and Thomas, 1964).

In neuropathy where degeneration of the axons occurs either as a result of toxic changes or of anterior horn cell atrophy, there is generally no significant impairment of nerve conduction velocity although marginal slowing may occur possibly due to loss of the more rapidly conducting fibres in the nerve trunk. On the other hand where segmental demylination has taken place very substantial falls in conduction velocity may occur and in these instances nerve conduction velocity measurement may provide diagnostic evidence of a peripheral neuropathy. Velocity is also slowed in pressure neuropathies where localized demyelination may occur and where conduction velocity studies may be of localizing value (Simpson, 1956).

One possible explanation for the slowing of nerve conduction velocity which occurs in demyelinated nerve is that there is interference with saltatory conduction so that conduction occurs continuously along the axon. However, Rasminsky and Sears (1972) have found that ventral root fibres in the rat which have

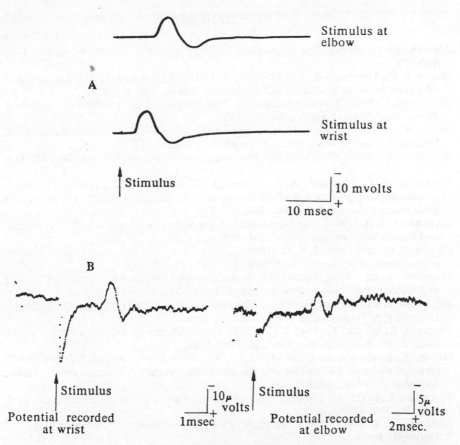

FIG. 3.9. Motor and sensory nerve conduction measurement in human ulnar nerve. A. Shows evoked potentials in abductor digiti minimi recorded with surface electrodes following stimulation of ulnar nerve at elbow and wrist. If the 2 latencies are subtracted the conduction velocity from elbow to wrist can be calculated. B. Shows action potentials recorded from ulnar nerve at wrist and elbow following stimulation of digital nerves at 5th finger with ring electrodes.

undergone demyelination following application of diphtheria toxin continue to show the stepwise increase in conduction latency which is characteristic of saltatory conduction. The slowing is likely to be related to delayed excitation at the nodes secondary to changes in the properties of the internodal myelin, particularly an increase in capacitance. It is of interest that demyelinated nerve also shows an increase in refractory period which appears to arise because the second of two stimuli fails to generate sufficient current to traverse a demyelinated internode.

REFERENCES

ADRIAN, E. D. (1914). The all-or-none principle in nerve. *J. Physiol. (Lond.)*, **47**, 460–474.

BAKER, P. F., HODGKIN, A. L. and SHAW, T. I. (1961). Replacement of the protoplasm of a giant nerve fibre with artificial solutions. *Nature*, **190**, 885–887.

BERNSTEIN, J. (1902). Untersuchungen zur Thermodynamik der bioloktrischen Ströme. *Enster Theil Pflügers Archiv.*, **92**, 521–562.

BERRY, C. M., GRUNDFEST, H. and HINSEY, J. C. (1944). The electrical activity of regenerating nerves in the cat. *J. Neurophysiol.*, **7**, 103—115.

BUNGE, R. P. (1968). Glial cells and the central myelin sheath. *Physiol. Rev.*, **48**, 197–251.

CALDWELL, P. C., HODGKIN, A. L., KEYNES, R. D. and SHAW, T. I. (1960). The effects of injecting 'energy-rich' phosphate compounds on the active transport of ions in the giant axons of loligo. *J. Physiol.*, **152**, 561–590.

CAVANAGH, J. B. (1964). The significance of the 'dying back' process in experimental and human neurological disease. *Int. Rev. exp. Path.*, **3**, 219–267.

CRAGG, B. G. and THOMAS, P. K. (1964). Changes in nerve conduction in experimental allergic neuritis. *J. Neurol. Neurosurg. Psychiat.*, **27**, 106–115.

DAWSON, G. D. (1965). The relative excitability and conduction velocity of sensory and motor nerve fibres in man. *J. Physiol. (Lond.)*, **131**, 436–451.

ERLANGER, J. and GASSER, H. (1937). *Electrical Signs of Nervous Activity*. Philadelphia: University of Pennsylvania Press, 2nd Edn. 1968.

GILLIATT, R. W. and TAYLOR, J. C. (1959). Electrical changes following section of the facial nerve. *Proc. roy. soc. Med.*, **52**, 1080–1083.

HODES, R., LARRABEE, M. G. and GERMAN, W. (1948). The human electromyogram in response to nerve stimulation and the conduction velocity of motor axons. *Archiv. Neurolog. Psychiat.*, **60**, 340–365.

HODGKIN, A. L. (1951). The ionic basis of electrical activity in nerve and muscle. *Biol. Rev.*, **26**, 339–409.

HODGKIN, A. L. (1964). *The Conduction of the Nervous Impulse*. Liverpool: Liverpool University Press.

HODGKIN, A. L. and HUXLEY, A. F. (1939). Action potentials recorded from inside a nerve fibre. *Nature*, **144**, 710–711.

HODGKIN, A. L. and HUXLEY, A. F. (1952). A quantitative description of membrane current and its application and excitation of nerve. *J. Physiol.*, **117**, 500–544.

HODGKIN, A. L. and HUXLEY, A. F. (1953). Movement of radioactive potassium and membrane current in a giant axon. *J. Physiol.*, **121**, 403–414.

HODGKIN, A. L. and KEYNES, R. D. (1955). Active transport of cations in giant axons from sepia and loligo. *J. Physiol. (Lond.)*, **128**, 28–60.

HUNT, C. C. (1954). Relation of function to diameter in afferent fibres of muscle nerves. *J. gen. Physiol.*, **38**, 117–131.

HUXLEY, A. F. and STÄMPFLI, R. (1949). Evidence for saltatory conduction in peripheral myelinated nerve fibres. *J. Physiol. (Lond.)*, **108**, 315–339.

KATZ, B. (1966). *Nerve Muscle and Synapse*. New York: McGraw-Hill.

KEYNES, R. D. (1951). The ionic movements during nervous activity. *J. Physiol.*, **114**, 119–150.

LANDAU, W. M. (1953). Duration of neuromuscular function after nerve section in man. *J. Neurosurg.*, **10**, 64–68.

LLOYD, D. P. C. (1943). Neuron patterns controlling transmission of ipsilateral hind limb reflexes in cat. *J. Neurophysiol.*, **6**, 293–315.

PAKKENBERG, H. (1966). The number of nerve cells in the cerebral cortex of man. *J. comp. Neurol.*, **128**, 17–19.

PIPER, H. (1908). Uber die Leitungsgeschwindigkeit in den markhaltigen, menschlichen Nerven. *Pflügers Arch. ges. Physiol.*, **124**, 591–600.

RASMINSKY, M. and SEARS, T. (1972). Internodal conduction in undissected demyelinated nerve fibres. *J. Physiol. (Lond.)* **227**, 323–350.

SIMPSON, J. A. (1956). Electrical signs in the diagnosis of carpal tunnel and related syndromes. *J. Neurol. Neurosurg. Psychiat.*, **19**, 275–280.

TASAKI, I. (1953). *Nervous Transmission*. Springfield: Thomas.

YOUNG, J. Z. (1936). The structure of nerve fibres in cephalopods and crustacea. *Proc. Roy. Soc. B.*, **121**, 319–337.

CHAPTER 4

Synaptic Transmission

INTRODUCTION

The site at which one nerve cell connects with another or with an effector organ such as a muscle is known as a synapse. Although the transmission of the nerve impulse along the nerve fibre is essentially an electrical process the action potential which arrives at the nerve ending is not in general adequate to depolarize the postsynaptic membrane. Although in certain invertebrates electrical transmission across the synapse has been shown to occur it is now recognized that synaptic transmission takes place almost universally through the passage of a chemical transmitter from one cell to another. The historical development of this concept has been summarized by Hubbard *et al.* (1969). The nature of the chemical transmitters at the autonomic nerve endings and the neuromuscular junctions is now clearly established although much remains to be learned of their mode of action. In the central nervous system although chemical transmission is generally assumed to occur, the nature of the transmitter substance at the majority of central synapses remains uncertain. In this chapter transmission at the neuromuscular junction and in the brain and spinal cord will be discussed. A further account of transmission in the autonomic system will be found in chapter 10.

THE STRUCTURE OF SYNAPSES

In certain invertebrates and in fish, synapses occur where transmission is by an electrical process. In these synapses it is not possible to identify a clear space between the adjoining cells and the pre and post synaptic membranes are fused (Pappas and Bennett, 1966). Synapses where transmission is by passage of a chemical substance show considerable variations in their structure but it is always possible to identify a presynaptic portion, with a terminal membrane which is separated from the postsynaptic membrane by a cleft or space which

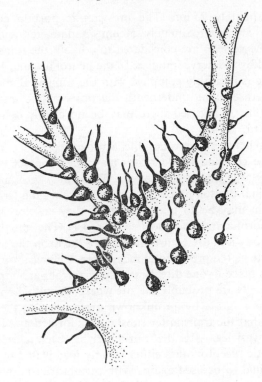

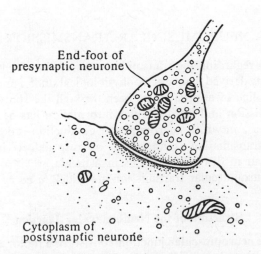

End-foot of
presynaptic neurone

Cytoplasm of
postsynaptic neurone

FIG. 4.1. (a) Dense collection of boutons termineaux on surface of neurone.
(b) Detail of junction between terminal bouton and post synaptic membrane.

measures approximately 25 nm. The presynaptic portion contains vesicular structures which are approximately 50 nm in diameter and also abundant mitochondria. The vesicles are considered to contain the transmitter substance which is liberated by the nerve impulse. In the neuromuscular junction the post-synaptic structure is relatively complex, with the subneural apparatus, which is rich in cholinesterase, lying underneath the postsynaptic membrane. At sites where noradrenaline is released there may be no clearly defined postsynaptic structure (Hubbard, 1970).

With synapses between neurones the arrangements may be very complex because the nerve cell and its dendrites may have contact with the terminal branches of very large numbers of axons. These may terminate by a swelling known as a terminal bouton and with certain neurones the terminal boutons in contact with them may be so numerous that they envelop nearly the entire surface of the neurone and its dendrites (Fig. 4.1). The impulses in a neurone arise in the cell body and are transmitted along the axon the terminal branches of which terminate as the presynaptic membrane. Chemical transmission across the synapse takes place in one direction only, viz. from axon to dendrite or cell body. The nerve cells are probably the site where the mitochondria and vesicles are formed. These migrate by an unknown mechanism to the nerve terminals where it is likely that the transmitter substance is formed and incorporated and stored within the vesicles. After the transmitter has been released and has acted on the postsynaptic receptors it is either rapidly inactivated or taken up by the presynaptic terminal to be used again. With certain transmitters, such as nora-drenaline, the uptake process is particularly important. Acetylcholine however is first broken down into choline and acetate and only the choline is taken up by the nerve terminal.

NEUROMUSCULAR TRANSMISSION

Our information regarding the transmission of impulses from nerve to muscle has been primarily derived from electrophysiological studies on nerve and muscle. A second useful line of approach has been through the study of the effects of drugs on transmission and thirdly, much information has been obtained from the study of disease in which neuromuscular conduction is defective. Clinically neuromuscular transmission is important because defects in neuromuscular transmission occur in disorders such as myasthenia gravis and because drugs which impair neuromuscular transmission are widely used as muscle relaxants in anaesthesia.

Structure of the Neuromuscular Junction

Anatomically the neuromuscular junction consists of a motor nerve ending and the postsynaptic membrane (Fig. 4.2). The postsynaptic membrane is that

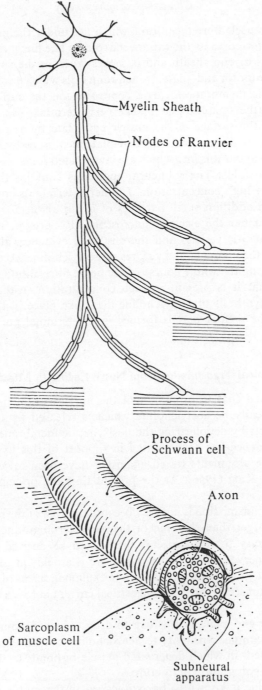

Myelin Sheath

Nodes of Ranvier

Process of
Schwann cell

Axon

Sarcoplasm
of muscle cell

Subneural
apparatus

FIG. 4.2. (a) Diagram of myelinated nerve branching to supply number of muscle fibres. (b) Junction between nerve terminal and muscle fibre.

portion of the muscle fibre membrane which lies under the nerve ending and it is sometimes referred to as the motor end–plate. The fine terminal of the nerve fibre has lost its myelin sheath and is separated from the surrounding tissues, but not from the motor end–plate, by Schwann cells which envelope the terminal. The postsynaptic membrane forms a depression on the surface of the muscle fibre known as the synaptic gutter. The nerve terminal lies within this gutter separated from the surface of the muscle end–plate by a space known as the synaptic cleft. Immediately under the end–plate membrane there is a zone known as the subneural apparatus into which are invaginated folds of surface membrane called junctional folds. The subneural apparatus contains the enzyme acetyl-cholinesterase in high concentration. The nerve terminals contain many mito-chondria and in addition small particles of up to about 50 nm diameter have been observed under the electron microscope (Robertson, 1956). These have been termed synaptic vesicles and there is good evidence, although as yet no absolute proof, that these contain stores of acetylcholine. Acetylcholine in fact can be found along the whole course of the nerve fibre although it is only in the nerve ending that it is present in high concentration. Although it has been suggested that synthesis of acetylcholine may take place in the nerve cell it is probable that the greater part is formed in the terminal portion of the nerve fibre (Hubbard, 1970).

Chemical Transmission from Nerve Ending to Muscle

It is now believed that transmission of the impulse from nerve to muscle is mediated chemically be acetylcholine which is released from the presynaptic terminals and acts by depolarizing the postsynaptic membrane at the end–plate zone. Much evidence has accumulated in support of this hypothesis and this evidence and the arguments raised against it have been reviewed in detail by del Castillo and Katz (1956). At the present time the principal evidence is as follows:

(1) Electrical transmission is unlikely because the area of the muscle membrane is many times larger than the area of the nerve terminal and a larger current would be necessary to depolarize it than could be derived from the action potential at the nerve ending. Moreover, there is a delay at the neuromuscular junction of about $\frac{1}{2}$ msec which is difficult to explain in terms of electrical spread. Attempts to demonstrate the flow of electrical current across a synapse have not been successful.

(2) The motor end–plate is sensitive to drugs which produce stimulation or paralysis. For example, sensitivity to acetylcholine can be demonstrated by the classical experiment in which denervated muscle responds to the application of acetylcholine by going into contracture.

(3) Acetylcholine is known to be synthesized in the motor nerve where it is present in bound form and released from the terminal portions during excitation.

(4) Cholinesterase inactivates acetylcholine and is present in high concentration in the subneural apparatus of the end–plate where it has been demonstrated histochemically.

(5) Direct evidence has been obtained that the external surface of the muscle fibre membrane has receptor molecules with which acetylcholine reacts. Electrophoretic application of acetylcholine through a micropipette is effective when the tip of the pipette is placed on the outer surface of the end–plate but becomes ineffective when the pipette enters the muscle fibre. The difference is not due to the high concentrations of cholinesterase that are found within the cell because the same events occur when carbaminylcholine, which is stable and resistant to cholinesterase is employed.

The Synthesis and Release of Acetylcholine

The synthesis of acetylcholine is brought about by the enzyme choline acetylase which catalyses the transfer of acetyl groups from coenzyme A to choline. ATP provides the energy for this reaction. Choline acetylase is present in the nerve in concentrations comparable to that of actylcholine but choline, although it is found in the extracellular fluid, is present in only very small amounts and there may be an active transport mechanism which moves choline from the extracellular fluid into the nerve. Acetylcholine is stored in protein bound form, possibly associated with choline acetylase, both inside and outside the synaptic vesicles. There is evidence that acetylcholine is liberated from the nerve ending in the form of discrete packets or quanta each containing many molecules of acetylcholine.

Acetylcholine release occurs spontaneously and continuously in small amounts even in the absence of a nerve impulse and this gives rise to what are known as miniature end–plate potentials. These are small potentials of about a $\frac{1}{2}$ mV amplitude which are recorded continuously if a microelectrode is inserted into the end–plate zone of a resting muscle (Fig. 4.3). The amplitude of these miniature end–plate potentials is increased by the application of an anticholinesterase and they are decreased in size by a competitive blocking agent such as curare. The response of the membrane to acetylcholine is thus graded rather than an all or nothing response and this is consistant with the quanta of acetylcholine containing a substantial number of molecules of transmitter.

Release of acetylcholine following nerve stimulation gives rise to a much larger potential which is known as the end–plate potential. The end–plate potential can most readily be recorded in curarized muscle because unless neuromuscular block is caused by curare or some other blocking agent, depolarization will proceed to the extent of giving rise to a propagated action potential. The incomplete depolarization which occurs in partially curarized muscle reaches a peak of about 30 mV in 1–1.5 msecs. A second nerve impulse a few msec after the first will cause a greatly augmented end–plate potential. The end–plate potential is thus a graded response and it does not have a refractory period. The effect of acetylcholine on the end–plate membrane is to increase the permeability of the membrane to ions, in particular sodium, potassium and ammonium. If this gives rise to partial depolarization of the cell membrane it will result in the end–plate potential. In the absence of curare the end–plate potential is associated with a fall in the membrane potential to the depolarization threshold which sets off the propagated action potential that spreads along the muscle fibre. As in the nerve fibre this is associated with passage of sodium and potassium across the cell membrane and it is possible that in muscle as in nerve there is a sodium pumping mechanism which restores the original ionic concentrations after activity.

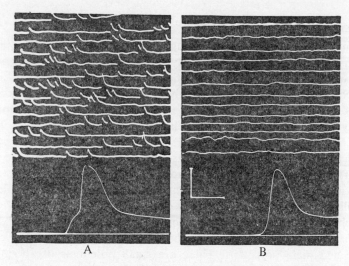

A   B

FIG. 4.3. Miniature end–plate potentials at end–plate zone of frog muscle. Left hand upper trace shows record with intracellular electrode from end–plate zone; right hand trace from elsewhere in muscle. Lower trace shows response to shock applied to motor nerve. Calibration 3.6 mV and 47 msec for upper trace, 50 mV and 2 msec for lower trace. Fatt P. and Katz B. (1952) *J. Physiol. (Lond.)* **117,** 109–128.

How the nerve impulse gives rise to the liberation of acetylcholine is not known but one factor may be the entry of calcium into the presynaptic axoplasm during the action potential. Calcium is necessary for the release of acetylcholine (Fatt and Katz, 1952) and it has been suggested that calcium may act, when it has entered the nerve ending, by disrupting the acetylcholine containing vesicles (MacIntosh, 1958). Magnesium has the opposite effect to calcium in this situation, reducing the amount of transmitter released. The manufacture of acetylcholine is interfered with by a group of quaternary bases known as hemicholiniums and these may act by inhibiting the carrier mechanism for transporting choline into the nerve (MacIntosh, Birks and Sastry, 1956). On the other hand botulinus toxin, which also interferes with the output of transmitter, has no effect on the formation of acetylcholine but interferes with its release (Burgen, Dickens and Zatman, 1949).

The propagated action potential spreads along the muscle fibre and in some way evokes the changes which initiate the muscle contraction. The mechanism is not wholly understood, but there is good reason to suppose (see chapter 5) that the walls of the transverse tubules, which may be in continuity with the muscle membrane, become depolarized as a result of the action potential and this excitation is transmitted to the sarcoplasmic reticulum in the region of the triads where calcium is released to diffuse to the region of the overlapping thick and thin filaments. This sets off the tension generating mechanism which is followed by relaxation when calcium moves back to be sequestered again within the reticulum.

Following excitation the muscle is refractory for a short period. The absolute refractory period is somewhat longer than that of nerve having a duration of between 1 and 2 msec. In much the same way as nerve, muscle can be excited by an external electrical stimulus, but muscle differs from nerve in its excitability to an electrical stimulus. To activate a muscle fibre a stimulus either of longer duration or of greater intensity than that necessary to excite nerve is required. On the other hand, a slowly rising pulse is more effective when applied to muscle than to nerve because the accommodation of muscle is less than that of nerve. These differences in excitability and accommodation are of clinical value (see chapter 5) as they may serve to distinguish denervated from innervated muscle.

Neuromuscular Block

Neuromuscular block can come about through a disturbance affecting either the presynaptic or the postsynaptic part of the neuromuscular junction. Presynaptic block may be due to failure of synthesis of acetylcholine, which occurs if the nerve is poisoned by hemicholinium, or failure of release of acetylcholine due to the action of magnesium ions or of a local anaesthetic such as procaine or resulting from the absence of calcium ions.

Postsynaptic block can be of the competitive variety, which is due to the presence of a substance which combines with the receptors for acetylcholine on the postsynaptic membrane to form an inactive complex. A block of this kind is produced by tubocurarine and gallamine. The effect of curare is to reduce the size of the end–plate potential so that it may fail to initiate the propagated action potential. Among the characteristics of competitive block are the following:

(1) The block is antagonized by acetylcholine and anticholinesterases.

(2) After a single dose of a competitive blocking agent the muscle shows increased sensitivity to subsequent doses.

(3) If tetanic stimulation is applied to partially blocked muscle the tetanus is not well sustained, but if single shot stimulation is restored there is a prolonged restoration of action potential size.

A second form of postjunctional block is known as depolarization block which is due to a substance producing prolonged depolarization of the motor end–plate. It can be produced by acetylcholine itself or by anticholinesterases such as neostigmine or by substances which have a similar action to acetylcholine in that they combine with the acetylcholine receptors and depolarize the postsynaptic membrane. Examples of this type of substance are decamethonium and suxamethonium.

The clinical importance of neuromuscular block lies in the study of disease such as myasthenia gravis where neuromuscular transmission is affected, and also in the clinical use of neuromuscular blocking agents particularly in connection with surgical anaesthesia. In myasthenia gravis the affected muscles are weak and fatigue readily. If myasthenic muscle is stimulated through its nerve it will fatigue rapidly but even when fatigued it will respond fully to electrical stimuli applied direct to the muscle, and the fatigue is rapidly relieved by anticholinesterase drugs such as neostigmine. Although it is clear from these observations that myasthenic weakness is due to neuromuscular block the site and nature of the block remains unknown. In some respects the block resembles the block which develops after the administration of curare to a healthy subject. In each instance if evoked potentials are recorded from a muscle during stimulation through its motor nerve, there is a progressive decrease in the size of the evoked potentials. There are however differences between myasthenic and curarized muscle. If myasthenic muscle is tetanized the tetanus is followed by a brief period of facilitation when the evoked potentials are larger than before the tetanus. This is similar to what is seen in curarized muscle and may be the result of facilitated release of acetylcholine from the motor nerve endings. However in myasthenic muscle this is followed by a later phase in which both the action potential and the twitch tension are depressed over about $\frac{1}{2}$ hour. Desmedt (1958) has suggested that this may be due to a pre-junctional failure of acetylcholine release, since it is similar to the effect which is seen when nerve is poisoned by hemicholinium when there is failure to synthesize acetylcholine.

Microelectrode studies on excised human intercostal muscle have provided further evidence that the neuromuscular block in myasthenia gravis may be prejunctional. In this preparation although miniature end–plate potentials occur at normal frequency their amplitude is much reduced (Elmqvist *et al.*, 1964). This would be interpreted as evidence that in myasthenia gravis the quanta of transmitter particles each contain a reduced amount of acetylcholine. An alternative explanation is that in myasthenia the muscle fibre membrane is abnormally insensitive to chemical transmitter.

Fatigue of electrically evoked potentials may also occur in other conditions besides myasthenia gravis, for example, in patients with lower motor neurone lesions such as those occurring in poliomyelitis and motor neurone disease. This effect can also be relieved by anticholinesterase indicating that here also there may be some disturbance at the neuromuscular junction (Mulder *et al.*, 1959). The mechanism here is unknown but a possible explanation may be that disease of the motor neurones can interfere with the synthesis of acetylcholine in the nerve cells and its transport along the axoplasm (Simpson, 1966).

Another condition where there is impairment of neuromuscular transmission is in the so-called myasthenic syndrome which can occur in association with bronchial carcinoma. Here there is muscular weakness and fatigue, but this does not respond to neostigmine, although it can be relieved by guanidine, a substance which promotes the release of acetylcholine. The effect of neuromuscular stimulation is of interest although the response to single shocks is a progressive fall in action potential size, during tetanic stimulation the evoked potentials increase in size progressively (Rooke *et al.*, 1960). This effect is similar to what occurs in poisoning with botulinus toxin and it may be that the defect in this syndrome is also prejunctional and the result of some interference with the release of acetylcholine.

SYNAPSES IN THE CENTRAL NERVOUS SYSTEM

Intracellular Recording from Nerones

The study of synaptic transmission in the central nervous system has been greatly advanced by electrophysiological methods, in particular the recording of intracellular potentials from neurones in the brain and spinal cord. Pharmacological methods have also yielded useful information, but at the present time it has only been definitely established in a few situations that transmission is mediated by particular transmitters, although much is known about the distribution of possible transmitter substances.

The technique of recording intracellularly from nerve cells has been to a large degree developed by Eccles and his associates. A clear description of the method of recording from spinal motoneurones in the cat was given by Brock, Coombs and Eccles in 1952. If a glass microelectrode is inserted through the surface of the spinal cord from which the pia–arachnoid has first been removed, an abrupt fall in potential of from 60–80 mV will signal the entry of the electrode into a cell. Since a resting potential can be recorded from many types of cell in addition to neurones, e.g. from neuroglia cells, it is necessary to confirm that the electrode is inside a nerve cell by showing that the cell can be excited to produce an action potential. This can be done by stimulating the nerve fibres which come out of the cord so as to excite the neurone antidromically. Other methods available for exciting a motor neurone are to stimulate an afferent nerve fibre so as to bring about a reflex discharge or to stimulate the neurone directly through the intracellular electrode. One method by which this can be done is to use a double barrelled electrode so that the stimulus is applied through one barrel while the second is connected to the recording apparatus.

Excitatory and Inhibitory Postsynaptic Potentials

Excitation of a motor neurone through its afferent nerve will give rise to a propagated action potential which can be registered as a spike by an intracellular electrode. A weaker stimulus which excites only a few afferent fibres

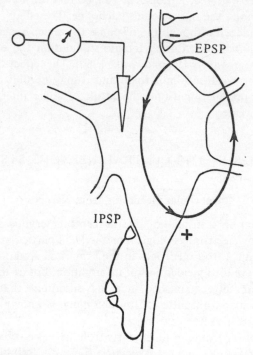

FIG. 4.4. Diagram of neurone to illustrate how excitatory postsynaptic potentials may give rise to local current flow which can lead to depolarisation at the axon hillock. A single nerve cell may be acted on by many excitatory and inhibitory fibres. In the nerve illustrated an inhibitory recurrent collateral is shown.

gives rise to partial depolarization of the nerve cell membrane. This is a localized response which is maximum at the site of the excitatory terminals and falls off exponentially with distance. This postsynaptic response has been termed the excitatory postsynaptic potential (EPSP) and in contrast to the spike, which is an all or nothing event, it is a graded response with no refractory period and in this way resembles the end–plate potential at the neuromuscular junction. The critical portion of the neurone for the development of a propagated action potential is the region of the axon hillock, and the nerve impulse is generated when local current flow resulting from summation of postsynaptic potentials in different parts of the neurone causes this part of the neurone to reach the depolarization threshold (Fig. 4.4).

It can be postulated that excitatory nerve terminals act by liberating an excitatory chemical transmitter which lowers the resting potential of the neurone by short circuiting the cell membrane. This short circuiting is probably brought about by increasing the permeability of the membrane to Na and K ions which gives rise to an inward flow of current. Some nerve fibres have an inhibitory action on the neurones with which they connect and their action may be brought about by the liberation of an inhibitory chemical transmitter. Stimulation of an inhibitory nerve is followed by an increase in the resting membrane potential of the neurone which it activates and this hyperpolarization is known as an inhibitory postsynaptic potential (IPSP). It is clear that a motoneurone may receive terminals from both excitatory and inhibitory nerves which act by producing opposite effects on the membrane potantial. It has been suggested that inhibitory transmitter acts by altering the permeability of the membrane to K and Cl ions so that entry of chloride into the cell results in an outward flow of current. Since the two types of transmitter produce opposite effects on membrane potential, it is clear that the development of an action potential as the result of depolarization caused by excitatory terminals can be effectively counteracted by inhibitory signals acting on other portions of the same neurone.

Presynaptic Inhibition

A second inhibitory mechanism has been shown to occur whereby a nerve is able to act on an excitatory nerve terminal and depress its output of transmitter.

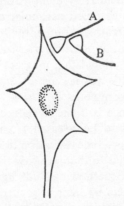

FIG. 4.5. Diagram to illustrate presynaptic inhibition by fibre from inhibitory interneurone B acting on presynaptic region of nerve fibre A.

This was first demonstrated by Frank and Fuortes (1957) who showed that stimulation of an afferent nerve could reduce the EPSP which could result from activation of neurones by neighbouring afferents. It was not clear originally whether this effect was due to depression of the presynaptic nerve endings or to inhibition of dendrites where hyperpolarization could not readily be demonstrated. It is now established that this form of inhibition is presynaptic (Eccles *et al.*, 1962) and comes about through the inhibitory nerve fibre acting on the presynaptic nerve ending to produce partial depolarization which in some way reduces the amount of transmitter liberated (Fig. 4.5). This form of inhibition occurs throughout the nervous system and has been shown to be particularly important in the spinal cord (see chapter 6).

It has also been shown that nerve fibres can act on the presynaptic terminals of other nerves to produce hyperpolarization and enhance their activity: presynaptic facilitation (Mendell and Wall, 1964).

CHEMICAL TRANSMITTERS IN THE CENTRAL NERVOUS SYSTEM

Methods of Study

Although the action of acetylcholine as a chemical transmitter has been clearly established at the neuromuscular junction (see above) and in the autonomic system (see chapter 10), and although it is widely distributed in the central nervous system, its status as a chemical transmitter has only been firmly established at one situation in the central nervous system, viz at the Renshaw cells in the spinal cord. Likewise noradrenaline is known to act as a transmitter in the autonomic system and is also present in the brain, but its action as a central transmitter has not been conclusively demonstrated. The action of chemical transmitters in the brain has assumed particular clinical significance since the introduction of drugs in the treatment of mental illness which may act by influencing chemical transmission, in particular, neuronal systems in the brain. Many substances have been isolated that may act as cerebral transmitters, but direct proof that they act in this way is generally lacking and knowledge of their site and mode of action is incomplete.

To establish that a substance is a chemical transmitter it must be shown to exist in nerve terminals and to be released from them after stimulation. In addition it must be shown to produce excitation or inhibition in neurones and to produce an overall effect similar to that resulting from physiological stimulation of nerve cells. An important method of studying the localization of possible transmitter substances has been by their histochemical identification. Thus the catecholamines can be identified histochemically. Early methods of identification of monoamines depended on biological assay, but a great deal of information

The orderly arrangement of spinal nerves whereby each is derived from one or more spinal roots, each formed from the union of an efferent ventral root and an afferent dorsal root, is of great clinical importance. Sherrington (1898) mapped the area of skin supplied by a single dorsal root by determining the area of sensation left after division of three roots above and below a single root left intact. This work was carried out in monkeys, but similar dermatomal maps have been prepared in man by this (Foerster, 1933) and other methods (Fig. 6.1). Since peripheral nerves generally contain fibres derived from more than a single segment, and since muscles may likewise be innervated by several segments, clinical examination of a part of the body where there is weakness or sensory loss may show whether the lesion corresponds to a peripheral nerve or segmental pattern. If the pattern is segmental, the distribution may localize it to particular roots or to a particular sector of the cord.

Afferent nerve fibres enter the spinal cord through the dorsal roots and the first sensory neurone lies within the dorsal root ganglion. Each dorsal root fibre, after it enters the cord, divides into an ascending and a descending branch. Some of the afferent fibres, and these tend to be larger myelinated fibres, have a relatively long ascending branch and a short descending branch. This long ascending branch enters the dorsal column of white matter on the same side of the cord and passes upwards to end in the gracile or cuneate nucleus in the medulla. Many of these fibres give off collaterals on the way to end in the dorsal grey matter, and some terminate in the grey matter of the cord, and so never reach the medulla. The medially situated gracile nucleus receives fibres from the lower parts of the body, the laterally placed cuneate nucleus from the upper limbs and trunk. The axons of the cells in the gracile and cuneate nuclei form the medial lemniscus which decussates in the medulla and passes up to end in the anterior part of the ventrobasal part of the thalamus.

Other smaller afferent fibres divide into short ascending and descending branches which pass upwards or downwards in a pathway known as the tract of Lissauer, an end by forming a synaptic connection with nerve cells in the substantia gelatinosa. The substantia gelatinosa lies at the apex of the dorsal horn of grey matter and it forms a column of nerve cells, which in the cervical region, becomes continuous with the spinal tract of the trigeminal nerve. The cells in the substantia gelatinosa give rise to axons that cross to ascend in the spinothalamic tract of the opposite side, which passes up the spinal cord and brainstem to end in the lateral and posterior parts of the ventrobasal complex of the thalamus. Only a proportion of the fibres in the spinothalamic tract reach the thalamus directly and many terminate in the reticular formation. Lamination occurs in the spinothalamic tract, so that fibres arising from the upper portions of the body are situated medially, and fibres arising caudally are displaced towards the lateral surface of the cord (Fig. 6.2).

It is well known that damage to the white matter of the spinal cord may give rise to dissociated sensory loss, in which the nature of sensory loss is dependent

D

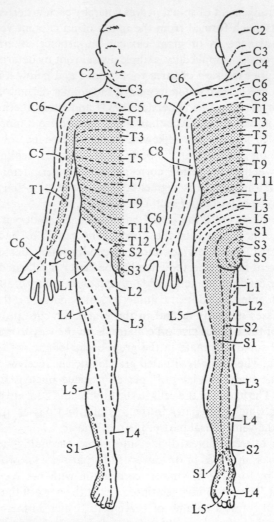

FIG. 6.1. Map of dermatomes according to Keegan. In this method of mapping skin sensibility information is based on area of sensory loss found in patients with root lesions due to an intervertebral disc protrusion. After Keegan, J. J. (1947), *J. Neurosurg.*, **4**, 115–139.

on which ascending pathways are affected. This has given rise to the concept that the fibres are grouped to travel in particular sensory pathways according to the modality of sensation which they carry, so that fibres carrying touch and proprioception pass up the posterior columns of the same side, whereas fibres carrying pain and temperature lie in the spinothalamic tracts of the opposite side. Although there is no doubt that there is functional specialization in the spinal pathways, so that certain portions of the cord are particularly important in relation to certain types of sensation, the precise separation of the white matter of the cord into defined sensory pathways, each responsible for a group of modalities, is an oversimplification which is misleading in many respects. Thus, there is no doubt that a hemisection of the cord will give rise to ipsilateral loss of touch and proprioception and to contralateral impairment of pain and temperature sensation. Moreover, cordotomy affecting the anterolateral portion of the cord will effectively relieve pain below the section, although the relief may not be permanent and a bilateral operation may be more effective than one restricted to one side. On the other hand, section of the dorsal columns in man

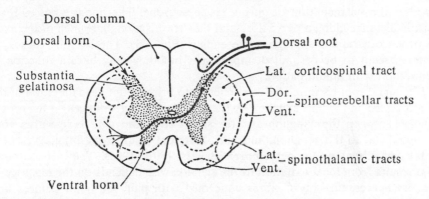

FIG. 6.2. Transverse section of spinal cord to show arrangement of uncrossed and crossed sensory pathways.

carried out to relieve the pain of a phantom limb (Cook and Browder, 1965) has been followed only by transient impairment of touch and proprioception. Although there is evidence that impulses conveying information about vibration are conveyed in the dorsal columns, there is also reason to believe that some follow other pathways such as the lateral columns (Calne and Pallis, 1966). Experimental dorsal column section in the monkey may give rise to a profound deficit in coordinated movement, particularly of an exploratory nature (Gilman and Denny-Brown, 1966). It would appear that the posterior columns are not the sole pathway for conveying information regarding touch and position, and it has been suggested that the posterior columns, which have become larger in relation to other tracts in the course of evolution, may have a particular function in providing the sensory information necessary for coordinated movement in space (Wall, 1970).

A striking feature of the spinothalamic tract is the relatively small number of fibres it contains (Glees, 1953, cited by Sinclair, 1967). Moreover, the cells of the substantia gelatinosa which give rise to the spinothalamic fibres receive converging afferents carrying different sensations (Wall and Cronly-Dillon, 1960). It is possible, therefore, that fibres in the spinothalamic pathway may carry information which has been derived from more than a single type of sensory stimulus, and that discrimination may be effected by the pattern of signal which is transmitted (see chapter 7).

THE AXON REFLEX

There is evidence that in certain situations, a reflex response occurs which involves the participation of only a single neurone. The impulse passes for a certain distance along a nerve fibre and then travels along a branch of the axon to produce a response at the nerve ending (Fig. 6.3). These axon reflexes, in general, seem to be of limited importance, but they may have a function in connection with inflammation.

If a dorsal root is stimulated, one effect is to bring about vasodilatation of the blood vessels in the part supplied by the root. This effect will occur if the root is divided between the ganglion and the spinal cord, but will be lost after root section distal to the ganglion, and must therefore result from impulses passing antidromically along the nerve fibres (Bayliss, 1901; 1902). The vasodilatation that results from local irritation to the skin likewise depends on the integrity of sensory nerves, possibly C fibres concerned with pain sensation (Hinsey and Gasser, 1930), and is probably due to impulses passing along branches of the sensory nerves that activate the small blood vessels, possibly by producing a vasodilator substance. In the triple response to a superficial scratch, described by Lewis, the flare which spreads from the red line at the site of the injury is considered to be due to an axon reflex. The triple response is associated with itch and pain and these sensations may be associated with the release of one or several chemical substances, including one which resembles histamine (Lewis, 1942).

Axon reflexes may also occur in the autonomic pathway (see chapter 10). Thus application of an alternating current to the skin results in piloerection and sweating over a distance extending several cm away from the stimulating electrode. Since this effect is abolished by postganglionic, but not by preganglionic sympathectomy, it is clearly the result of an axon reflex in the sympathetic pathway (Lewis and Marvin, 1927; Wilkins *et al.*, 1938).

Nerve conduction studies have shown that in patients with peripheral nerve lesions, it is sometimes possible to evoke muscle potentials which have a latency long enough to imply a reflex response, but too short to allow for transit of the impulse to the spinal cord and back again. This could be explained by an axon reflex occurring in recovering nerve fibres where axonal branching is taking place (Fullerton and Gilliatt, 1965).

GENERAL CHARACTERISTICS OF REFLEX ACTION

The principal characteristics of spinal reflexes were worked out in detail by Sherrington and his colleagues, and have been very fully described by Sherrington (1906) and Creed *et al.* (1932). Much of this work was carried out in the dog using a chronic spinal preparation in which the cord was divided below the cervical segments which give rise to the phrenic nerve. In this preparation,

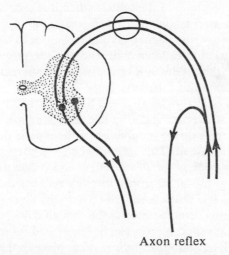

Axon reflex

FIG. 6.3. Diagram to show pathway for axon reflex in which efferent arc is formed by branching of afferent pathway.

reflexes may be studied by attaching a muscle tendon to a myograph and observing the tension developed following sensory stimulation or electrical stimulation of afferent nerves. The recording of reflexly evoked potentials in ventral roots (Lloyd, 1943a) has provided quantitative information concerning reflex activity and made it possible to distinguish between monosynaptic and polysynaptic reflex arcs. More recently, the application of microelectrodes into the grey matter of the cord and into individual neurones has made it possible to understand some of the general aspects of reflex activity in terms of what is known about synaptic transmission. The clinical study of reflexes in the human subject has not always reproduced the findings in experimental animals, and it is important to bear this in mind when applying the results of experimental work to the understanding of human disease.

The principal reflexes which were studied by Sherrington and his colleagues included the flexor reflex, which is a withdrawal response to unpleasant stimuli, generally applied to the skin, the stretch reflex and the scratch reflex. Study of these reflexes reveals important characteristics that distinguish the effect of a stimulus that excites a reflex, from one which is applied to an isolated nerve. Thus, a reflex response does not observe the all-or-nothing law but is *graded*, the strength of response depending on the strength of the stimulus. The response is graded because the effect of an afferent stimulus depends on how large a part of the motor neurone pool it excites. In the same way, if a muscle is able to be excited through several afferent nerves, each nerve can excite only part of the motor neurone pool which supplies the muscle, so that the reflex response is always less than the response of the muscle when it is excited through its motor nerve. This is known as *fractionation*. The *latent period* of a reflex also depends on the stimulus intensity, the latency becoming shorter as the stimulus intensity is increased. This variation in latency depends on the properties of the central reflex pathway, since the conduction velocities of the afferent and efferent nerves are not affected by stimulus intensity. If the conduction time along the nerve trunks is known, the central reflex time can be calculated from the latent period. If a muscle is activated reflexly the muscle may continue to twitch after the stimulus is over, whereas direct stimulation of the muscle through its nerve will produce only a single twitch. This *after-discharge* is particularly prominent in polysynaptic reflexes such as the flexor reflex, and is due to the fact that some impulses travelling to motor neurones through reflex arcs may be delayed in internuncial bypaths. If a reflex is elicited repeatedly, there is a falling off in the response. This is readily demonstrated in the scratch reflex, which fatigues more rapidly than the flexor reflex. Nerves can be stimulated for long periods without showing signs of fatigue and *reflex fatigue* takes place in the central part of the reflex arc (see chapter 5). A reflex can only be elicited through its afferent pathway. In other words, conduction along a reflex arc is in one direction only and, in this way also, it differs from a nerve which can conduct either orthodromically or antidromically.

If a single stimulus is inadequate to evoke a reflex response, two such stimuli applied within a short interval to one another may do so. This process of *summation* can come about in two ways. Firstly, two stimuli set up within the same afferent nerve may summate, provided the second is not so close to the first as to be within its refractory period. Secondly, spatial summation may occur where several afferent fibres activate an overlapping part of the motor neurone pool. Summation implies an enduring excitatory condition established by the stimulus. This has been called a 'central excitatory state'. In spatial summation a single afferent may fail to produce an adequate central excitatory state in the overlapping field of the motor neurone pool, but if both afferents are excited together, the excitatory state may become adequate so that two afferent fibres may excite a larger number of efferent fibres than can be accounted for by the additive effect of each fibre's area of excitation.

Many movements which occur reflexly depend on the interaction of different muscles, and it is necessary for the contraction of certain muscles to be accompanied by the relaxation of others. Thus, if a reflex movement is not to be interfered with by the contraction of the muscles opposing it, there must be some means whereby that contraction can be inhibited. So if afferent impulses arise at the skin to initiate a coordinated contraction of the flexor muscles, which occurs in the flexor reflex, a spread of impulses will occur at the same time to inhibit the neurones activating the extensor muscles, which are antagonistic to the flexors. The expression 'central inhibitory state' was originally applied to processes of this kind at a time when little information was available regarding the underlying mechanism. The mechanism whereby the antagonist relaxes as the protagonist contracts in a reflex movement is known as *reciprocal innervation*. It implies that the afferent nerves must establish a central excitatory state in one group of neurones while initiating a central inhibitory state in a different portion of the motor neurone pool (see below).

SPINAL AND POSTURAL REFLEXES

The Flexor Response

The natural response to a painful stimulus is to withdraw the affected part. This withdrawal response is well illustrated in the flexor reflex which has been studied in detail in the spinal dog. Application of a painful stimulus to the foot results in flexion and withdrawal of the limb, while at the same time the opposite limb extends and takes the weight of the body. This extension of the contralateral limb is termed the crossed extensor response. The afferent impulses concerned in the flexor response appear to arise from the skin, and the reflex can readily be elicited by electrical stimulation of nerves which arise from the skin. The flexor reflex is subserved exclusively by a polysynaptic central pathway. It illustrates many of the characteristics described above that can only be explained on this basis. Thus, it has a latency which may vary considerably with the strength of the stimulus and the after-discharge may be prolonged.

The Extensor Thrust Reflex

In the spinal dog pressure on the plantar surface of the foot or separation of the toepads evokes an extensor movement of the limb. This reflex is probably important in respect of reflex standing and walking. It cannot be elicited by electrical stimulation of the plantar nerves.

The Stretch Reflex

If the tendon of an extensor muscle is tapped, the muscle responds by a brisk contraction known as a tendon jerk. The contraction is set up by a reflex which originates in receptors in the muscle that respond to stretch, and the afferents of which connect with motor neurones in the sqinal cord, and excite them to bring about a contraction in the muscle that will oppose the stretch. A muscle will not only contract in response to a sudden brief stretch, such as a tap on its tendon, but will also contract steadily to oppose a slowly applied stretching force, such as may occur if a limb is moved passively. The tendon jerk is an example of a phasic stretch reflex. The response to passive movement is a tonic stretch reflex. In each instance, the stretch receptor in the muscle is a complex structure known as a muscle spindle. The stretch reflex has a short latency which does not vary in the manner that the latency of the flexor reflex varies and after discharge is not a feature. It is clear that in the case of the phasic stretch reflex, the reflex arc is a simple two neurone monosynaptic pathway, but the tonic stretch reflex probably includes a polysynaptic central pathway.

Although the stretch reflex can be obtained from flexor muscles, it is much more prominent in the extensors and has been thoroughly studied in animals in association with *decerebrate rigidity*. This condition may be produced by separating the cerebral hemispheres from the brainstem by a section between the anterior and posterior colliculi. The animal assumes a rigid posture with limbs extended and head erect that is due to a sustained contraction of the extensor muscles. These muscles are the antigravity muscles, and the effect of decerebrate rigidity in the cat or dog is to hold it in an erect posture if placed upright on its feet. This rigidity is due to sustained activity of the tonic stretch reflex and it is abolished by section of the posterior roots. If the attempt is made to flex the extended limb there is at first resistance, but then the resistance suddenly gives and the limb flexes without resistance. This clasp knife effect has been termed the 'lengthening reaction'. It carries the implication that there is a second proprioceptive mechanism which is inhibitory and enables a muscle to yield to a pull which is so severe that it might be injurious. There is evidence that this inhibitory pathway arises from the golgi receptors in the tendons. Sometimes the lengthening reaction is accompanied by extension of the contralateral limb; this is the *crossed extensor reflex of Philippson*.

Muscle Tone

In the human subject, injury to the corticospinal pathway, particularly in the internal capsule, is accompanied by hyperactive stretch reflexes in the extensor muscles. This is known as spasticity and in its complete form, this includes marked resistance of the muscles to passive flexion of the limb, with a well marked lengthening reaction and exaggerated tendon reflexes. The excitability of the phasic stretch reflex is not always affected to the same degree as the tonic stretch reflex. The expression *muscle tone* is used in clinical practice to describe the resistance of a muscle to passive stretch. In spasticity, the normal degree of resistance to passive movement is increased and muscle tone is increased. In a lesion of the lower motor neurone where the stretch reflex arc may be interrupted, the muscle is flaccid to passive movement and muscle tone is reduced. When a muscle is completely relaxed no contraction of muscle fibres is taking place, but continuous contractions can be recorded from muscles which are maintaining a body posture. The term postural tone is also used to denote this continued contraction, which is distinct from the resistance to passive movement of clinical tonus.

THE ANALYSIS OF REFLEX ACTION

The detailed analysis of spinal reflexes has been made possible by the development of electrophysiological methods for exciting and recording reflexes and for studying the behaviour of single neurones within the cord. Important advances have also come about through study of the structure and function of stretch receptors in muscle and tendon.

The Electrical Recording of Reflexes

The train of events in a spinal reflex can be recorded on an accurate time scale if a dorsal root is stimulated and the reflexly potentials are recorded from electrodes applied to the ventral root (Lloyd, 1943a). If the intensity of the stimulating pulses is progressively increased, it is found that whereas a weak stimulus will evoke a potential with a very short latency, of the order of 0.50 msec, stronger pulses will evoke potentials which start later and persist for several msec (Fig. 6.4). A latency of 0.50 msec only allows sufficient time for an impulse to cross a single synapse, so it is evident that the low threshold afferents are concerned in a two neurone reflex arc, whereas the higher threshold afferents form part of a polysynaptic arc. The low threshold fibres are large diameter (more than 20 μm) rapidly conducting fibres not normally found in cutaneous nerves, and the high threshold fibres are of smaller size. Lloyd was able to show that the low threshold fibres concerned in the monosynaptic reflex were derived from muscular nerves, whereas the afferents for the polysynaptic reflexes came from the skin.

This technique can be applied to the study of the tendon reflex by recording dorsal and ventral root potentials after a tendon tap. The difference between the latencies recorded at the dorsal and ventral roots indicates the central reflex latency, and in the spinal cat Lloyd (1943b) has shown by this technique that the tendon jerk is subserved by a two neurone arc.

In the human subject a monosynaptic reflex can be evoked by electrical stimulation which appears to follow the same central pathway as the ankle jerk. This was first described by Hoffmann (1918) and is known as the H reflex and was later described in detail by Magladery *et al.* (1950). It is obtained by stimulating the posterior tibial nerve and recording evoked potentials from the triceps surae. A stimulus too weak to excite the efferent fibres will evoke a late potential, the latency of which lengthens as the stimulating electrode is moved distally, and disappears as the stimulus intensity is increased and an early directly evoked potential appears. Magladery and his associates used electrodes inserted into the

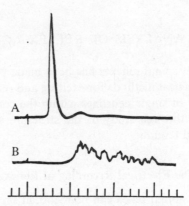

FIG. 6.4. A. Short duration response recorded from ventral root following stimulus to afferent nerve from muscle. The short latency indicates that the reflex follows a 2 neurone arc. B. Complex long duration response of longer latency following stimulus to afferent nerve from skin which has given rise to polysynaptic discharge. Time scale 1 msec. After Lloyd, D. P. C. (1943), *J. Neurophysiol.*, **6**, 111–119.

lumbar theca to record spinal root potentials. They recorded a latency of 1.50 msec between dorsal and ventral root potentials which, allowing for conduction in the afferent and efferent fibres, allows sufficient time only for passage through a single synapse (Fig. 6.5.) The H reflex, under normal circumstance, can only be demonstrated after stimulation of the posterior tibial nerve, but in patients who show spasticity it can be evoked by stimulation of other peripheral nerves. The ease with which it can be evoked depends on many variables, including the excitability of the motor neurone pool. A single H reflex is followed by several hundred msec of altered excitability (Fig. 6.6). The time course of this altered excitability can be recorded by evoking the reflex with paired stimulating pulses, and altered responses occur both in spastic paralysis and in Parkinsonian rigidity (see chapter 10) (Olsen and Diamantopoulos, 1967).

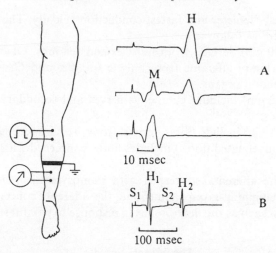

FIG. 6.5. Arrangement for evoking monosynaptic reflex (H response) from posterior tibial nerve in human subject. In a it is seen that as stimulus strength is increased the reflex response (H wave) decreases in amplitude as the directly evoked response (M wave) appears. In b, two H responses are evoked by stimuli 80 msec apart and the second response is smaller than the first.

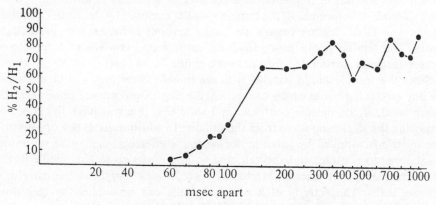

FIG. 6.6. Recovery of excitability of H reflex when it is evoked by paired stimuli.

Afferent Nerve Fibres

Motor and sensory nerves have been classified into A, B, and C fibres in respect of conduction velocity following analysis of the compound action potential (see chapter 3). Reflex afferent nerves have been classified in terms of threshold stimulus required to excite them. In general, this classification corresponds to one based on fibre size and conduction velocity, the fibres of lowest threshold having the largest diameter and fastest conduction velcoity. The principal afferent fibre types are as follows:

Group I (13–20 μm) derived from muscles and tendons. Of these Group IA include the primary afferents from muscle spindles and Group IB afferents from Golgi tendon organs.

Group II (4–12 μm) includes cutaneous nerves and secondary afferents from muscle spindles.

Group III (1–4 μm) include fibres derived from pressure receptors.

Group IV (unmyelinated fibres) includes fibres concerned with ischaemic pain in muscle.

In general, the afferents concerned with monosynaptic reflexes belong to Group I. The remaining groups contribute the afferents concerned with polysynaptic reflexes, such as the flexor reflex in response to painful stimuli.

The Muscle Spindle

The muscle spindles and the Golgi tendon organs are the principal structures sensitive to stretch which are found in muscles and tendons. The spindles are particularly profuse in the limb muscles and lie embedded in the muscles in parallel with the muscle fibres. A single spindle measures up to 4 mm in length and 200 μm in diameter, and consists of a bundle of intrafusal muscle fibres, about 10 in number in the human spindle, enclosed by a capsule of fibrous tissue. The Golgi tendon organs lie in the tendons in series with the muscle fibres. The tendon organ has a fusiform capsule and consists of a bundle of tendon fasciculi surrounded by a network of fine nerve fibres.

Since the spindles lie in parallel with the muscle fibres they will be stretched by any stretching force which causes lengthening of the muscle fibres. On the other hand, if the muscle contracts and shortens, this will have the effect of removing the stretching force from the spindle. In addition to its sensory supply, the spindle is supplied by small motor nerves, γ efferents, that cause the intrafusal fibres to contract and shorten, and so apply tension to the spindle in the same manner as an external stretching force, which lengthens the extrafusal muscle fibres. The activity of a muscle spindle can be studied by recording potentials from its afferent nerves. This can be done both during an applied stretch to a muscle and during stimulation applied to the γ motor system. Spindles will respond to two types of stretching force, viz., a continuously maintained, tonic or static stretch and secondly an incremental, dynamic or phasic stretch. A spindle afferent which responds to static stretch will discharge for so long as a given length of the extrafusal muscle fibres in proportion to that of the intrafusal fibres is held constant. A spindle afferent responding to dynamic stretch does not register a particular length of the muscle fibres, but fires so long as the length is changing and the firing frequency is in proportion to the rate of change. The response to dynamic or phasic stretch is clearly seen in the tendon jerk. The tendon organs which are in series with the muscle fibres respond to muscle tension, and there is no efferent pathway from the central nervous system by which their sensitivity may be adjusted. The stretch reflexes are thus mediated by three types of receptor, viz, the tonic and phasic receptors in the spindles which respond to changes in muscle length, and the tendon organs which respond to changes in muscle tension. The spindles, however, have a particular importance in connection with the control of movement. This is because they are not merely passive receptors but are exposed to continual control and adjustment by the central nervous system through the fusimotor system.

The intrafusal fibres of the spindles have a central excitable zone rich in nuclei and a peripheral zone which is the actively contractile zone. The fibres are of two kinds; the first are called nuclear bag fibres due to the dense collection of nuclei in the central zone; in the second or nuclear chain fibres, the nuclei are arranged in a single central row. The sensory innervation consists also of two types of nerve fibre. The first are rapidly conducting Group IA fibres and arise from primary or annulospiral endings which are situated in the central part of each intrafusal fibre. The second are more slowly conducting Group II fibres which arise from more peripherally situated secondary, or flower spray endings, which are found mainly on the nuclear chain fibres. The motor innervation through the γ efferent fibres supplies the muscles through two types of nerve ending. The plate endings resemble motor end–plates, are more numerous on the nuclear bag fibres and give rise to a propagated type of response on the muscle fibre. The trail endings form a diffuse network over both types of fibre and the response at a trail ending is a localized response resembling an end–plate potential (Fig. 6.7).

If the primary sensory endings are activated, it is seen that they are sensitive to the rate of change which takes place in muscle length, and therefore participate in the dynamic or phasic stretch reflex. The secondary endings, are sensitive to a sustained alteration in the length of the muscle, and are therefore concerned in the tonic or static stretch reflex (Cooper, 1961). The γ efferents can also be divided into dynamic and static efferents. The present evidence suggests that the efferents which end on the trail endings are the dynamic efferents, whereas the efferents which end in the plate endings are concerned with the tonic stretch reflex. It is not yet clear whether the nuclear bag and nuclear chain fibres can be differentiated functionally on this basis (Boyd, 1966).

The Group IA afferents from the spindles connect directly with the motor neurones in the spinal cord and thus subserve the monosynaptic reflex arc of the tendon reflex. At the same time, some collaterals pass to interneurones which inhibit the motor neurones supplying the antagonist muscle. The afferent fibres from the Golgi tendon organs are Group IB afferents and these connect with the motor neurones through a single inhibitory interneurone. The central connections for the static or tonic stretch reflex are complex and less fully understood, but it appears that the central reflex pathway for this reflex is polysynaptic.

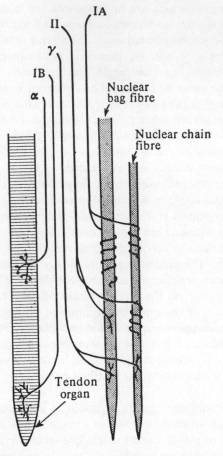

FIG. 6.7. Diagram to show principle connections of muscle spindle, skeletal muscle fibre and Golgi tendon organ.

The Servo Control of Muscular Contraction

In addition to its role in postural mechanisms through the stretch reflex, the muscle spindle is also important in the control of voluntary movement. Although a muscle contraction can be initiated and maintained by descending impulses activating the α motor neurones in the spinal cord, an alternative pathway is provided by the small motor neurones that give rise to the γ efferents. Impulses which pass down the γ efferents by exciting the intrafusal fibres may cause the spindle to shorten so that it is stretched, and the resulting afferent discharge activates the α neurones to cause contraction of the muscle. There is evidence that stimulation of structures in the forebrain, including the motor cortex, will alter the rate of spindle discharge, but it is uncertain how far a voluntary contraction is initiated indirectly in this way through a reflex servo loop. Direct recording from human spindle afferents with fine tungsten electrodes inserted into a peripheral nerve has confirmed that there is a greatly increased discharge from spindles during a voluntary contraction, but this does not precede the onset of the contraction. Although this confirms the close relationship between α and γ discharge it does not provide evidence that activation of α neurones is initiated indirectly through activation of the γ efferents (Hagbarth and Vallbo, 1969; Vallbo, 1970 and 1971). In a normal movement it may be more appropriate to consider the γ loops as providing servo assistance rather than servo control (Matthews, 1964 and 1972).

In a sustained contraction against a load the close relationship between α and γ discharge is particularly important. When a muscle contracts against a load it is unable to shorten, so that the spindles remain under stretch, and the spindle discharge continues to activate the α neurones. The role of α–γ linkage in the reflex proprioceptive control of movement has been studied particularly in connection with the action of the respiratory muscles. These muscles exert an especially accurate control of movement, not only in connection with rhythmic respiratory activity, but also in connection with sound production and speech. A small movement of the intercostal muscles exerts a relatively powerful effect and their servo adjustment is particularly elaborate and complex. There is a very close linkage between α and γ discharge to the intercostals, and the spindles have an important function in adjusting the force of contraction to match the variations in load. In the conscious human subject the process has been shown to be still more elaborate. Thus, a sudden increase in load is not followed immediately by the expected effect of increased muscle contraction due to spindle activation, but there is first a brief period in which the muscle is inhibited. This inhibition is apparently the result of a reflex arising from the tendon organs and it allows time for more precise voluntary adjustment (Newsom Davis and Sears, 1970).

The diaphragm differs from the intercostals in that the contractions are largely isotonic with a relatively large excursion of movement. Spindles and fusimotor γ fibres are few in number, and in contrast to the intercostals, the control of movement is largely through the α pathway, and proprioceptive control is less elaborate (von Euler, 1966; Granit, 1970).

The relative role of the two descending pathways, the one activating the small motor neurones, the other activating the α motor neurones, is determined to some extent by the cerebellum. Decerebrate rigidity depends, under normal circumstances, upon the stretch reflexes and on their facilitation by descending influences from the brain stem. If the dorsal roots to a limb affected by decerebrate rigidity are divided, the limb at once becomes flaccid (Sherrington, 1906). This is not the case if the animal, in addition to being decerebrate has the cerebellum, in particular the anterior lobe, also removed. This was clearly shown by

Pollock and Davis (1927 and 1931), who produced a form of decerebrate rigidity by ligation of the carotid and basilar arteries. In this preparation, necrosis of the anterior lobe of the cerebellum occurred and the decerebrate rigidity which followed was unaffected by posterior root section.

These observations could be explained if removal of the cerebellum were considered to bring about a 'switching off' of the stretch reflexes, while other influences became more efficient than usual in exciting the anterior horn cells. Granit and his colleagues (1955) have shown that the removal of the cerebellum is associated with a reduction in the activity of the γ efferents which supply the

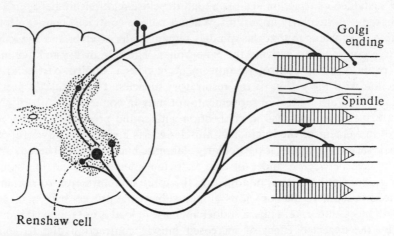

FIG. 6.8. Diagram to show principle components of stretch reflex arc and of Renshaw loop. The primary afferent fibre from the muscle spindle makes direct connection with the anterior horn cell whereas the afferent from the golgi tendon organ is separated from it by an inhibitory interneurone.

muscle spindles. Loss of the servo assistance provided by the fusimotor system could account for the impaired co-ordination seen in cerebellar disease (Granit, 1970).

If the γ loop provides the main servo system for the smooth control of voluntary contraction, a further arrangement in the α neurones provides a possible further servo loop which may also exert an important controlling influence. This is the system provided by the Renshaw cells (Renshaw, 1941) which are inhibitory neurones that act on the α motoneurones. They are themselves excited by recurrent collaterals which arise from the motor nerve fibres. The Renshaw system thus provides a feedback loop which prevents excessive discharge rates in motor neurones and possibly reduces synchronous firing. (Fig. 6.8).

Central Excitation and Inhibition

Sherrington's concepts of central excitatory state and central inhibitory state have been clarified by information derived from the use of intracellular recording techniques on neurones in the spinal cord, a field of study which has been very largely developed by Eccles and his associates. Nerve cells in the spinal cord have been found to have a membrane potential of about 70 mV. Stimulation of an impaled nerve cell can be effected either antidromically by stimulating the motor axon or orthodromically by stimulating the sensory nerve that connects with it.

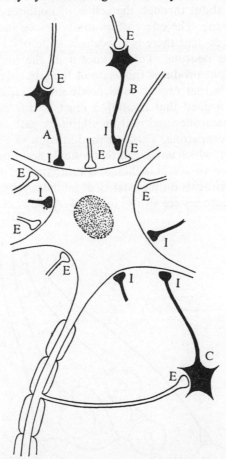

FIG. 6.9. Diagram to illustrate how motor neurone is acted on by many nerve terminals each of which may produce an EPSP or IPSP. Three modes of inhibition are illustrated. A. Inhibition applied from one neurone to another through an intermediate inhibitory cell. B. Inhibition occurring through action of inhibitory neurone on presynaptic terminal of excitatory neurone. C. Recurrent inhibition through collateral branch of axon exciting inhibitory neurone.

Excitation of a nerve cell results in a reduction of the membrane potential. This is a localized nonpropagated and graded response without refractory period, and thus allows successive stimuli to summate. This localized depolarization of the nerve cell is known as an excitatory postsynaptic potential (EPSP). Since a single nerve cell may receive synaptic connections from many thousands of nerve fibres, the swollen terminals of which are situated close together along the post-synaptic membrane, spatial summation readily occurs so that the summated EPSP from adjacent synaptic areas may become adequate to cause the neurone to discharge (Fig. 6.9, see chapter 4).

Inhibition comes about through the action of inhibitory nerve fibres on the postsynaptic membrane. The effect of an inhibitory impulse is to increase the membrane potential so that there is a localized hyperpolarization that opposes the discharge of the neurone. This is known as the inhibitory postsynaptic potential (IPSP). What produces this state of hyperpolarization is not known, but one possibility is that excitation is produced by separate humoral trans-mitters. Eccles has argued that inhibition must always be brought about by separate inhibitory neurones and that an inhibitory pathway must always con-tain at least one interneurone. This is a modification of Sherrington's original concept of inhibition, which envisaged that a single nerve might exert excitatory action through some of its branches and inhibitory actions through others (Eccles, 1969). Experiments on the latency of inhibitory reflexes tend to support the view that interneurones are always involved (Araki *et al.*, 1960).

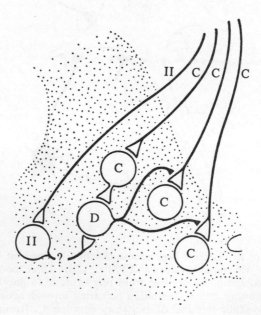

(A)

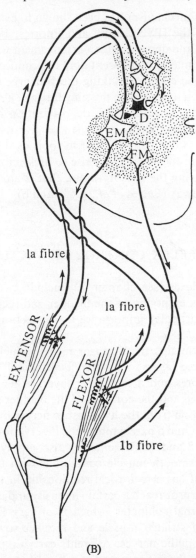

(B)

FIG. 6.10. (a) Schematic diagram illustrating the suggested pathway for pre-synaptic inhibitory action on a cutaneous primary afferent fibre. Three cutaneous afferent fibres (C) and one muscle afferent fibre Group II (II) with their mono-synaptic endings on interneurones are shown. D symbolizes the interneurone which has presynaptic connexions on cutaneous primary afferent fibres. (b) Schematic diagram illustrating the suggested pathways for presynaptic inhibitory action on a primary afferent fibre (1a fibre) of an extensor muscle by afferent volleys in 1a (from annulospiral (AS) endings on muscle spindles) and 1b (from Golgi tendon organs) afferent fibres of a flexor muscle. EM and FM symbolize extensor and flexor motoneurones, while D is the interneurone that has presynaptic connexions on primary muscle afferent fibres. Eccles, J. C., Kostyuk, P. G. and Schmidt, R. F. (1962), *J. Physiol. (Lond.)*, **161**, 237–257.

A second inhibitory mechanism has been shown to exist that does not depend on the production of the IPSP (Frank and Fuortes, 1957). This is known as presynaptic inhibition and depends on an arrangement whereby an interneurone connects with the terminal of an afferent fibre to produce partial depolarization. (Fig. 6.10). This has the effect of making the discharge of the afferent fibre less effective by an unknown mechanism, possibly through a reduction in the amount of transmitter substance released. This depolarization may, at the same time, lead to a discharge of the afferent neurone and give rise to the slow potential change that can be recorded from the dorsal roots as the dorsal root potential. The inhibitory interneurones which give rise to presynaptic inhibition constitute a feedback loop, reducing the sensory input, that is analagous to the Renshaw loop in the motor pathway (Eccles *et al.*, 1963a and b).

THE REFLEX CONTROL OF MICTURITION

Autonomic spinal reflexes (see chapter 10) include vasomotor reflexes, reflex sweating and the reflex emptying of the bladder and rectum. The reflex control of micturition is of particular importance in connection with disease affecting the spinal cord.

The bladder wall contains the detrusor muscle which consists of unstriped fibres arranged in three layers; an outer longitudinal layer, a thick layer of circularly arranged fibres and a thin inner layer. When this muscle contracts, the sphincters may open and the contents of the bladder are expelled. It receives a sympathetic innervation from the hypogastric nerves that are derived from the upper lumbar segments and a parasympathetic innervation from the pelvic nerves which come from S2, 3 and 4. These nerves also supply the internal sphincter, which is made up of smooth muscle continuous with the middle layer of the detrusor, with which it has a reciprocal relationship in that it relaxes when the contractions of the detrusor reach a certain intensity and allows urine to pass into the urethra. The external sphincter, which is of very little importance in the female, is made up of striated muscle and receives somatic innervation from S3 and 4 through the pudic nerves. Afferents carrying pain sensation travel in the hypogastric nerves, those concerned in reflex emptying of the bladder in the pelvic nerves (Fig. 6.11).

In the investigation of bladder reflexes in the human subject, the cystometrogram has provided a particularly useful technique (Denny-Brown and Robertson, 1933). In this method the bladder is filled by means of a double lumen catheter and the vesical pressure can be recorded continuously by means of an isometric cystometer. The slope of the pressure–volume curve obtained in this way gives a measure of bladder tonus, and the contraction waves that occur as the pressure in the bladder rises can be recorded. Other methods of study that have proved useful have included the recording of the sequence of events during bladder filling by cineradiology and by intravesical cinematography through a cold light cystoscope.

The bladder responds to distension by rhythmical contractions of the bladder wall, that are in part dependent on the properties of smooth muscle. The contractions are not directly dependent on the distending pressure, but depend much more closely on the rate at which it is applied. A rapid distension of the bladder may evoke strong contractions, but the bladder can adapt to slow

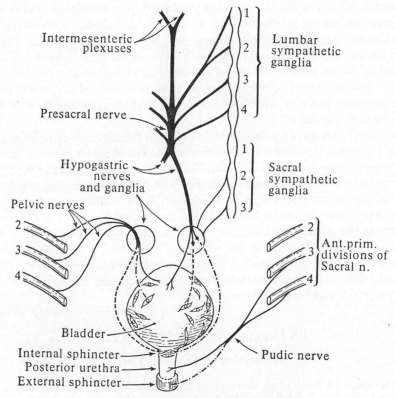

FIG. 6.11. The innervation of the bladder (after Learmonth).

distension to contain a large volume of fluid in a relatively relaxed state. Distension of the bladder also evokes a stretch reflex through the pelvic nerves, which in the absence of inhibition from higher centres, can bring about emptying of the bladder. Normally, reflex emptying of the bladder is under voluntary suppression, but this is not the case in the infant, where the bladder empties automatically as it becomes distended. The same situation may occur in some patients with spastic paraplegia, where the bladder is isolated from voluntary control. In tabes dorsalis, on the other hand, where the afferent arc of the bladder reflex is affected, the bladder reflex may be lost and the bladder becomes progressively enlarged with overflow incontinence. The action of the sympathetic innervation of the bladder appears to be less important than that of the parasympathetic, since division of the hypogastric nerves seems to have little effect on bladder function, although pain sensation is lost.

In the adult, micturition normally occurs voluntarily after distension of the bladder has given rise to the desire to micturate. The voluntary process appears to be one of 'letting go' so that the sacral reflex brought about by stretching of the smooth muscle of the bladder wall is released from inhibition. At the onset of micturition, strong contractions of the detrusor muscle occur, these contractions also causing the internal sphincter to relax. At the same time there is relaxation of the perineum and there is inhibition of the tonic contraction of the external sphincter with relaxation of the urethra. The external sphincter is not essential for the control of micturition, since bladder control is possible even if it is denervated, but it is capable of preventing bladder emptying if the internal sphincter is damaged.

The central pathways for the control of bladder function are complex and not wholly understood. Stimulation experiments show that many areas of the cerebral cortex may be concerned in micturition, but the medial surface of the frontal lobe appears to be particularly important, and although complex, the overall effect of the cortex appears to be inhibitory. Both inhibitory and excitatory centres have been located in the brain stem and hypothalamus. The descending pathway in the spinal cord concerned with micturition has been found to be in the lateral column situated on an equatorial plane which passes through the central canal (Nathan and Smith, 1958). The control of bladder function in man, both in health and in disease of the nervous system, has been extensively reviewed by Plum (1962) and by Guttmann (1973).

PARAPLEGIA AND SPASTICITY

Transection of the Spinal Cord

If the spinal cord is divided, there is an immediate loss of all voluntary movement below the level of the section and all perception of sensation below the level of the lesion is lost. Initially after the section all reflex activity below the section ceases, an event which was termed spinal shock by Marshall Hall in 1850. The stage of spinal shock is succeeded by a gradual return of reflex activity, many of the reflexes eventually becoming hyperactive, so that eventually a stage of spastic paraplegia or tetraplegia is reached.

Spinal Shock

The depression of reflex activity which follows section of the spinal cord is of relatively short duration in the simpler forms of vertebrate life. Thus, in the frog spinal shock passes off in a few minutes, whereas in the cat or dog it will persist for several hours, and in the monkey it may be several weeks before reflexes return. In man, there is considerable variation in the duration of reflex depression and reflexes may return earlier in younger subjects. Some return may occur as early as three or four days after transection but may be delayed for as long as six weeks (Guttmann, 1970). Although as a general rule, spinal shock occurs immediately after cord section in man, it is sometimes possible to obtain certain of the reflexes, such as the ankle jerks and the plantar responses for a limited period of time after the injury. Spinal shock is more complete and severe in the segments of the body nearest to the lesion. This is reflected in the order in which the return of reflex activity occurs, reflexes frequently recovering first in the more caudally situated segments. The loss of reflexes occurs in the segments distal to the cord lesion, but again, this rule is not an absolute one since there may be an increase in reflex excitability above the lesion (Schiff–Sherrington phenomenon) and sometimes there may be a transient upward spread of reflex depression (Guttmann, 1970).

The loss of reflexes in spinal shock also affects autonomic responses. Thus the vasoconstrictor reflexes, which are mediated by the sympathetic, may be depressed so that after a high cord transection the blood pressure may fall, and tilting the patient, may result in severe postural hypotension. Generally, the vasoconstrictor reflexes return as the other features of spinal shock pass off. The bladder reflexes are also lost after transection of the cord so that the bladder becomes distended, and if the distension is not relieved an overflow incontinence will occur when the pressure inside the bladder rises sufficiently to overcome the internal sphincter.

Spinal shock is not due to the physical trauma of the cord section since it will develop if the spinal cord is cooled and passes off again after rewarming; moreover, if the distal segment of cord is divided after recovery from spinal shock there will be no further development of spinal shock (Sherrington, 1906). The most important factor in the development of spinal shock is that the affected part of the spinal cord is cut off from descending, mainly excitatory impulses from higher centres and the pathways which are of paramount importance are the vestibulospinal, reticulospinal and corticospinal tracts. One mechanism by which this may come about is through loss of excitation through the γ efferent pathway so that the intrafusal fibres in the spindles relax and afferent discharge from the spindles ceases. Little is known regarding the physiological changes which accompany spinal shock at a cellular level. If a posterior root is divided, the boutons termineaux that are derived from it and from synaptic contact with an anterior horn cell degenerate. At the same time, there occurs a marked disorganization in the arrangement of boutons termineaux derived from neighbouring intact axons, which is maximal after about 24 hours and is reversible. If similar changes were to occur after cord transection, this could account for some of the transient features of spinal shock as well as the abnormal reflex patterns which develop during recovery (Illis, 1967).

Recovery of Reflex Activity

The first reflexes to return during recovery from spinal shock are flexor reflexes evoked by stimulation of the skin. In the dog, the crossed extension reflex, which is associated with reflex flexion, recovers early, extensor thrust appearing later (Sherrington, 1906). In man, the flexion reflexes appear first and are followed later by the reappearance of tendon reflexes. A feature of this withdrawal response is dorsiflexion of the great toe and this may occur in isolation in the presence of relatively minor lesions of the corticospinal system. For this reason, it is a valuable sign in clinical neurology and is known as the sign of Babinski (see below). As the flexor reflex recovers, it gradually comes to be more easily excited and from wider areas of skin. In some cases a stage is reached where reflex withdrawal of the limbs is accompanied by emptying of the bladder and rectum and sweating in the segments below the transection. This sequence of events where reflex flexion is accompanied by spread of the reflex discharge to the autonomic outflow has been termed the mass reflex.

In the 1914–18 war many patients became paraplegic as a result of spinal injuries. Many of these patients died due to bedsores and urinary tract infections while in a state of paraplegia in flexion. The reflex changes in these patients have been fully described by Riddoch (1917). After the 1939–45 war, improved methods of treatment made it possible to secure not only prolonged survival, but also the active rehabilitation of these patients and it became clear that the stage of predominantly flexor activity was succeeded by a stage of alternating flexor and extensor spasms, with an ultimate development in long surviving cases, of a stage of predominantly extensor activity (Kuhn, 1950). In 1917 Riddoch suggested that it may be possible to distinguish between complete and partial spinal cord lesions by the pattern of reflex activity, since extensor reflexes tend to predominate in partial lesions, whereas, at that time it appeared that paraplegia in flexion was the invariable state in complete transections of the cord. Subsequent experience has shown that this distinction cannot be made and that paraplegia in extension is frequently present as the final clinical state in patients with complete cord lesions. Guttmann (1952) has pointed out that the posture of the limbs in the early period following injury is an important factor in determining the eventual reflex pattern. Thus, if the limbs are held for a prolonged period in adduction and semiflexion this will tend to promote flexor spasms and lead to paraplegia in flexion. This posture results in facilitation of the stretch reflex of the flexor muscles and by overstretching the extensors, leads to weakening of the reflexes in those muscles. The reverse effect is obtained if the limbs are fixed in extension and abduction and extensor responses are facilitated if the patient is nursed prone and encouraged to stand between parallel bars.

Bladder reflexes may return after about three weeks so that the retention of urine, which is present initially, passes off and the patient may become incontinent. In some patients, an automatic bladder will develop, which will empty itself when the pressure within the bladder reaches a certain level. Distension of the bladder is accompanied by a discharge of the sympathetic below the level of the transection. This leads to reflex vasoconstriction and sweating, the distribution of which depends on how much of the sympathetic outflow is below the level of the transection. With a lesion below T6 there is vasoconstriction of the lower limbs and vasodilatation of the fingers. With higher lesions, there is vasoconstriction also of the fingers, and a rise in blood pressure will occur along with vasodilatation of the face, neck and nasal mucosa. These changes may indicate to the patient, who has no sensation of bladder distension, that automatic voiding is about to take place (Guttmann and Whitteridge, 1947).

Incomplete Transection of the Cord

Incomplete lesions of the spinal cord are commoner than complete transections and occur not only as a result of trauma, but in many diseases affecting the central nervous system. They are generally associated with spasticity and marked hyperexcitability of the reflexes. A complete lateral hemisection of the cord is known as the Brown–Sequard syndrome. In this condition, motor power is lost on the side of the lesion, but sensation is affected differently on the two sides, due to the anatomical arrangement of the sensory tracts in the spinal cord. Thus, pain and temperature sensation is lost on the side opposite to the lesion, since fibres carrying these modalities cross soon after entering the cord causing pain and temperature to be carried up in the ventrolateral columns of the opposite side. On the other hand, touch and proprioception are affected on the same side as the lesion, since fibres carrying touch sensation pass upwards on the same side and do not cross until they reach the brain stem. This is an example of dissociated anaesthesia which occurs in lesions in the central nervous system where fibres carrying particular modalities of sensation are damaged.

Spasticity

In an earlier section, muscle tone was described as the resistance of a muscle to passive stretch. Spasticity may be regarded as the excessive resistance to passive movement which occurs when spinal reflexes are released from supraspinal control. The clinical situation, however, is more complex, since in spastic paralysis the stretch reflex is not necessarily the only reflex to be hyperactive. In many cases there is a marked preponderance of flexor activity which is evoked by painful stimuli exciting cutaneous receptors. Moreover, the characteristics of spasticity are strongly influenced by the level of the lesion in the central nervous system. In patients who have lesions above the midbrain, for example in the cortex or the internal capsule, there is hypertonus affecting the limbs contralateral to the lesion. The hypertonus in the upper limbs affects predominantly the adductors of the shoulder and the flexors of the elbows and wrist, whereas in the lower limbs the hypertonus affects particularly the extensor muscles. The condition has features in common with experimental decerebrate rigidity in which there is continuous spasm of the antigravity muscles. In lesions at the midbrain in man, a condition very closely resembling decerebrate rigidity can occur with opsisthotonos and fixed extension of all four limbs. In lesions of the spinal cord, the situation may be very complex with some patients showing marked hypertonus of the extensors, while in others, the flexor reflex is predominant.

Spasticity in man resembles experimental decerebrate rigidity in that the affected muscles show the lengthening reaction or clasp knife phenomenon, and the hypertonus can be abolished by section of the dorsal roots (Förster, 1911). Rushworth (1960) has shown that if the peripheral nerve to a spastic muscle is infiltrated with dilute procaine, spasticity may be abolished without causing paralysis. This may be due to selective blockade of the small motor nerve fibres and suggests that the hyperexcitability of the stretch reflex in spasticity is mediated through the γ efferents. In one patient he studied, hemiplegia resulted from thrombosis of the left vertebral artery and in this patient, infiltration with procaine did not reduce spasticity until power was also lost, suggesting that the rigidity was not dependent on the γ system but maintained by an 'α' discharge like the Pollock and Davis preparation (see above). Cases of this kind are rare, and it is likely that in nearly all cases of human spasticity the hypertonus is maintained through the stretch reflex, which is rendered hyperexcitable through the gamma pathway.

In spinal spasticity, the excitability of reflexes in the affected part of the cord may be so great that organized reflex activity is lost, and features so clearly demonstrated in the spinal animal, such as reciprocal innervation and the crossed extensor reflex, are seldom seen. If the flexor reflex is evoked on one side, the likely effect will be a flexion movement of both limbs. A reason for this difference between man and the experimental animal is that in the spinal animal the sensory inflow has generally been effectively reduced by extensive deafferentation, and it is clear that in man, measures to reduce the sensory inflow will restore reciprocal innervation (Dimitrijevic and Nathan, 1967). Partial lesions of the spinal cord tend to be associated with more severe spasticity than complete transverse section (Pedersen, 1969).

While it is clear that spasticity is the result of release of spinal reflex activity from supraspinal control there is much uncertainty about how this supraspinal control is mediated. Lesions of the corticospinal (pyramidal) tracts are generally associated with spasticity, but section of the pyramids where there is relatively little mixing of corticospinal fibres with other descending fibres may be followed by flaccid paralysis (Tower, 1940). Although the evidence regarding the effects of corticospinal lesions is conflicting, it is clear that subcortical centres such as the vestibular nucleus, the reticular formation and the cerebellum are all important in the regulation of spinal reflexes, and damage to the descending pathways associated with these centres contributes significantly to disturbances of muscle tone which are seen in patients with disease of the brain and spinal cord.

SEGMENTAL REFLEXES IN MAN

Two groups of segmental spinal reflexes are of particular value in clinical localization. These are the tendon reflexes, which are evoked by a brisk tap applied to a muscle tendon and certain superficial reflexes, which are elicited by stimulation of the skin. The tendon reflexes arise from stimulation of the muscle spindles and are short latency monosynaptic reflexes. The superficial reflexes arise from stimulation of the skin. They are polysynaptic reflexes and include the so-called nociceptive responses to painful stimulation.

The Tendon Jerk and Related Reflexes

The Tendon Jerk

The tendon jerks correspond to the phasic component of the stretch reflex (Creed *et al.*, 1932). The peripheral receptor for the reflex is the muscle spindle, and the latency of the reflex is such that it can only be subserved by a two neurone arc. If the muscle tension is recorded at the same time as the electromyogram during a tendon reflex, it is seen that there is a sharp burst of electrical activity immediately before the tension develops. During the period when tension is increasing and levelling off, there is electrical silence, which is followed by a further electrical discharge as the tension declines. This 'silent period' (Fig. 6.12) is due to the release of tension from the muscle spindles as the muscle fibres shorten during contraction (Creed *et al.*, 1932). It has also been shown to occur if a muscle is made to contract suddenly by an electrical stimulus during a voluntary contraction (Merton, 1951). The duration of the silent period depends on the intensity of the voluntary contraction, but is generally of the order of 100 msec, and it may be followed by a rebound of increased muscular contraction. Another way to produce it is to allow a muscle contracting isometrically suddenly to shorten when it is spoken of as the 'unloading reflex' (Angel *et al.*, 1965).

Under certain circumstances a kind of oscillation may be set up in the reflex arc so that the reflex is repeated regularly if tension is maintained on the tendon. The tap on the tendon evokes a jerk contraction, as a result of which the tension is taken off the spindles and the silent period occurs. As the muscle relaxes, the spindles are again put under tension and a further tendon jerk occurs. If the jerk continues to repeat itself in this way the process is known as clonus. A few beats of clonus may occur in healthy subjects, but clonus is not normally sustained unless the reflexes are hyperactive. In patients with spasticity, the silent period is well developed. In Parkinson's disease it is little influenced by rigidity but is frequently prolonged when resting tremor is conspicuous (McLellan, 1972).

A tendon jerk may be increased if a strong voluntary contraction is carried out in a different limb at the moment when the tendon is tapped. This is known as reinforcement (Jendrassik, 1885), and is a useful method of demonstrating reflexes which are depressed. The mechanism is unknown, but must be due to some downwardly transmitted facilitatory impulse acting on the motor neurone pool.

Absence of tendon jerks may be evident in spinal shock, in disease affecting the peripheral nerves or the anterior horn cells and is a valuable localizing sign, if the reflex arc is interrupted by disease affecting the segment subserved by a particular tendon reflex. In spasticity, not only are the tendon reflexes frequently abnormally brisk, sometimes with sustained clonus, but certain tendon jerks which cannot normally easily be obtained, such as the jaw jerk and the finger jerks may be readily elicited. There is, however, considerable variation in the excitability of the tendon jerks not only between different individuals, but also in the same person at different times. Thus in physically healthy individuals, they may appear abnormally lively after strenuous exercise or in association with anxiety. The character of the reflexes as a clinical sign must therefore be interpreted with caution and asymmetry may be the most significant feature.

The Hoffmann response and the tonic vibration reflex

The monosynaptic reflex, described by Hoffman in 1918, which can be evoked by electrical stimulation of the posterior tibial nerve, has been termed the H reflex, and is subserved by the same reflex pathway as the ankle jerk. This reflex has been more fully described in an earlier section (see above pp. 98-99).

If a muscle or its tendon is stimulated mechanically by high frequency vibration (100–150 Hz) this will result in sustained contraction of the muscle exposed to vibration and relaxation of its antagonist. This tonic vibration reflex (TVR) is subserved on the afferent side by Group IA afferents activated by the primary endings in the muscle spindles. Vibration thus excites endings which are concerned with phasic as well as tonic stretch reflexes, but the effect of sustained vibration is to excite a tonic response. The tonic vibration reflex is frequently reduced in patients with spastic paralysis but in these patients it may nevertheless enhance the strength of a voluntary contraction, an effect which has been made use of in rehabilitation procedures. The reflex is of normal intensity in patients with Parkinson's disease but may be somewhat reduced in patients with cerebellar disorders (Hagbarth and Eklund, 1966 and 1968; Lance *et al.*, 1966).

Superficial Reflexes

The flexor reflex, by which the whole limb is withdrawn from a painful stimulus applied to the skin, and which has been so fully analyzed by Sherrington, is the most striking example of a cutaneous reflex. It is clear, however, that extensor muscles may also participate in cutaneous reflexes, a well known example being the extensor thrust reflex in response to pressure applied to the toe pads. Hagbarth (1952) has shown that in the cat's hind limb, extensor reflexes may be elicited from specific sites on the skin and that in particular, extensor reflexes can be evoked by stimulating the skin overlying the extensor muscles. In a later study (Hagbarth, 1960), reflex responses were studied in human lower limbs by stimulating the skin with electrical pulses and recording action potentials from muscles under study by needle electrodes. Stimulation of the foot produced contraction of the flexor muscles with inhibition of the extensors, but the extensors were, in general, excited by stimulation of the skin immediately overlying. In each case, the effect was to produce a withdrawal movement either of the limb as a whole, or of the affected part, from the offending stimulus. Activation of a group of muscles in this way is generally accompanied by relaxation of the corresponding muscles on the opposite side of the limb. In spinal man this pattern of reflex response to cutaneous stimulation is altered. This is largely because the flexor reflex is much more easily elicited, and from a wider area, so that stimulation of almost any part of the skin gives rise to a movement of generalized flexion (Dimitrijevic and Nathan, 1968).

The cutaneous reflexes of most general clinical application are the abdominal reflexes and the plantar response.

The Abdominal Reflexes

These are elicited by stroking the skin of the abdomen with a blunt object. The reflex response is a brisk contraction of the abdominal muscle. They probably have the same functional significance as the gluteal and cremasteric reflexes. Their clinical significance lies in the fact that they may be lost in the presence of a lesion affecting the segments through which they are subserved. More important, they are frequently lost when there is a lesion of the corticospinal tract, particularly in multiple sclerosis. Since they are frequently lost in people with a lax abdomen, whether due to obesity, multiparity or surgical operations, their total absence is of doubtful significance, and greater importance attaches to unilateral loss or asymmetry of the reflexes.

The dependence of the reflex on the integrity of the corticospinal tracts has led to the suggestion that it must depend on a long loop pathway extending up the spinal cord into the brain. However, Kugelberg and Hagbarth (1958) have measured its latency by recording the muscle potentials in the abdominal wall evoked by electrical stimulation of the skin, and have shown that although the latent period is variable, like that of the flexor reflex and other polysynaptic reflexes, the shortest latency of the reflex corresponds with a central delay of less than 5.0 msec, long enough for a polysynaptic reflex, but too short for anything but a segmental spinal reflex. Further studies (Hagbarth and Kugelberg, 1958) have shown that although it readily habituates, disappearing after repreated stimulation, it can always be reinforced by a sufficiently painful stimulus. Moreover, in patients with corticospinal lesions in which it is absent after light cutaneous stimulation, it can always be elicited by a strong stimulus to the intercostal nerves. The conclusion seems inescapable that the abdominal reflex following a painful stimulus is a simple polysynaptic withdrawal response. The reflex response to the relatively light stimulation of the clinical reflex is dependent on a conditioning or sensitization process in turn dependent on cerebral events.

The Plantar Response

If the sole of the foot in a healthy subject is stimulated, there occurs a movement of flexion and adduction of the toes. In the presence of disturbed function of the corticospinal tract, the same stimulus may evoke dorsiflexion of the great toe, which is sometimes associated with dorsiflexion or fanning of the other toes. This abnormal plantar response was originally described by Babinski in a series of papers, the first in 1896. Both the normal and the abnormal plantar response may be accompanied by dorsiflexion of the ankle and flexion of the knee and hip. In clinical practice, the most effective site for eliciting the pathological plantar response is the lateral border of the sole of the foot. When a pathological plantar response is evoked flexion of the affected limb may, on occasion, be accompanied by an extension movement of the contralateral limb with plantar flexion of the toes. This was, in fact, the first example of the crossed extensor reflex to be noted in man (Bramwell, 1911).

The terminology whereby the normal plantar response is spoken of as flexor and the pathological as extensor, has given rise to some confusion, since in physiological terms flexion means any movement which approximates the limbs to the trunk, and extension as any movement which lengthens the limb. The fact that the pathological plantar response includes what in this sense, is flexion of the toes, has led to the view that the so called extensor plantar response is part of the abnormally excitable flexor reflex which occurs in patients with lesions affecting the corticospinal pathway (Marie and Foix, 1912; Walshe, 1914, 1954). Kugelberg *et al.* (1960) have studied the matter by investigating the nociceptive reflexes of the lower limbs using electrical stimuli to activate the skin receptors and recording the reflex responses with needle electrodes inserted in the muscles. They found that stimulation of all parts of the foot in the healthy subject was followed by flexion of the proximal limb muscles, but that plantar flexion (physiological extension) of the toes occurred with stimulation at every site except the ball of the toe when dorsiflexion of the toe (physiological flexion) occurred. This can be explained as a natural adaptation whereby stimulation of the foot provokes withdrawal from the offending stimulus. Thus, if the toe is stimulated, the natural reaction is one of generalized flexion with dorsiflexion of the toes. If the heel is stimulated, the reaction is to raise it from the ground, a movement which is assisted by plantar flexion (extension) of the toes. When these experiments were carried out in patients with spastic paraplegia, it was found that stimulation of the ball and hollow of the foot and of the heel now produced dorsiflexion to the toes. One can therefore postulate that, in the healthy subject, the response of the limb to painful stimulation of the foot is one of generalized flexion of the limb, which includes local extensor reflexes to stimulation of parts of the foot. In spastic paralysis, the local extensor reflexes are lost, as their field of excitation is encroached on by that of the hyperactive flexor responses.

The Blink Reflex

If a light tap is given to the forehead the subject blinks. This is known as the glabellar tap reflex and it was first described by Overend in 1896. It readily habituates in healthy subjects, but in patients with Parkinson's disease it continues with repeated tapping. Reflex blinking can be elicited by stimulation of the cornea and of many parts of the face. Although the most important afferent pathway is along the trigeminal nerve, there is evidence, also, that of the afferent fibres a proportion may be carried in the facial nerve. The reflex can be readily elicited by electrical stimulation of the supraorbital nerve, and reflex blinking may also follow flashes of light or sudden noise.

The electrical responses of the orbicularis oculi in reflex blinking were first studied by Kugelberg (1952) and subsequently by Rushworth (1962). If the response of orbicularis oculi is recorded electromyographically following glabellar tap or stimulation of the supraorbital nerve, it is seen that the reflex response has two components, an early response with a latency of the order of 15 msec, and a late response with a latency which may be about 30 msec. Following electrical stimulation of the supraorbital nerve, the early response occurs on the same side only, but the late response can be recorded bilaterally. On repeated stimulation, the early response is persistant, but in the healthy relaxed subject the late response habituates rapidly (Fig. 6.12). It has been suggested, that the early component is a proprioceptive reflex and that the later response is a nociceptive reflex arising from stimulation of the skin. However, both components of the blink reflex can be obtained by electrical stimulation of the skin, and spindles have not been described in facial muscles. Shahani (1968) has suggested that the two components of the blink reflex may be analagous to the two components of the flexor reflex, which can be demonstrated by recording from tibialis anterior when the skin of the foot is stimulated electrically.

In patients with lesions of the trigeminal nerve, the first component of the blink reflex may be reduced in amplitude and have a prolonged latency. In patients with Bell's palsy, both components may be delayed. In patients with hemiplegia, the first component is frequently exaggerated with a small late component, whereas in Parkinson's disease both components may be of high amplitude and the second component does not habituate. Although almost invariably present in Parkinson's disease, a persistant glabellar reflex is not specific for this condition, since it has been observed in a wide variety of disorders where there is atrophy or loss of cerebral substance (Pearce *et al.*, 1968).

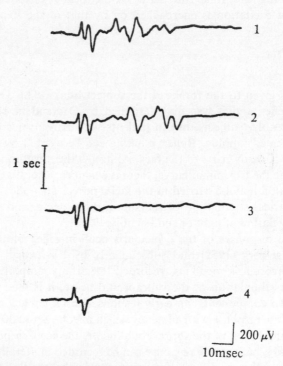

Fig. 6.12. Electrical record of blink reflex evoked by repetitive taps over the glabella at 2 sec intervals. On this occasion habituation of the second phase of the reflex occurs after the second tap.

REFERENCES

Angel, R. W., Eppler, W. and Iannone, A. (1965). Silent period produced by unloading of muscle during voluntary contraction. *J. Physiol.* (*Lond.*), **180**, 865–870.

ARAKI, T., ECCLES, J. C. and ITO, M. (1960). Correlation of the inhibitory post-synaptic potential of motoneurones with the latency and time course of inhibition of monosynaptic reflexes. *J. Physiol. (Lond.)*, **154**, 354–377.

BAYLISS, W. M. (1901). On the origin from the spinal cord of the vaso-dilator fibres of the hind-limb and on the nature of these fibres. *J. Physiol. (Lond.)*, **26**, 173–209.

BAYLISS, W. M. (1902). Further researches on antidromic nerve-impulses. *J. Physiol. (Lond.)*, **28**, 276–299.

BOYD, I. A. (1966). Discussion on muscle spindles. In: *Muscular Afferents and Motor Control*. Ed. Granit, R. New York: John Wiley & Sons, pp. 115–119.

BRAMWELL, B. (1911). Note on the crossed plantar reflex. *Rev. Neurol. and Psychiat.* **IX**, 49–53.

CALNE, D. B. and PALLIS, C. A. (1966). Vibratory sense: a critical review. *Brain*, **89**, 723–746.

COOK, A. W. and BROWDER, E. J. (1965). Functions of posterior columns in man. *Arch. Neurol. (Chicago)*, **12**, 72–79.

COOPER, S. (1961). The response of the primary and secondary endings of muscle spindles with intact motor innervation during applied stretch. *Quart. J. exp. Physiol.*, **46**, 389–398.

CREED, R. S., DENNY-BROWN, D., ECCLES, J. C., LIDDELL, E. G. T. and SHERRINGTON, C. S. (1932). *Reflex Activity of the Spinal Cord*. Oxford: Clarendon Press.

DENNY-BROWN, D. and ROBERTSON, E. G. (1933). On the physiology of micturition. *Brain*, **56**, 149–190.

DIMITRIJEVIĆ, M. R. and NATHAN, P. W. (1967). Studies of spasticity in man. I. Some Features of Spasticity. *Brain*, **90**, 1–30.

DIMITRIJEVIĆ, M. R. and NATHAN, P. W. (1968). Studies of spasticity in man. 3. Analysis of reflex activity evoked by noxious cutaneous stimulation. *Brain*, **91**, 349–368.

ECCLES, J. C., SCHMIDT, R. F. and WILLIS, W. D. (1963a). The mode of operation of the synaptic mechanism producing presynaptic inhibition. *J. Neurophysiol.*, **26**, 523–538.

ECCLES, J. C., SCHMIDT, R. F. and WILLIS, W. D. (1963b). Depolarization of the central terminal of cutaneous afferent fibres. *J. Neurophysiol.*, **26**, 646–661.

ECCLES, J. C. (1969). *The Inhibitory Pathways of the Central Nervous System*. Liverpool: University Press.

VON EULER, C. (1966). Proprioceptive control in respiration. In: *Muscular Afferents and Motor Control*. Nobel Symposium I. Ed. Granit, R. New York: John Wiley & Sons, pp. 197–207.

FÔRSTER, O. (1911). Resection of the posterior nerve roots of the spinal cord. *Lancet*, **ii**, 76–78.

FÖRSTER, O. (1933). The dermatomes in man. *Brain*, **56**, 1–39.

FRANK, F. and FUORTES, M. G. F. (1957). Presynaptic and postsynaptic inhibition of monosynaptic reflexes. *Fed. Proc.*, **16**, 39–40.

FULLERTON, P. M. and GILLIATT, R. W. (1965). Axon reflexes in human motor nerve fibres. *J. Neurol. Neurosurg. Psychiat.*, **28**, 1–11.

GILMAN, S. and DENNY-BROWN, D. (1966). Disorders of movement and behaviour following dorsal column lesions. *Brain*, **89**, 397–418.

GLEES, P. (1953). The central pain tract (tractus spino-thalamicus). *Acta neuroveg.* (Wien), **7**, 1–4 and 160–174, cited by Sinclair (1967).

GRANIT, R. (1970). *The Basis of Motor Control*. London: Academic Press.

GRANIT, R., HOLMGREN, B. and MERTON, P. A. (1955). The two routes for excitation of muscle and their subservience to the cerebellum. *J. Physiol. (Lond.)*, **130**, 213–224.

E

GUTTMANN, L. (1952). Studies on reflex activity of isolated cord in spinal man. *J. Nervous and Mental Disease*, **116**, 957–972.

GUTTMANN, L. (1970). Spinal shock and reflex behaviour in man. *Paraplegia*, **8**, 100–110.

GUTTMANN, L. (1973). *Spinal Cord Injuries*. Oxford: Blackwell.

GUTTMANN, L. and WHITTERIDGE, D. (1947). Effects of bladder distension on autonomic mechanisms after spinal and injuries. *Brain*, **70**, 361–404.

HAGBARTH, K. E. (1952). Excitatory and inhibitory skin areas for flexor and extensor motoneurones. *Acta Physiol. scand.*, Vol. 26, suppl. **94**, 1–58.

HAGBARTH, K. E. (1960). Spinal withdrawal reflexes in the human lower limbs. *J. Neurol. Neurosurg. Psychiat.*, **23**, 222–227.

HAGBARTH, K. E. and EKLUND, G. (1968). The effects of muscle vibration in spasticity rigidity and cerebellar disorders. *J. Neurol. Neurosurg. Psychiat.*, **31**, 207–213.

HAGBARTH, K. E. and KUGELBERG, E. (1958). Plasticity of the abdominal skin reflex. *Brain*, **81**, 305–318.

HAGBARTH, K. E. and VALLBO, Å. B. (1969). Single unit recordings from muscle nerves in human subjects. *Acta physiol. scand.*, **76**, 321–334.

HINSEY, J. C. and GASSER, H. S. (1930). The component of the dorsal root mediating vaso-dilatation and the Sherrington contracture. *Amer. J. Physiol.*, **92**, 679–689.

HOFFMANN, P. (1918). Über die Beziehungen der Sehnenreflexe zur willkürlichen Bewegung und zum Tonus. *Zeitschrift für Biologie (Z. Biol.)*, **68**, 351–370.

ILLIS, L. S. (1967). The motor neurone surface and spinal shock. In: *Modern Trends in Neurology*. 4. Ed. Williams, D. London: Butterworths, pp. 53–68.

KUGELBERG, E. (1948). Demonstration of A and C fibre components in the Babinski plantar response and the pathological flexor reflex. *Brain*, **71**, 304–319.

KUGELBERG, E., EKLUND, K. and GRIMBY, L. (1960). An electromygraphic study of the nociceptive reflexes of the lower limb. Mechanism of the plantar responses. *Brain*, **83**, 394–410.

KUGELBERG, E. and HAGBARTH, K. E. (1958). Spinal mechanism of the abdominal and erector spinae skin reflexes. *Brain*, **81**, 290–304.

KUHN, R. A. (1950). Functional capacity of the isolated human spinal cord. *Brain*, **73**, 1–51.

LANCE, J. W., DE GAIL, P. and NIELSON, P. D. (1966). Tonic and phasic spinal cord mechanisms in man. *J. Neurol. Neurosurg. Psychiat.*, **29**, 535.

LEARMONTH, J. R. (1931). A contribution to the neurophysiology of the urinary bladder in man. *Brain*, **54**, 147–176.

LEWIS, T. (1942). *Pain*. New York: Macmillan.

LEWIS, T. and MARVIN, H. M. (1927). Observations upon a pilomotor reaction in response to faradism. *J. Physiol. (Lond.)*, **64**, 88–106.

LLOYD, D. P. C. (1943a). Reflex action in relation to pattern and peripheral source of afferent stimulation. *J. Neurophysiol.*, **6**, 111–119.

LLOYD, D. P. C. (1943b). Conduction and synaptic transmission of the reflex response to stretch in spinal cats. *J. Neurophysiol.*, **6**, 317–326.

McLELLAN, D. L. (1972). Levodopa in Parkinsonism: reduction in the electromyographic silent period and its relationship with tremor. *J. Neurol. Neurosurg. Psychiat.* **35**, 373–378.

MAGLADERY, J. W. and McDOUGAL, D. B. Jr. (1950). Electrophysiological studies of nerve and reflex activity in normal man. I. Identification of certain reflexes in the electromyogram and the conduction velocity of peripheral nerve fibres. *Bull. Johns Hopk. Hosp.*, **86**, 265–290.

MARIE, P. and FOIX, Ch. (1912). Les reflexes d'automatisme medullaire. *Rev. Neurol.* **23**, 657–676.

MATTHEWS, P. B. C. (1964). Muscle spindles and their motor control. *Physiol. rev.*, **44**, 219–288.

MATTHEWS, P. B. C. (1972). Mammalian muscle receptors and their central actions. *Monographs of the Physiological Society Number* 23. London: Arnold.

MERTON, P. A. (1951). The silent period in a muscle of the human hand. *J. Physiol. (Lond.)*, **114**, 183–198.

NATHAN, P. W. and SMITH, M. C. (1958). The centrifugal pathway for micturition within the spinal cord. *J. Neurol. Neurosurg. Psychiat.*, **21**, 177–189.

NEWSOM DAVIS, J. and SEARS, T. A. (1970). The proprioceptive reflex control of the intercostal muscles during their voluntary activation. *J. Physiol. (Lond.)*, **209**, 711–738.

OLSEN, P. Z. and DIAMANTOPOULOS, E. (1967). Excitability of spinal motor neurones in normal subjects and patients with spasticity, Parkinsonian rigidity and cerebellar hypotonia. *J. Neurol. Neurosurg. Psychiat.*, **30**, 325–331.

PEARCE, J., AZIZ, H. and GALLAGHER, J. C. (1968). Primitive reflex activity in primary and symptomatic Parkinsonism. *J. Neurol. Neurosurg. Psychiat.*, **31**, 501–508.

PEDERSEN, E. (1969). *Spasticity: Mechanism, measurement, management.* Springfield: Thomas.

PLUM, F. (1962). Bladder Dysfunction. In: *Modern Trends in Neurology.* 3. Ed. Williams, D. London: Butterworths.

POLLOCK, L. J. and DAVIS, L. (1927). The influence of the cerebellum upon the reflex activities of the decerebrate animal. *Brain*, **50**, 277–312.

POLLOCK, L. J. and DAVIS, L. (1931). Studies in decerebration. VI. The effect of deafferentation upon decerebrate rigidity. *Amer. J. Physiol.*, **98**, 47–49.

RENSHAW, B. (1941). Influence of discharge of motoneurones upon excitation of neighbouring motoneurones. *J. Neurophysiol.*, **4**, 167–183.

RIDDOCH, G. (1917). The reflex functions of the completely divided spinal cord in man, compared with those associated with less severe lesions. *Brain*, **40**, 264–402.

RUSHWORTH, G. (1960). Spasticity and rigidity: an experimental study and review. *J. Neurol. Neurosurg. Psychiat.*, **23**, 99–118.

RUSHWORTH, G. (1962). Observations on blink reflexes. *J. Neurol. Neurosurg. Psychiat.*, **25**, 93–108.

SHAHANI, B. (1968). Effects of sleep on human reflexes with a double component. *J. Neurol. Neurosurg. Psychiat.*, **31**, 574–579.

SHERRINGTON, C. S. (1904). Correlation of reflexes and the principle of the final common path. *Nature*, **70**, 460–466.

SHERRINGTON, C. S. (1898). Experiments in examination of the peripheral distribution of the fibres of the posterior roots of some spinal nerves. Part II. *Philos. Trans*, CXC, b, 45–186.

SHERRINGTON, C. S. (1906). *The Integrative Action of the Nervous System.* Cambridge: University Press. New York, reprinted 1947.

SINCLAIR, D. (1967). *Cutaneous Sensation.* London: Oxford University Press.

TOWER, S. (1940). Pyramidal lesion in the monkey. *Brain*, **63**, 36–90.

VALLBO, Å. B. (1970). Slowly adapting muscle receptors in man. *Acta physiol. scand.* **78**, 315–333.

VALLBO, Å. B. (1971). Muscle spindle response at the onset of isometric voluntary contractions in man. Time difference between fusimotor and skeletomotor effects. *J. Physiol. (Lond.)*, **318**, 405–431.

WALL, P. D. (1970). The sensory and motor role of impulses travelling in the dorsal columns towards cerebral cortex. *Brain*, **93**, 505–524.

WALL, P. D. and CRONLY-DILLON, J. R. (1960). Pain, itch and vibration. *Arch. Neurol. Psychiat. (Chicago)*, **2**, 365–375.

WALSHE, F. M. R. (1914). The physiological significance of the reflex phenomena in spastic paralysis of the lower limbs. *Brain*, **37**, 269–336.

WALSHE, F. M. R. (1956). The Babinski plantar response, its forms and its physiological and pathological significance. *Brain*, **79**, 529–556.

WILKINS, R. W., NEWMAN, H. W. and DOUPE, J. (1938). The local response to faradic stimulation. *Brain*, **61**, 290–297.

CHAPTER 7

Sensation

Information from the external environment is received by the nervous system through a system of specialized organs that act as transducers, which convert the energy derived from an external stimulus into coded signals that are transmitted along nervous pathways. These signals are ultimately organized into perceptions of objects in the external world. Sensory organs may be highly specialized structures, such as the eye, and the organs concerned with smell, hearing and balance, or they may comprise a single encapsulated nerve ending, such as the Pacinian corpuscle, or simply a network of free nerve endings. In general, the organs of sensation are highly specific, responding only to particular forms of energy, such as light or sound, particular chemical substances, or the application of warmth or pressure. It is also clear that certain receptors will respond to more than one type of stimulus, with perhaps a particularly low threshold for one modality.

Although there are wide differences in structure between different sensory receptors, they have in common a single transducer mechanism. In each case, the energy of the stimulus gives rise to a depolarization, which is not an all or nothing event, but a graded response, the magnitude of which depends on the intensity of the stimulus. This generator potential in turn gives rise to a repetitive discharge along the nerve fibre, the frequency of which is dependent on the amplitude of the generator potential and hence the intensity of the stimulus. A major difficulty in the study of sensation is that most of the direct recording experiments on sensory nerves have been carried out on animals, but only the conscious human subject can describe the quality and intensity of the perceived sensation. However, it has been found that if a subject is asked to distinguish the smallest differences in intensity of a sensation which he can perceive, the relationship to the intensity of the stimulus is broadly similar to that between the amplitude of the generator potential and the stimulus intensity in an experimental preparation. The relationship is a complex one, but in general, it is true that the intensity of the sensation, or the amplitude of the generator potential, is related to the log of the stimulus intensity.

125

GENERAL PROPERTIES OF SENSATION

Specific Nerve Energies

The existence of five distinct senses, vision, hearing, taste, smell and touch, was recognized by Aristotle, and it is common knowledge that the major sense organs are specifically adapted to subserve particular varieties of sensation. Moreover, stimulation of a sense organ, or of a particular sensory nerve, by a variety of different stimuli will generally give rise to only a single sensation. For example, stimulation of the retina by pressure or of the optic nerve by an electric current will produce a visual sensation. These observations have been given formal recognition in Müller's law of specific nerve energies, which states that stimulation of a specific end organ will give rise to a specific sensation and to no other, no matter what the nature of the stimulus.

This concept does not imply that there is any specific quality in the nerves which carry different sensations or in the type of signal that they carry. It is, in fact, clear that a similar frequency code is generally applicable to sensory nerves carrying different sensations. It does imply that sensory receptors have a specific transducer mechanism which will respond preferentially to energy of a particular kind. In its most rigid form, it implies that each modality of sensation has a specific receptor from which sensation is transmitted along a specific pathway to end in specific cells in the central nervous system.

Detailed examination of sensory processes has thrown doubt on how far the law of specific nerve energies can be universally and rigidly applied. Certain receptors can subserve more than one modality of sensation and, in some situations, there is evidence that different receptors may converge on a single sensory pathway. In the skin, different forms of sensation appear to be subserved by undifferentiated nerve endings that cannot be distinguished anatomically, although they may well have specific transducing properties at a molecular level. While it has been generally held that pain is due to excitation of specific receptors, it has also been argued that pain may come about through over-stimulation of any receptor, or from excessive stimulation of many fibres subserving different modalities. Microelectrode studies have shown that it is possible to record evoked potentials from single cortical cells following stimulation of sensory receptors, but it is also clear that sensory signals may be filtered and modified in their passage through central pathways.

The Generator Potential

The application of a stimulus to a receptor results in a steady potential change in the cell membrane of the receptor cell. It is this steady potential change or generator potential, which sets off a repetitive discharge in the sensory nerve fibre. The generator potential is a graded response dependent on the intensity of the stimulus, that does not obey the all-or-nothing law, and in this way resembles the end–plate potential which initiates the propagated action potential in a muscle fibre.

In the muscle spindle the generator potential can be recorded by placing an electrode on the primary afferent fibre close to the muscle spindle, with a second indifferent electrode on the muscle tendon. On stretching the muscle, a slow potential is recorded due to depolarization of the sensory nerve where it joins the spindle. This is followed by a repetitive discharge of impulses along the afferent fibre (Katz, 1950 a and b). The generator potential has been very thoroughly studied in the Pacinian corpuscle. This is a receptor which is found in the skin and subcutaneous tissues, in the fascial planes and in the mesentery and which is responsive to pressure. It is an oval structure up to 4 mm in length, and consists of concentric laminae derived from the flattened processes of connective tissue cells which surround a single nerve terminal. This is the terminal of a myelinated nerve, which loses its myelin sheath after entering the capsule, so that the final part of the nerve ending within the capsule consists of bare unmyelinated nerve. If the corpuscle is stimulated by applying pressure to the capsule, the pressure is transmitted to the unmyelinated nerve terminal that is partially depolarized. A repetitive spike discharge can then be recorded, which is propagated along the nerve fibre and appears to start at the first node of Ranvier (Gray and Sato, 1953).

Generator potentials have been recorded from a wide variety of sense organs, and a particularly useful preparation has been the eye of the horse shoe crab, Limulus. In this preparation incident light causes a generator potential in light sensitive retinula cells which surround a neurone, known as an eccentric cell. Depolarization of the eccentric cell, due to direct spread from the retinula cells, can be recorded by an intracellular microelectrode. This depolarization in turn gives rise to a repetitive spike discharge (Fuortes, 1959) (Fig. 7.1).

Stimulus Intensity, Sensation and Discharge Frequency

Early observations on the changes in stimulus intensity, which were necessary to produce a just noticeable difference in a subject's estimate of the magnitude of a sensation, led to the formulation of Weber's law. This can be expressed in the terms that the increase in stimulus necessary to produce an appreciable increase in sensation always bears the same relation to the whole stimulus. This ratio of stimulus increment to total stimulus intensity, which is necessary to produce a just noticeable difference in sensation, varies with different sense organs. Thus, for the ear it is greater than 1/20, whereas for the eye it is less than 1/150. This law is only applicable in the middle ranges of intensity and does not apply to very strong or very weak stimuli.

If just noticeable differences in sensation are assumed to be equal, a sensory scale can be derived which can be plotted against stimulus intensity. This gives rise to Fechner's law, which states that the subjective intensity of a sensation is proportional to the log of the stimulus intensity. Studies that have been carried out on the eye of Limulus have shown that the frequency of discharge is directly related to the amplitude of the generator potential, but that both are proportional to the log of the stimulus intensity (Fuortes 1959). Subsequent work has shown that the just noticeable difference tends to increase in size as the magnitude of the sensation increases and that both the subjective sensation and the discharge

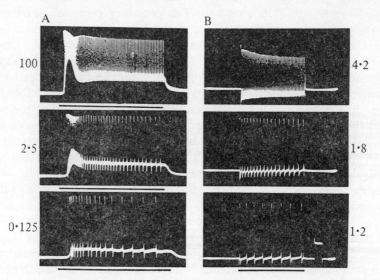

FIG. 7.1. Responses of impaled eccentric cell of Limulus ommatidium to light and depolarizing currents. A. Shows generator potential with superimposed spikes both of which are proportional to the log of the light intensity. B. Shows the spike discharge which follows the application of a depolarizing current and in this case the spikes are linearly related to the current intensity. Figures on left give relative intensity of light used. Figures on right give intensity of current in nA. Time scale 1 sec. Fuortes, M. G. F. (1959), *J. Physiol. (Lond.)*, **148**, 14–28.

frequency can be better expressed as proportional to the stimulus intensity raised to the power of n. If the log of the stimulus intensity is plotted against the log of the response, a linear relationship may be obtained (Werner and Mountcastle, 1965).

Adaptation

It is common knowledge that a person becomes unaware of certain forms of stimulus if they are applied over a long period. Thus, one is not normally consciously aware of the continuous contact of clothing on the body or of the pressure of a watch strap on the wrist or the temperature of the environment. This is partly due to the fact that attention is easily diverted from a continuing stimulus and there are complex central mechanisms which determine the degree of awareness given to different forms of stimulus at a given time.

An important peripheral factor is the fact that the discharge frequency of sensory fibres tends to decrease with time if the stimulus is continued. This is known as adaptation. Since there is considerable variation between sensory nerves in this respect sensory fibres can be classified according to whether they are rapidly adapting or slowly adapting. The change that takes place in discharge frequency appears to depend on changes that take place in the generator potential, since, with a rapidly adapting fibre there is a rapid fall in the size of the generator potential, which, on the other hand, is well maintained in a slowly adapting fibre.

The Pacinian corpuscle is a particularly rapidly adapting receptor and if pressure is applied to one it will evoke a discharge lasting only a few msec. On the other hand, the afferent fibre from a muscle spindle will continue to discharge for long periods if stretch is maintained. A rapidly adapting response may be spoken of as a dynamic in contrast to a static or slowly adapting response. It is uncertain how far adaptation is due to change in the receptor and how far to one in the afferent nerve fibre. With the Pacinian corpuscle, it appears that the structure of the receptor is particularly important. Its structure is such that sustained pressure on a corpuscle produces only a transient deformation of the nerve ending. It has been found, that if the nerve ending is dissected free of the capsule, sustained mechanical stimulation will give rise to a generator potential which subsides relatively slowly (Loewenstein and Mendelson, 1965).

With certain forms of sensation there is still doubt as to how far adaptation occurs. This applies particularly to pain, where the evidence is conflicting, but it does appear that many forms of artificially induced pain will become less evident if the stimulus is maintained. There is not, however, always a close correlation between the degree at which awareness of a sensation will fall off and the extent to which peripheral receptors show adaptation. With smell, for example, it is well known that the sense of smell may fatigue rapidly, so that after a short time an odour may cease to be perceived altogether, and yet the receptors are slowly adapting (Ottoson, 1963).

CUTANEOUS SENSATION

Specialized Nerve Endings

The law of specific nerve energies gained strong support from the observation of Blix (1884) that careful stimulation of the skin will reveal discrete spots where the sensations of touch, cold, warmth and pain can be preferentially evoked. Von Frey (1906) suggested that these sensations were appreciated by specific receptors situated under the sensitive spots. Meissner's corpuscles were considered to subserve touch, Ruffini's end organs warmth, Krause's end-bulbs cold and free nerve endings pain.

However, detailed study of the anatomy of the skin has failed to show any correlation between specific receptors and sensory spots. Moreover, the specialized end organs described above are only present in specialized areas of skin such as the palms, soles and certain areas of exposed mucous membrane. In the hairy skin, which represents the greater part of the body surface, there are only two types of sensory ending which occur frequently, viz, the endings which innervate hair follicles and free nerve endings which ramify in a complex network (Hagen *et al.*, 1953). Since the hairy skin subserves the principal varieties of cutaneous sensation, it is not possible to explain the different modalities of cutaneous sensation on the basis that they are subserved by morphologically distinct receptors. Nevertheless, it is possible that nerve endings subserving particular sensations have a distinctive molecular structure not recognizable by the light microscope. The subject has been reviewed in detail by Sinclair (1967).

An important concept was introduced by Head (1905) who made a study of the return in sensation in his own arm after a cutaneous nerve had been sectioned. He found that during recovery a zone of impaired sensation developed in which painful stimuli had a peculiarly unpleasant quality and were poorly localized. He called this protopathic sensibility as distinct from epicritic sensibility, which returned after full recovery, in which light touch was perceived with accurate localization and changes in temperature could be clearly defined. He postulated separate nervous pathways for protopathic and epicritic sensibility. He explained the findings during the recovery of sensation on the basis that protopathic fibres regenerate more rapidly than epicritic. This hypothesis has not been confirmed by anatomical evidence, and the evidence against it has been marshalled by Walshe (1942). However, the concept of protopathic sensation may still usefully be applied to pain. Bishop (1959) has advanced the view that small fibres are concerned with a poorly localized form of sensation, which is more primitive in evolutionary terms and that the more elaborate forms of sensation that provide finer discrimination depend on more recently evolved and larger nerve fibres.

Weddell and his colleagues have put forward the view that the law of specific nerve energies is no longer valid for cutaneous sensation, and that the modality of a sensation is determined by the spatio temporal pattern of excitation in the nerves and not by specific nerve terminals subserving particular cutaneous modalities. They argue that the frequency of discharge may determine whether stimulation of cutaneous fibres give rise to a sensation of touch or pain, and that cold and warmth can be explained by a differential rate of firing between deep and superficial fibres (Lele *et al.*, 1954).

Melzack and Wall (1962) recognize that receptors are specialized as transducers of particular kinds of stimulus. Indeed, in physiological terms of threshold to different varieties of stimulus and rates of adaptation, they show more specialization than was envisaged by von Frey. They argue, however, that it is incorrect to imagine a point to point relationship between the response of a specialized receptor and the psychological sensory experience. This must depend on the spatial and temporal patterns of impulses arising from skin receptors and the manner in which they are filtered and coded in the central nervous system. In an earlier study, Wall (1960) showed that fibres responding to many different modalities of skin sensation converge on cells in the dorsal horn of the spinal cord and give rise to a pattern of discharge that depends on the nature of the stimulus.

Innervation of the Skin

The innervation of the skin is derived from a deep and superficial plexus of myelinated and unmyelinated fibres. The superficial plexus is derived from the deep plexus which consists of larger fibres.

In all types of skin, a very large proportion of the sensory endings consist of morphologically undifferentiated nerve endings. In addition, there are endings which can be distinguished under the light microscope according to whether they have a clearly defined capsule or simply an expansion of the tip. Endings with expanded tips include Merkel's discs and Ruffini end organs. Encapsulated endings include Meissner corpuscles, Krause end-bulbs and Pacinian corpuscles. Ruffini endings and Pacinian bodies are widely distributed in the deep sub-cutaneous tissues. In the superficial skin a wide variety of differentiated endings, including Merkel's discs and Meissner corpuscles, are present, but in hairy skin the only morphologically specialized organs are located in relation to the hair follicles.

There is very little certainty as to the receptor function of the different organs. With the Pacinian corpuscle, there is little doubt that the main function is as a mechanoreceptor, the adequate stimulus with the lowest threshold being deformation of the capsule. It is likely that the deformation produced by bending a hair is the principal exciting factor at a hair follicle. Although the apparently bare nerve endings are similar in appearance, there is now abundant electrophysiological evidence that many fibres respond preferentially to a single type of stimulus.

Tactile Sensation

The sensations that can be appreciated following stimulation of the skin include light touch, pressure, vibration, tickle, itch, temperature and pain. The perception of pain and temperature is described below. It is clear that the perception of touch can take place through a wide variety of receptors which include the hair follicles in the hairy skin, Meissner corpuscles in the glabrous skin and in all areas free nerve endings. It is clear also, that the sensation is mediated by a wide variety of afferent nerve fibres, including both rapidly conducting A fibres and small diameter C fibres. Some of the receptors responsive to touch are rapidly adapting, others are slowly adapting. For perception of pressure, it is clear also that more than a single type of receptor is important. The Pacinian corpuscle is traditionally associated with deep pressure, but is rapidly adapting and can hardly be concerned with sustained pressure (Fig. 7.2).

In the clinical testing of sensation, tactile sensation is frequently carried out by lightly touching the skin with cotton wool or a camel hair brush, and finer discrimination by the ability to distinguish between one and two points of a blunt compass. A more accurate assessment of sensation is obtained by measurement of the threshold. This is done by estimating the mean of the ascending and descending thresholds. The ascending threshold is obtained by applying stimuli

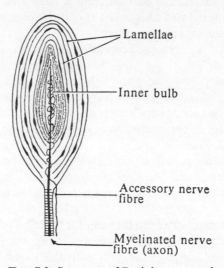

Lamellae

Inner bulb

Accessory nerve fibre

Myelinated nerve fibre (axon)

FIG. 7.2. Structure of Pacinian corpuscle.

of progressively increasing strength until the stimulus is strong enough to be felt. The threshold is taken as the mean of the last two stimuli in the series. The descending threshold is obtained by moving progressively from a strong stimulus until the stimulus can no longer be felt. Accurate pressure can be achieved by using nylon thread on an electrically controlled diaphragm or a kinohapt, which is a stylus released by a solenoid to produce a known pressure (Sinclair, 1967).

Two point discrimination depends on the receptive area of individual nerve fibres. Where the skin is richly innervated by many fibres, each with a small receptive zone, two points can be identified even when they are close together. Where the receptor fibres are sparse and each is responsive to a wide area of stimulation, the capacity for two point discrimination is correspondingly limited. Two point discrimination is most highly developed over the tongue. On the finger pads two points can be distinguished if they are about 1–2 mm apart, over the back and trunk they can only be distinguished if they are separated by several cm. The clinical value of testing two point discrimination lies in the fact that it is not only a test for the innervation of the skin, but also tests the integrity of the sensory cortex. Discrimination between two points not only requires intact sensation, but the subject must make a judgment regarding the quality of the sensation for which the sensory cortex is necessary.

The ability to detect vibration probably depends on more than a single type of receptor. In man, the highest frequency of vibration that can be perceived when applied to the skin is about 1000/sec over the fingers, but less elsewhere on the body. Clinically, vibration sense is generally tested by applying a 128 cycles tuning fork over a bony point. A bony surface is not strictly necessary and vibration can still be appreciated if the subcutaneous tissues are infiltrated with local anaesthetic down to the periosteum. If the skin is infiltrated with anaesthetic, vibration can be felt provided the deeper tissues are not infiltrated at the same time (Newman *et al.*, 1949). For the lower frequencies of vibration, it is likely that many of the relatively slowly adapting receptors in the skin and sub-cutaneous tissues are adequate. For high frequency vibration, a rapidly adapting receptor is clearly necessary. Much evidence points to the rapidly adapting Pacinian corpuscle, which is found both in superficial tissues and in periosteum, as an important receptor for the appreciation of vibration (Hunt, 1961). The mode of perception for tickle and itch is not fully understood but there are grounds for regarding these sensations as related to the sensation of pain.

Temperature

The observation that discrete spots sensitive to warmth and cold can be identified on the skin lends support to the view that there are specific nerve endings respon-sible for mediating these sensations, although it has not been possible to identify morphologically distinct receptors underneath the spots. Thermal sense is unevenly distributed over the body, the exposed surfaces tend to be less sensitive and cold spots are more numerous than warm. Sensitivity to changes in tempera-ture varies according to the condition of the skin and the prevailing temperature, and is particularly acute when the temperature is around 30°C. If the skin is cold, warming it to this temperature gives rise to an apparent increase in the number of cold spots. If a hot ending is placed on a cold spot, it will give rise to a sensation of cold. This phenomenon has been termed paradoxical cold and perhaps accounts for the fact that extremes of temperature may give rise to similar sensations.

Weber (1846) put forward the theory that temperature receptors respond only to changes in temperature, cold endings being stimulated by a fall in temperature and hot endings by a rise in temperature. This does not explain the common observation that if a cold object is placed on the skin and then removed the sensation of cold persists in spite of the fact that the temperature of the skin is rising. The work of Zotterman and his colleagues, who recorded from single nerve fibres during the application of warmth and cold to the tongue of the cat, has shown that temperature receptors do indeed respond to changes of temperature. However, over a limited range of temperature, both warm and cold receptors react with a steady discharge at different temperatures so that the system is also, in a sense, analagous to a thermometer.

In a series of experiments, recordings were made from small filaments of the lingual nerve while the tongue was stimulated by a copper probe, known as a thermode, through which water circulated at a known temperature. It was found that fibres responsive to cold would discharge steadily between temperatures of 10° and 40°C, a maximum steady discharge rate of about 10/sec occurring at a

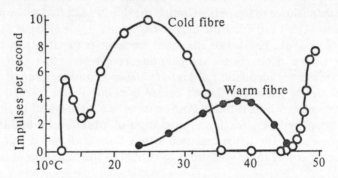

FIG. 7.3. Frequency of discharge recorded from cold fibre and warm fibre following exposure of receptors on cat's tongue to constant temperatures. Zottermann, Y. (1953), *Ann. Rev. Physiol.*, **15**, 357–372.

temperature of 30°C. A second, but lesser, peak occurs at about 10°C, and a third at 45–50°C. This third peak at a relatively high temperature is consistant with the observation of paradoxical cold. Fibres responsive to warmth also give a steady discharge between the temperatures of 20° and 45°C, with a peak at about 37°C, but the maximum steady discharge rate is considerably slower than that of the cold fibres and does not exceed 4/sec. With both types of fibre there is a characteristic discharge frequency for each level of temperature (Fig. 7.3).

Both cold and warm receptors respond to a change in temperature with a rise in discharge frequency to many times the resting discharge rate. With cold sensitive fibres this occurs if there is a fall in temperature, with warm sensitive fibres if the temperature rises (Dodt and Zotterman, 1952a and b; Zotterman 1953).

Landgren (1957a and b) has recorded from the tongue projection area of the infraorbital surface of the hemisphere of the cat using extracellular microelectrodes to record evoked potentials from single cells. Of these, a number of cells responded only to cooling of the tongue, others to different forms of stimulation such as touch or pressure, while a number responded to more than a single type of stimulation. There is thus strong evidence for specific fibre systems responding to particular forms of stimulation, including changes in temperature, but there is also evidence that fibres responsive to different sensations may converge on the same cortical cells.

CHEMICAL SENSATION

The senses of smell and taste are each responsive to chemical stimulation. The sense of taste is relatively specialized, being concerned largely with the identification of food, while smell is capable of providing complex information concerning the environment. Smell is able to discriminate a very much wider range of substances than taste and in very much lower concentrations. In man it is much less important as a general form of sensation in relation to other senses than in simpler forms of life.

Taste

Taste receptors are situated on the dorsal surface of the tongue, with the exception of the central part. The receptors for taste are known as taste buds and these are found in the papillae which are seen on the surface of the tongue and give rise to its roughened appearance. These papillae have been described as fungiform, filiform, circumvallate and foliate. Four primary taste sensations may be recognized, viz, sweet, sour bitter and salt and it is the combination of these primary sensations, together with the many olfactory sensations which food may give rise to, that account for the varieties of flavour which may be experienced. The tip of the tongue is able to appreciate all four sensations of taste but is particularly sensitive to sweet and salt; sour is most easily appreciated on the lateral borders of the tongue and bitter at the base.

Each taste bud is an oval structure consisting of a cluster of receptor cells, the tips of which project on the surface to form a gustatory pore which makes contact with the dissolved substances that give rise to taste. The taste bud is innervated from its base by small myelinated fibres. A single axon may innervate up to about 8 taste cells and some cells are innervated by more than a single axon.

The innervation of the taste buds provides an interesting example of the trophic function of nerve. The life span of a taste cell is less than 5 days, so that as they degenerate new cells are continuously being formed and reinnervated. If the sensory nerve is divided, the taste buds disappear in the course of about 7 days but are reformed as the nerve regenerates (Beidler, 1963). The sensory pathway for taste from the anterior two thirds of the tongue is via the chorda tympani, and from the posterior third by the glossopharyngeal nerve. Most taste fibres end in the nucleus tractus solitarius where a relay passes to the thalamus in close association with the medial lemniscus and the quintothalamic tract. The cortical area for taste is in the area of sensory cortex associated with other modalities derived from the tongue.

It is possible to record a generator potential from single taste cells using an intracellular microelectrode. If this is done, it is found that although taste cells will generally respond to more than a single variety of taste stimulus, there is considerable variation between different receptors in their sensitivity to different tastes (Beidler, 1963).

Single fibre potentials can be recorded from the chorda tympani following stimulation of the taste receptors in the tongue. This has been done by Zotterman and his colleagues on a variety of animals, including the cat, dog, monkey and frog, and also in birds and fish (Fig. 7.4.). It was found that the response of

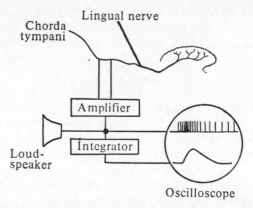

Fig. 7.4. Arrangement for recording impulses from chorda tympani. Zottermann, Y. (1967), *Progress in Brain Research*, **23**, 139–154.

nerves concerned with taste was highly specific, fibres showing a definite pattern of sensitivity to different substances, some responding to a single class of substances only. There is also a considerable range of species difference. Thus the cat responds very poorly to sweet (Beidler, 1963) and the carp shows a marked sensitivity to human saliva (Konishi *et al.*, 1963).

Observations have also been made on the human chorda tympani, exposed at operations to mobilize the stapes. Although it has not been possible to record from single fibres and determine their specificity, it was possible in this way to confirm the general pattern of evoked response to different sensory stimuli. It is of interest that water, which will evoke a response in a number of mammals including cats, dogs and rhesus monkeys, evokes no gustatory response when applied to the human tongue (Diamant *et al.*, 1963; Zotterman, 1967).

In cases of paralysis of the facial nerve, the sense of taste is sometimes affected if the facial nerve is inflamed or damaged above the point where the chorda tympani leaves it. It has been suggested that this is particularly liable to occur in cases of Bell's palsy if the lesion is severe enough to cause partial denervation, so that testing the sense of taste may possibly give information that is of prognostic value. Taste may be tested clinically by application to the tongue of solutions of salt, sugar, acid and quinine. A simple clinical method for estimating the threshold is to apply a small electrical current (less than 100 μ amperes) to the tongue through the anode of a battery generator. In the presence of intact sensation a sour taste is experienced (Peiris and Miles, 1965; Robertson, 1970).

Smell

In man, the sense of smell is relatively unimportant in obtaining information about the environment in comparison with vision and hearing, but in many of

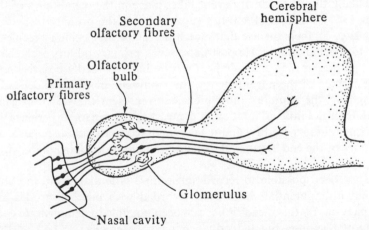

FIG. 7.5. Organization of vertebrate olfactory system. After Nieuwenhuys, R. (1967), *Progr. Brain Res.*, **23**, 1–64.

the earlier forms of life this is not the case. Thus, in fish a predominant part of the higher brain may be concerned with olfaction and in insects a large part of the information necessary for food seeking, homing and reproduction is derived from chemical stimuli. In mammals, other than primates, the size of the olfactory bulbs are very much larger than in man in proportion to total brain size. Even in the human subject, however, the sense of smell is highly specific, so that it is possible to distinguish by this means perhaps several thousand distinct substances. The sensitivity is such that certain substances can be identified in concentrations in air of less than parts/10^6.

The receptive cells concerned with smell are nerve cells which are situated in the mucosa of the nasal cavity (Fig. 7.5). The peripheral part of this cell is a dendrite which ends in a terminal vesicle on the surface of the nasal cavity where it gives off a group of hairs or cilia. The central part is a small unmyelinated axon. These axons pass to the olfactory bulb where they form a ramifying network of fibres which make contact with the dendrites of the second order olfactory neurones or mitral cells. The junction between the axon of the primary olfactory neurone and the dendrite of the mitral cell is a complex plexus of nerve fibres known as a glomerulus. In man, the axons of the mitral cells travel along the olfactory tract to end in the cortex of the prepyriform area and the adjacent amygdaloid nucleus. The primary olfactory receptors are embedded in a mass of supporting or sustentacular cells. There is evidence that these cells may have more than a supporting function, and are possibly concerned with the removal of odoriferous molecules or the secretion of enzymes concerned at the receptor site (Ottoson and Shepherd, 1967).

Little is known about the receptor mechanism of the primary olfactory cell. It seems likely that the primary event takes place in the membranes of the cilia (Ottoson, 1963). Amoore (1963) has suggested that the primary receptors have receiving sites on their surface that match the shape of specific molecules which give rise to specific odours. He postulates seven primary odours each characterized by a particular molecular shape. Ottoson has recorded a negative potential from the surface of the nasal mucosa, the amplitude of which is dependent on the strength of the stimulus and which may represent the olfactory generator potential. It shows little adaptation in contrast to the general experience that the sense of smell adapts readily, and it may be that adaptation as regards smell is not a feature of the end organ, but depends on inhibition taking place within the bulb.

It has not been possible to record single fibre potentials from the olfactory nerves, but unit potentials have been recorded with microelectrodes inserted into the mucosa. By this means it has not been possible to demonstrate complete specificity of response, but individual unit responses seem to be preferentially evoked by particular stimuli, although generally more than one type of stimulus is effective. This could mean that each receptor cell carries more than one type of receptor site and different receptors vary in the proportions in which the different receptor type sites are distributed (Gesteland *et al.*, 1963).

Electrical recording from the bulb using fine extracellular electrodes has shown spike discharges in response to different odours with a tendency for particular odours to evoke discharge from localized regions of the bulb (Adrian, 1950). Intracellular electrode studies of the bulb have shown a complex pattern both of evoked response and inhibition by different sensory stimuli (see review by Ottoson and Shepherd, 1967).

Clinically, the sense of smell is frequently lost as a result of head injuries. The site of damage is not known and is probably variable, but the filaments of the olfactory nerves would appear to be particularly vulnerable as they pass through the cribriform plate of the ethmoid to enter the anterior cranial fossa. Loss of sense of smell may also occur as a result of local pressure on the bulb or tract by frontal lobe tumours or a meningioma arising in the olfactory groove. This loss of sense of smell, if it is due to local pressure, may be unilateral and the patient is unlikely to be aware of it unless it is disclosed by formal testing. The hippocampus is a common site of origin for an epileptic discharge. Although it is no longer regarded as containing the cortical centre for smell, it is likely that spread of the epileptic disturbance from the hippocampus to the adjacent brain is responsible for the hallucination of smell which sometimes constitutes the aura of a temporal lobe seizure.

Pain

Many people have in the past argued that pain depends solely on the intensity of stimulation and not on stimulation of a particular pathway with specific receptors. There is much that can be said for this view, in particular, the fact that pain can be evoked by stimulation by a variety of different stimuli. Thus, excessive warmth or excessive cold can give rise to a sensation of pain and the effects of bright light or excessive noise can also be felt as unpleasant. On the other hand, the observation that pain sensitivity can be localized in discrete spots in the skin, separate from touch and temperature, led von Frey (1894) and others to argue that pain is subserved by separate nerve endings. This is supported by the observation that stimulation of touch and pressure organs, even if excessive, can be applied without producing pain (Cattell and Hoagland, 1931). Moreover, the dissociation between pain and other sensations, which can follow peripheral nerve blocks, and the selective abolition of pain that may follow anterolateral cordotomy, cannot readily be explained unless there is a pathway in some degree specific for pain.

Von Frey postulated that fibres sensitive to pain were free nerve endings. Sherrington (1906) argued that free nerve endings, relatively undifferentiated and responsive to a variety of stimuli, were well adapted to responding to intense potentially damaging stimuli. These nociceptive fibres which carried signals capable of causing the psychological reaction of pain also provided the afferent arc for reflex withdrawal.

Although it cannot be said that any groups of nerve fibres are specific for the transmission of pain, there is now strong physiological evidence that painful impulses from the skin are, for the most part, carried in small nerve fibres, either group A δ fibres or unmyelinated C fibres. Direct recording from nerve fibres in the cat, following the application of different stimuli to the skin, has shown that action potentials corresponding to small myelinated and C fibres can be recorded following painful stimulation (Zotterman, 1939). If action potentials are recorded following the application of stimuli to the hind limb muscles, it has been found that, if pain is produced by squeezing muscle or injecting saline, potentials are recorded in small myelinated fibres that can also apparently respond to stimulation of pressure receptors (Paintal, 1960). In patients undergoing cordotomy, Collins and his associates (1960) recorded nerve action potentials while applying various stimuli to the sural nerve. Activation of δ fibres gave rise to pain which became unbearable when C fibres were activated. The application of nerve blocks to human peripheral nerve has been of interest in this connection, since different blocking agents affect nerve fibres in a different order. If a nerve is blocked by procaine, the smallest diameter fibres are affected first and clinically, the perception of pain is lost before touch. On the other hand, if a nerve is blocked by pressure, the myelinated fibres fail before un-myelinated and the sensation of touch is lost before pain (Sinclair and Hinshaw, 1950). The study of nerve fibre recovery after injury has been less informative, since although awareness of pain returns before touch, the order in which different fibres recover is not known (Napier, 1952).

To show that painful stimuli are, for the most part, conveyed in particular classes of nerve fibre in no way explains the clinical aspects of pain, much less the psychological attributes of unpleasant experience. These aspects will be further discussed below.

Pain Threshold

The clinical testing of pain sensation is normally carried out by the application of painful stimuli to the skin, which can be done most easily by the application of a prick with a sharp point. By this means, it is possible to distinguish from normal pain perception total sensory loss to pain and various degrees of hypo-algesia and hyperalgesia.

Accurate measurement of the pain threshold requires careful standardization of the experimental conditions, since variables such as skin temperature, if not properly controlled, will produce marked alterations. Pain can be evoked by various stimuli, such as direct contact with weighted needles, or contact with a probe of known temperature or by electrical stimulation. All these methods have disadvantages. One technique which has been widely employed is the application of a pure thermal stimulus by radiant heat. This can be applied by irradiating the skin from a dolorimeter for a predetermined period, the skin having been previously blackened with India ink to promote absorption of heat. The result can be expressed quantitatively in terms of cal/cm^2 of skin/sec and provided care is taken to maintain constant conditions, consistent thresholds for a given individual can be obtained (Hardy *et al.*, 1952).

The pain threshold is lowered if the skin is hyperaemic or inflamed, as it may be after exposure to ultra-violet radiation. Another form of hyperalgesia may arise if pain is referred to the skin from a deeply situated site of inflammation, or if there is disease affecting the central pathways for pain, as in the thalamic syndrome. When this occurs, although when pain is felt it is abnormally intense, the pain threshold is not lowered. In a peripheral neuropathy the threshold for sharp pain, which is rapidly conducted is raised, but there may be a lowered threshold for burning pain which is more slowly transmitted (see below). Analgesic drugs may markedly raise the pain threshold (Wolff and Wolf, 1948).

First and Second Pain

In 1874 Remak and others noted that in certain patients with tabes dorsalis the response to pain was delayed. This led to the discovery that in a healthy subject a painful stimulus may be followed almost immediately by a sharp pain, and after an interval of a second or longer by a second pain, somewhat more intense and less clearly localized. The matter was studied in detail by Lewis and Pochin (1937) and Pochin (1938). They found that the latency for second pain was longest the further the stimulus from the spinal cord, being maximal if the stimulus was applied to the toe. This suggested that slow and fast pain were mediated by different sets of peripheral nerve fibres. Additional evidence was obtained from experiments in which pain was elicited after block of a peripheral nerve with cocaine or by ischaemia. Cocaine blocks small nerve fibres first and in a cocaine block slow pain was lost before fast pain. The opposite effect was observed in ischaemic block in which the more rapidly conducting fibres are affected first. Studies on patients with tabes dorsalis showed that the latency of the pain corresponded with that of second pain in healthy subjects, indicating that in tabes there may be selective loss of rapidly conducting fibres which transmit pain.

Subsequent studies have tended to confirm that pain is conducted by two peripheral pathways, pain which is experienced after a short latency being conveyed in group A δ fibres, slow pain in unmyelinated C fibres. The difference in quality between first and second pain is of interest, since the burning character of slow pain is in some respects similar to the protopathic sensation which Head described during regeneration of peripheral nerve.

The Nature of Pain

Although physiological studies have made it possible to identify particular classes of nerve fibre that are especially important for the transmission of painful stimuli, and there is clinical evidence that painful sensations are carried along particular pathways in the spinal cord, there are many things that make it difficult to accept that pain is a specific modality subserved by specific nervous connections which have no other function. Although the operation of anterolateral cordotomy for the relief of pain would seem to support the view that pain is a specific modality carried in the spinothalamic tract, it is difficult to explain on this basis the failure of this operation to relieve the pain of such conditions as causalgia, post herpetic neuralgia, and the pain of phantom limb. The variability in sensitivity to pain, which occurs not only between different individuals, but in the same individual in different circumstances, requires explanation. Thus, mentally defective persons may sometimes show little sensitivity to pain. The same individual may show heightened sensitivity in a state of anxiety or complete insensitivity under hypnosis or in a state of hysterical dissociation or in the excitement of the field of battle. A number of cases have been described of individuals, who are of normal intelligence and who are completely insensitive to pain, although the nervous system is clinically intact (Ogden *et al.*, 1959; Magee, 1963). Complete universal insensitivity of this kind is not observed with the sensations of touch and temperature. On the other hand, there is evidence that pain and temperature make use of the same pathway. Thus, extremes of warmth and cold will give rise to pain, whereas touch will not unless there is also hyperalgesia. Likewise, pain and temperature sensation are both lost in disease affecting the spinothalamic system, such as syringomyelia, and may both also be affected in peripheral disorders such as hereditary sensory radiculopathy. Moreover, if an animal is allowed to stimulate itself through electrodes implanted in the brain, it will stimulate itself repeatedly with the electrode in certain situations as though the stimulus gives rise to pleasure. With the electrode elsewhere it will avoid stimulation, apparently because the stimulus is unpleasant (Olds, 1958). It appears that the appreciation of pain depends in some measure on the activation of particular anatomical structures within the brain.

Melzack and Wall (1965) have put forward a hypothesis to account for cutaneous pain, which takes into account the existence of a degree of specificity in peripheral receptors and nerve fibres, but suggests a mechanism whereby painful stimuli can determine the intensity of activation of central pathways. It has been shown (Wall, 1960) that cells in the dorsal horn of the cord receive converging fibres responding to different sensory modalities. In the gate control theory that they put forward, it is suggested that central transmission (T) fibres receive touch and other signals through large afferent fibres, and signals derived from painful stimuli through small afferent fibres (Fig. 7.6). Both these groups of afferent fibres also converge on cells in the substantia gelatinosa which give off fibres to inhibit both the large and small afferent terminals by presynaptic inhibition. The action of the large fibres, however, is to excite, whereas the small afferent fibres inhibit the substantia gelatinosa cells. The effect of this arrangement is that signals in the large afferent fibres decrease the total sensory inflow by increasing presynaptic inhibition, whereas signals in the small afferents reduce presynaptic inhibition and hence increase the total sensory inflow. It can be argued that when the total inflow along this pathway reaches a certain level, it gives rise to the sensation of pain. Mendell and Wall (1965) have recorded from dorsal cord cells in the cat and shown that stimulation of group A afferents can arrest the discharge of these cells, whereas stimulation of C afferents may enhance it.

The idea that the psychological response is the result of excessive activation of the nervous system has an obvious advantage in terms of evolution. A gate mechanism which is opened by a lack of balance between C fibre and A fibre activation is capable of explaining some of the clinical difficulties in connection with pain. For example, in post herpetic neuralgia there may be intense pain, although tactile sensation is diminished. However, the presence of discharge in C fibres could cause an excessive sensory inflow if the inhibitory feedback from tactile signals is lost. It is of interest that post herpetic neuralgia, causalgia and the pain of a phantom limb may all be relieved in certain individuals by external massage or the application of a vibrating stimulus to the affected part.

Nordenboos (1959) has suggested that much of pain is transmitted, not along a direct spinothalamic pathway, but along a multisynaptic afferent system which is exposed along its course to activation from slow afferent fibres and inhibition

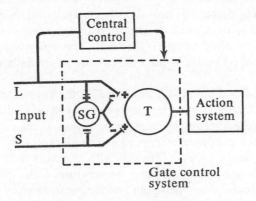

FIG. 7.6. Diagram to show postulated input arrangement in substantia gelatinosa in gate control theory of pain. Melzack, R. and Wall, P. D. (1965), *Science*, **150**, 971–979.

by fast afferents. Anatomical evidence is gradually accumulating that there are two anatomical pathways for pain in the spinal cord, one a direct pathway to the ventrobasal nuclei of the thalamus, the other an interrupted pathway having many connections with the brain stem reticular formation (see chapter 6). This makes it possible for the information to be filtered and also exposed to the influence of descending inhibitory pathways. Damage to this system could account for some of the phenomena of central pain.

Paraesthesiae

Paraesthesiae are sensations which arise in a limb as a result of changes affecting the nerve supply and not arising from peripheral stimuli. They are a common symptom of disease affecting both the peripheral and the central nervous system, and considerable interest therefore applies to nervous pathways that convey them. They can readily be produced by pressure on a peripheral nerve which gives rise to a tingling sensation while pressure is maintained, ischaemic paraesthesiae, and to a succession of abnormal sensations which develop after the pressure is removed, post ischaemic paraesthesiae.

If a sphygmomanometer cuff is inflated around a limb to a pressure above the systolic blood pressure, a tingling sensation develops below the cuff after about 2 mins and lasts for 3–4 mins. If inflation of the cuff is maintained for 5 mins, or preferably longer, and then released, return of the circulation is immediately followed by changing sensations of warmth and cold. These thermal paraesthesiae persist for about a minute and are followed by three distinct sensations that are felt simultaneously. The first is a tingling sensation resembling vibration, the second a feeling of tension in the distal part of the limb as though a movement of flexion is taking place, this sensation has been called pseudo-cramp (Lewis *et al.*, 1931), and lastly a pricking sensation. The sensation of tension lasts till about four minutes after release of the cuff. The other two sensations persist longer, up to about 15 mins if the cuff has been kept inflated for as long as 30 mins.

Merrington and Nathan (1949) have studied the source and transmission of these sensations in a series of experiments carried out on healthy subjects and on patients with disease affecting the sensory pathways. If the experiment is carried out with one of the peripheral nerves to a limb blocked either by local pressure with a clamping device or by infiltration with procaine (with a pressure block touch sensation is lost before pain and temperature, with a procaine block pain is lost first), it is found that when pain and temperature sensation are selectively lost, then all types of paraesthesiae can be experienced, except thermal paraesthesiae, but when touch sensation is lost selectively then only thermal paraesthesiae can be felt. It appears, therefore, that all paraesthesiae except thermal are carried in nerve fibres which transmit touch sensation. If the cuff is inflated above the stump of an amputated limb, the paraesthesiae are felt in the phantom limb, so it is evident that the sensations arise in the compressed segment of nerve and are not dependent on cutaneous receptors. If the experiment is carried out on a patient with loss of pain and temperature sensation due to syringomyelia or a lateral medullary syndrome, only thermal paraesthesiae are lost in the anaesthetic part. It is of interest that in patients who were studied who had a marked loss of vibration sense, pseudo-cramp was particularly impaired, although there was some loss also of tingling and pricking. The conclusion was therefore reached, that all varieties of postischaemic paraesthesiae are transmitted in that part of the spinal cord which is concerned with the transmission of touch, vibration and proprioception. The conclusion can perhaps be extended further to say that when disease of the spinal cord or brain stem gives rise to tingling or pricking paraesthesiae, the irritative lesion is likely to be along one of these pathways.

Pain Producing Substances

If a blister is made on the skin and the surface removed, the effect of chemical substances in producing pain can be studied by applying known concentrations of different agents to the exposed raw surface of the base. Substances which produce pain include acid and alkaline solutions, potassium ions, acetylcholine, histamine and 5–hydroxytryptamine. The action of histamine is of interest in that low concentrations will give rise to itch, pain resulting from higher concentrations. Of particular interest has been the study of the pain producing effects of tissue extracts. Thus, tissue extracts prepared from areas of skin where experimental burns have been produced will produce intense pain when injected intradermally. Blister fluid will also produce pain, but only if it is activated by contact with an activating substance such as glass.

The pain producing substances in blister fluid are probably polypeptides derived from plasma by the action of proteolytic enzymes. The active substances are considered to be kinins such as bradykinin and kallidin and in addition to producing pain, may give rise to contraction of smooth muscle, vasodilatation and a fall in blood pressure. The clinical importance of these substances is not known, but they may contribute to the pain of local inflammation and possibly conditions such as migraine (Keele and Armstrong, 1964).

If an area of skin is injured, the area of injury is hypersensitive to pain. This zone of *primary hyperalgesia*, where the pain threshold is low, may be conditioned by the effect of pain producing substances. After an interval, this zone may become surrounded by an area of *secondary hyperalgesia* where the pain threshold is not lowered, but where the sensation of pain is abnormally intense. This secondary hyperalgesia is probably due to central spread of excitation from the fibres innervating the primary zone (Hardy *et al.*, 1950).

Visceral Sensation and Referred Pain

Deep pain is characteristically dull in quality and poorly localized and may be associated with autonomic accompaniments such as nausea and sweating. It may be felt in the general location of the affected part or it may be referred to other parts of the body which share the same segmental innervation.

Some abdominal viscera give rise to sensory impulses in somatic nerves innervating the adjacent parts of the abdominal wall or diaphragm, but in general, their sensory innervation is through sympathetic and parasympathetic pathways. Unlike autonomic efferent fibres, the sensory nerves do not have a cell station in peripheral ganglia, but have their first sensory neurone in the dorsal root ganglia along with somatic afferent nerves. The afferent fibres carrying painful sensations, for the most part, travel along with the sympathetic nerves, whereas the afferents subserving visceral reflexes as well as organic sensations, such as hunger and thirst, are associated with parasympathetic nerves.

Faulty localization and distant reference of pain occurs from a wide variety of subcutaneous structures including not only the heart, parietal peritoneum and abdominal viscera but also skeletal muscles, ligaments and periosteum. Frequently the character of pain derived from viscus has two qualities, viz, a dull aching quality poorly localized to the site of the viscus and a relatively sharp quality localized in a corresponding cutaneous segment. There are several reasons for the faulty localization of deep pain. One is its relative infrequency, another is that it is not possible to use vision to verify the source of stimulation and a third is that visceral afferents are less numerous than those from the skin.

To explain the segmental reference of deep pain, Mackenzie (1893) suggested that impulses from the viscera set up an 'irritable focus' in the segment in which they enter the spinal cord. This lowers the threshold for impulses from the surface of the body that enter the same segment of the cord. Pain may be localized to the skin of the affected segment and at the same time, hyperalgesia may develop at the site of referral. This theory of facilitation of subliminal painful stimuli arriving at the appropriate segment of the cord has been developed by others (Hinsey and Phillips, 1940). Ruch (1965) has argued that facilitation is not necessary to account for referred pain and that it is adequate to postulate that visceral afferents converge on the same nerve cells in the cord as cutaneous pain afferents. Since afferent stimuli affecting these neurones commonly come from the skin, false localization of visceral stimuli as coming from the skin readily occurs. Melzack (1973) has developed the idea that small visceral afferents converging on T cells in the substantia gelatinosa, which are also activated by fibres from the skin, may give rise to pain in the affected segments if the input is adequate. This may also occur if the gate is opened by other mechanisms, such as a relative loss of large afferent fibres or by a central biassing mechanism. An alternative explanation put forward by Sinclair *et al.*, (1948) is that branching of pain afferents occurs so that a single axon may send fibres to the site of origin of the pain and other branches to the site of referral.

It is evident from clinical studies of pain reference that the mechanism is not always the same. Under different circumstances referred pain may be associated with either primary or secondary hyperalgesia. If saline is injected into interspinous ligaments, referred pain develops which may be associated not only with hyperalgesia, but also with muscle spasm and may be abolished by local injection with procaine (Hockaday and Whitty, 1967). On the other hand, if pain is produced by immersing one finger in ice cold water it will spread to a neighbouring finger even if this is rendered anaesthetic (Dalessio, 1972). It is possible that the first effect is due to liberation at the site of referral of a pain producing substance, but this will not explain the second effect, which must be due to some form of central spread. Although pain is referred according to a segmental pattern, it is not always confined to the segments giving rise to the pain. With muscle pain, which can be produced by local infiltration of muscles with saline, the area of reference is not always consistant with dermatomes but may conform more to the innervation of deeply situated organs. Thus, infiltration of multifidus muscle opposite first and second lumbar spines gives rise to testicular pain (Kellgren, 1938).

Central Pain

The expression central pain in the strict sense refers to pain arising from lesions in the central nervous system which give rise to spontaneous unpleasant sensations. A very important instance is provided by the thalamic syndrome (Déjerine and Roussy, 1906) in which the posterolateral ventral nucleus is damaged, usually by a vascular lesion. This gives rise to a contralateral sensory impairment which is, however, accompanied by spontaneous pains and unpleasant sensations. Although the threshold for all forms of sensation is raised, any adequate stimulus, whatever its nature, is liable to evoke unpleasant sensations which may be of agonizing intensity. This combination of sensory impairment with hyperpathia and dysesthesiae is sometimes spoken of as anaesthesia dolorosa, a condition which can arise as a rare but intractable complication after the treatment of trigeminal neuralgia by sensory root section.

Similar syndromes may arise in spinal cord disease, in particular in syringomyelia. There are also a number of peripheral causes of intractable pain, which although they are not associated with a clearly defined central pathological focus, have a number of characteristics which commonly occur in central pain. These include spontaneous pain, sensory impairment, abnormal overreaction to stimuli and failure to be relieved by operations designed to divide the sensory pathway for pain such as cordotomy. Conditions which fulfil these criteria include post herpetic neuralgia, the phantom limb syndrome and causalgia.

Causalgia (Mitchell, 1872) is of interest in a number of respects. It is a rare complication of peripheral nerve injury and in addition to giving rise to severe spontaneous pain, as well as unpleasant sensations evoked by stimuli not normally painful to the healthy subject, there is a marked associated autonomic disturbance. The limb may be cyanosed with profuse sweating and eventually the skin becomes smooth and glossy with brittle nails. A number of cases obtain conspicuous benefit from sympathectomy. Barnes (1953) has suggested that the mechanism of the disturbance is that the injury has led to a connection or artificial synapse forming between sympathetic and afferent nerve fibres, so that a discharge in the autonomic fibres activates the sensory nerves to give rise to pain. Noordenbos (1959) has argued that the mechanism is one of loss of myelinated fibres, so that pain results from an imbalance between the discharge of rapid and slowly conducting afferent fibres. He explains the autonomic disturbance by suggesting that some afferent fibres travel, for part of their course, along the sympathetic pathway in a similar manner to that of visceral afferents. The concept of lack of balance between fast and slow conducting fibres is one that can be applied also to the pain of post herpetic neuralgia and the phantom limb syndrome, and has been further developed by Melzack and Wall (1965; see above). Pain arising from damage to the thalamus and other central structures may be related to interference with corticofugal impulses which have a controlling action on the sensory input. Attempts have been made to relieve intractable central pain by destructive lesions to thalamic nuclei made stereotactically but in many instances the benefit is not permanent (Hankinson, 1969).

Headache

The sensitivity to pain of the various structures has been studied by applying painful stimuli to different tissues inside and outside the skull during neurosurgical operations. It is evident that the structures covering the skull, particularly the arteries, are generally sensitive to pain. Within the cranium, pain sensitive structures include the venous sinuses and their tributaries, the arteries at the base of the brain, the fifth, ninth and tenth cranial nerves and the dura covering the base of the skull. The brain substance, most of the dura and pia arachnoid and the ependyma lining the ventricles are insensitive to pain (Wolff and Wolf, 1948).

The site of headache may have some localizing significance in terms of the situation of the underlying pathology. With lesions above the tentorium, reference of pain is generally within the distribution of the ophthalmic division of the fifth cranial nerve. With lesions below the tentorium, pain may be referred in the distribution of the ninth and tenth cranial nerves or the upper three cervical nerves and is generally felt over the back of the head and in the neck. If headache is due to a brain tumour, the pain is produced by traction on neighbouring structures which are sensitive to pain and the headache may be of localizing value since it not infrequently overlies the tumour. If the headache is unilateral it is generally on the same side as the tumour.

If the pressure of cerebrospinal fluid is lowered by withdrawal of fluid, 20 ml is sufficient if the subject is sitting in an upright position, headache will develop which becomes more intense the more fluid is removed and may be relieved if the subject lies with head down. The cause of this headache is not so much the fall in pressure as the loss of the cushioning effect of cerebrospinal fluid, which leads to downward displacement of the brain with traction on the intracranial veins and other pain sensitive structures. This loss of cerebrospinal fluid is the reason for the headache which may follow lumbar puncture and air encephalography. Experimental headache produced in this way may be relieved by replacement of the fluid with intrathecal sterile saline. If the intracranial pressure is increased by injecting larger quantities of saline headache does not occur. It is of interest that if headache is induced by the injection of histamine, which gives rise to dilatation and overdistension of the intracranial arteries, the headache can be relieved by increasing the intracranial pressure which gives external support to the walls of the arteries (see review by Wolff and Wolf, 1948).

In clinical practice, many headaches are due to referred pain from structures innervated by the fifth, ninth and tenth cranial nerves and the upper cervical nerves. Headache can thus arise from disease affecting the teeth, paranasal sinuses, eyes, ears and cervical spine. Many headaches are accompanied by continued contraction of the muscles of the scalp and suboccipital region. In these headaches, which are often described as a diffusely experienced dull ache, it is possible that the continued muscle contraction contributes to the discomfort, but these headaches are frequently complicated by psychological factors.

Migraine headache has been shown to be related to dilatation and pulsations occurring in the branches of the external carotid artery (Graham and Wolff, 1937). In classical migraine, the headache is unilateral and is preceded by focal neurological symptoms on the other side, usually a visual disturbance such as a scotoma in the contralateral visual field. The headache may be accompanied by nausea, vomiting and photophobia. It is generally held that the prodromal phase is due to cerebral ischaemia resulting from spasm of the pial vessels, whereas the headache is due to dilatation of extracranial vessels. This view is supported by the relief which may follow vasoconstriction brought about by administration of ergotamine tartrate. However, although it is generally agreed that migraine is a condition in which vascular disturbance is a prominent and possibly the paramount feature, it is clear that other factors are also important. If pressure is applied to the scalp vessels during a headache they are not only prominent, but may also be tender. This led Chapman and his co-workers (1960) to collect samples of fluid from the subcutaneous tissues at the site of pain during a migraine headache. They found that this fluid contained a pain producing substance which had many properties in common with bradykinin and they named this 'headache stuff' neurokinin. Migraine headaches can frequently be prevented by regular medication with methysergide which is a serotonin antagonist. 5–hydroxytryptamine itself appears to have little pain producing action, but it can be shown to potentiate the action of bradykinin (Sicuteri *et al.*, 1965). Further evidence for the importance of biological amines in migraine includes the finding of an increased output of 5-hydroxyindoleacetic acid and other catechol amine breakdown products in the urine of patients during a migraine attack. If reserpine, which depletes the tissues of 5-hydroxytryptamine, is given to a person liable to have migraine attacks, it may induce an attack. Many patients subject to migraine find that their attacks are brought on by taking foods which are rich in tyramine. (See reviews by Keele, 1967; Curzon, 1967 and Dalessio, 1972).

THE THALAMUS

All forms of sensation, with the exception of the sense of smell, are relayed through the thalamus before reaching the cerebral cortex. In addition to its sensory function, the thalamus is clearly important as an integrating centre since it contains nuclei which receive no fibres from the sensory afferent pathways, but project to wide areas of the cerebral cortex. In addition, there are nuclei which have subcortical connections only, and others which relay to different parts of the cortex from hypothalamic nuclei and from the cerebellum.

In its development, the nuclei of the thalamus become differentiated from a fairly homogeneous collection of cells which surrounds the third ventricle. The important sensory relay stations are the geniculate bodies that lie on the lower surface of the pulvinar which is a prominent mass forming the dorsal portion of the thalamus. The lateral geniculate bodies are a relay station for vision and the medial geniculate bodies for hearing. The medial lemniscus, the spinothalamic tracts and the trigeminal lemniscus all project into the ventrobasal complex of the thalamus. This is one of the two major relay stations situated in the ventral portion of the thalamus. The other is the lateroventral nucleus, which receives fibres from the dentate nucleus in the cerebellum and projects to the cortex of the frontal lobe. The ventrobasal complex consists of posteromedial and postero-lateral nuclei. In these the body is represented topographically, but is inverted from side to side so that sensory impulses from the lower limb end in the lateral part, whereas impulses from the head terminate medially.

REFERENCES

ADRIAN, E. D. (1950). The electrical activity of the mammalian olfactory bulb. *Electro-enceph. clin. Neurophysiol.*, **2**, 377–388.

AMOORE, J. E. (1963). Stereochemical theory of olfaction. *Nature*, **198**, 271–272.

BARNES, R. (1953). The role of sympathectomy in the treatment of causalgia. *J. Bone Jt. Surg.*, **35-B**, 172–180.

BEIDLER, L. M. (1963). Dynamics of taste cells. In: *Proc. 1st Int. Symp. Olfaction and Taste.* Ed. Zotterman, Y. Oxford: Pergamon Press, pp. 133–144.

BISHOP, G. H. (1959). The relation between nerve fibre size and sensory modality: phylogenetic implications of the afferent innervation of cortex. *J. Nervous and Mental disease*, **128**, 89–114.

BLIX, M. (1884). Experimentelle Beitrage zur Lösung der Frage über die specifische Energie der Hautnerven. *Z. Biol.*, **20**, 141–156.

CATTELL, McK. and HOAGLAND, H. (1931). Response of tactile receptors to inter-mittent stimulation. *J. Physiol. (Lond.)*, **72**, 392–404.

CHAPMAN, L. F., RAMOS, A. O., GOODELL, H., SILVERMAN, G. and WOLFF, H. G. (1960). A humoral agent implicated in vascular headache of the migraine type. *Arch. Neurol. (Chicago)*, **3**, 223–229.

COLLINS, W. F., NULSEN, F. E. and RANDT, C. T. (1960). Relation of peripheral nerve fibre size and sensation in man. *Arch. Neurol. Psychiat. (Chicago)*, **3**, 381–385.

CURZON, G. (1967). Amine changes in migraine. In: *Background to Migraine.* Proc. First Migraine Symposium. Ed. Smith, R. London: Heinemann, pp. 134–143.

DALESSIO, D. J. (1972). *Wolff's Headache and Other Head Pain.* 3. New York: Oxford University Press.

DÉJERINE, J. and ROUSSY, G. (1906). Le syndrome thalamique. *Rev. neurol.*, **14**, 521–532.

DODT, E. and ZOTTERMAN, Y. (1952a). Mode of action of warm receptors. *Acta physiol. scand.*, **26**, 345–357.

DODT, E. and ZOTTERMAN, Y. (1952b). The discharge of specific cold fibres at high temperatures (the paradoxical cold). *Acta physiol. scand.*, **26**, 358–365.

DIAMANT, H., FUNAKOSHI, M., STROM, L. and ZOTTERMAN, Y. (1963). Electrophysiological studies on human taste nerves. In: *Proc. 1st Int. Symp. Olfaction and Taste*. Ed. Zotterman, Y. Oxford: Pergamon Press, pp. 193–203.

FREY, M. VON (1894). Beitrage zur Sinnesphysiologie des Schmerzsinns. *Ber. sachs Ges. Wiss. math. phys. Cl.*, **46**, 185–196 and 283–296.

FREY, M. VON (1906). The distribution of afferent nerves in the skin. *J. Amer. med. Ass.*, **47**, 645–648.

FUORTES, M. G. F. (1959). Initiation of impulses in visual cells of limulus. *J. Physiol. (Lond.)*, **148**, 14–28.

GESTELAND, R. C., LETTVIN, J. Y., PITTS, W. H. and ROSAS, A. (1963). Odor specificities of the frog's olfactory receptors. *Proc. 1st Int. Symp. Olfaction and Taste*. Wenner-Gren Center. Ed. Zotterman, Y. Oxford: Pergamon Press. **1**, 19–34.

GRAHAM, J. R. and WOLFF, H. G. (1937). Mechanism of Migraine Headache and Action of Ergotamine Tartrate. *Res. Publ. Ass. nerv. ment. Dis.* Baltimore: Williams & Wilkins Co., **18**, 638–669.

GRAY, J. A. B. and SATO, M. (1953). Properties of the receptor potential in Pacinian corpuscles. *J. Physiol. (Lond.)*, **122**, 610–636.

HAGEN, E., KNOCHE, H., SINCLAIR, D. C. and WEDDELL, G. (1953). The role of specialized nerve terminals in cutaneous sensibility. *Proc. roy. Soc. B.*, **141**, 279–287.

HANKINSON, J. (1969). Stereotactic surgery. In: *Recent Advance in Neurology and Neuropsychiatry*. Ed. Lord Brain and Marcia Wilkinson. London: Churchill.

HARDY, J. D., WOLFF, H. G. and GOODELL, H. (1950). Experimental evidence on the nature of cutaneous hyperalgesia. *J. clin. Invest.*, **29**, 115–140.

HARDY, J. D., WOLFF, H. G. and GOODELL, H. (1952). *Pain Sensations and Reactions*. Baltimore: Williams & Wilkins.

HEAD, H. (1905). The afferent nervous system from a new aspect. *Brain*, **28**, 99–115.

HINSEY, J. C. and PHILLIPS, R. A. (1940). Observations upon diaphragmatic sensation. *J. Neurophysiol.*, **3**, 175–181.

HOCKADAY, J. M. and WHITTY, C. W. M. (1967). Patterns of referred pain in the normal subject. *Brain*, **90**, 481–496.

KATZ, B. (1950a). Action potentials from a sensory nerve ending. *J. Physiol. (Lond.)*, **111**, 248–260.

KATZ, B. (1950b). Depolarization of sensory terminals and the initiation of impulses in the muscle spindle. *J. Physiol. (Lond.)*, **111**, 261–282.

KEELE, C. A. and ARMSTRONG, D. (1964). Substances producing pain and itch. *Physiol. Soc. Monograph No*. 12. London.

KEELE, C. A. (1967). Polypeptides and other substances which may produce vascular headache. In: *Background to Migraine*. Proc. First Migraine Symposium Ed. Smith, R. London: Heinemann, 126–133.

KELLGREN, J. H. (1938). Observations or referred pain arising from muscle. *Clin. Sci.* **3**, 175–190.

HUNT, C. C. (1961). On the nature of vibration receptors in the hind limb of the cat. *J. Physiol. (Lond.)*, **155**, 175–186.

LANDGREN, S. (1957a). Cortical reception of cold impulses from the tongue of the cat. *Acta physiol. scand.*, **40**, 202–209.

152   *Clinical Neurophysiology*

LANDGREN, S. (1957b). Convergence of tactile, thermal, and gustatory impulses on single cortical cells. *Acta physiol. scand.*, **40**, 210–221.

LELE, P. P., WEDDELL, G. and WILLIAMS, C. M. (1954). The relationship between heat transfer, skin temperature and cutaneous sensibility. *J. Physiol.* (*Lond.*), **126**, 206–234.

KONISHI, J. and ZOTTERMAN, Y. (1963). Taste functions in fish. In: *Proc. 1st Int. Symp. Olfaction and Taste.* Ed. Zotterman, Y. Oxford: Pergamon Press. 215–233.

LEWIS, T., PICKERING, G. W. and ROTHSCHILD, P. (1931). Centripetal paralysis arising out of arrested blood flow to the limb. *Heart*, **16**, 1–32.

LEWIS, T. and POCHIN, E. E. (1937). The double pain response of the human skin to a single stimulus. *Clin. Sci.*, **3**, 67–76.

LOEWENSTEIN, W. R. and MENDELSON, M. (1965). Components of receptor adaptation in a Pacinian corpuscle. *J. Physiol.* (*Lond.*), **177**, 377–397.

MACKENZIE, J. (1893). Some points bearing on the association of sensory disorders and visceral disease. *Brain*, **16**, 321–354.

MAGEE, K. R. (1963). Congenital indifference to pain. *Arch. Neurol. Psychiat.* (*Chicago*). **9**, 635–640.

MELZACK, R. (1973). *The Puzzle of Pain.* Harmondsworth: Penguin.

MELZACK, R. and WALL, P. D. (1962). On the nature of cutaneous sensory mechanisms. *Brain*, **85**, 331–356.

MELZACK, R. and WALL, P. D. (1965). Pain mechanisms: a new theory. *Science*, **150**. 971–979.

MENDELL, L. M. and WALL, P. (1965). Responses of single dorsal cord cells to peripheral cutaneous unmyelinated fibres. *Nature*, **206**, 97–99.

MERRINGTON, W. R. and NATHAN, P. W. (1949). A study of post-ischaemic paraesthesia *J. Neurol. Neurosurg. Psychiat.*, **12**, 1–18.

MITCHELL, S. W. (1872). *Injuries of Nerves and their Consequences.* Philadelphia: Lippincott.

NAPIER, J. R. (1952). The return of sensibility in full thickness skin grafts. *Brain*, **75**, 147–166.

NEWMAN, H. W., DOUPE, J. and WILKINS, R. W. (1939). Some observations on the the nature of vibratory sensibility. *Brain*, **62**, 31–40.

NOORDENBOS, W. (1959). *Pain.* Amsterdam: Elsevier.

OGDEN, T. E., ROBERT, F. and CARMICHAEL, E. A. (1959). Some sensory syndromes in children: indifference to pain and sensory neuropathy. *J. Neurol. Neurosurg. Psychiat.*, **22**, 267–276.

OLDS, J. (1958). Selective effects of drives and drugs in 'reward' systems of the brain. *Ciba Foundation Symposium on Neurological Basis of Behaviour.* Ed. Wolstenholme G. E. W. and O'Connor, C. M. London: Churchill, 124–141.

OTTOSON, D. (1963). Generation and transmission of signals in the olfactory system. *Proc. 1st Int. Symp. Olfaction and Taste.* Wenner-Gren Centre. Ed. Zotterman, Y. Oxford: Pergamon Press. **1**, 35–44.

OTTOSON, D. and SHEPHARD, D. M. (1967). Experiments and concepts in olfactory physiology. *Progress in Brain Research. Vol. 23. Sensory Mechanisms.* Ed. Zotterman, Y. Amsterdam: Elsevier. 83–138.

PAINTAL, A. S. (1960). Functional analysis of group III afferent fibres of mammalian muscles. *J. Physiol.* (*Lond.*), **152**, 250–270.

PEIRIS, O. A. and MILES, D. W. (1965). Galvanic stimulation of the tongue as a prognostic index in Bell's palsy. *Brit. med. J.*, **ii**, 1162–1163.

POCHIN, E. E. (1938). Delay of pain perception in tabes dorsalis. *Clin. Sci.*, **3**, 191–196.

ROBERTSON, M. A. H. (1970). Simple instrument for measuring the sense of taste. *Brit. med. J.*, **2**, 109.

RUCH, T. C. (1965). Pathophysiology of pain. In: *Physiology and Biophysics*. Ed. Ruch, T. C. and Patton H. D., 19th Edn. Philadelphia: Saunders.

SHERRINGTON, C. S. (1906). *The Integrative Action of the Nervous System*. Cambridge: University Press. Reprinted 1947, New York: Charles Scribner's Sons.

SICITURI, F., FRANCHI, G., FANCIULLACCI, M. and DEL BIANCO, P. L. (1965). Serotonin-bradykinin potentiation on the pain receptors in man. *Life Sciences*, **4**, 309–316.

SINCLAIR, D. (1967). *Cutaneous Sensation*. London: Oxford University Press.

SINCLAIR, D. C. and HINSHAW, J. R. (1950). A comparison of the sensory dissociation produced by procaine and by limb compression. *Brain*, **73**, 480–498.

SINCLAIR, D. C., WEDDELL, G. and FEINDEL, W. H. (1948). Referred pain and associated phenomena. *Brain*, **71**, 184–211.

WALL, P. D. (1960). Cord cells responding to touch, damage and temperature of skin. *J. Neurophysiol.*, **23**, 197–210.

WALSHE, F. M. R. (1942). The anatomy and physiology of cutaneous sensibility: a critical review. *Brain*, **65**, 48–112.

WEBER, E. H. (1846). Temperatursinn. In: *Handwörterbuch der Physiologie*. Vol. 3. Ed. Wagner, R. pp. 100–110. Braunschweig.

WERNER, G. and MOUNTCASTLE, V. B. (1965). Neural activity in mechanoreceptive cutaneous afferents: stimulus-response relations, Weber functions, and information transmission. *J. Neurophysiol.* **28**, 359–397.

WOLFF, H. G. (1963). *Headache and Other Head Pain*. 2nd Edn. London: Oxford University Press.

WOLFF, H. G. (1972). *Headache and Other Head Pain*. 3rd Edn., revised by Donald J. Dalessio. New York: Oxford University Press.

WOLFF, H. G. and WOLF, S. (1948). *Pain*. Illinois: Charles C. Thomas.

ZOTTERMAN, Y. (1953). Special senses: thermal receptors. *Ann. Rev. Physiol.*, **15**, 357–372.

ZOTTERMAN, Y. (1939). Touch, pain and tickling: an electrophysiological investigation on cutaneous sensory nerves. *J. Physiol. (Lond.)*, **95**, 1–28.

ZOTTERMAN, Y. (1967). The neural mechanism of taste. *Progress in Brain Research*. Vol. 23. Sensory Mechanisms. Amsterdam: Elsevier, 139–154.

CHAPTER 8

Vision

THE STRUCTURE OF THE EYE

The human eye is a specialized sensory organ that is sensitive to electromagnetic radiation within a limited bandwidth that extends from approximately 400–700 nm. Its structure follows the same general plan as that of other vertebrate eyes (Fig. 8.1).

The eyeball, or globe of the eye, is a hollow structure with an anterior opening through which light passes. The light is focused by a lens to form an inverted image on the light sensitive retina that forms the inner surface of the globe. The two outer layers of the eyeball are the choroid, which forms the highly vascular middle coat and is continuous with the ciliary body and the iris, and the outer protective coating which is made up of the sclera and cornea. The cornea is transparent to allow entry of light into the eye. The interior of the eye is filled with a transparent fluid, the aqueous humour, and a transparent jelly, the vitreous humour. The aqueous humour lies in the anterior chamber of the eye, which is situated between the cornea and the iris, and in the posterior chamber of the eye that lies between the iris and the anterior surface of the lens. The vitreous humour lies behind the lens and occupies the greater part of the cavity of the eyeball.

The iris is a circular structure surrounding a central aperture which is known as the pupil. Contractile elements within the iris enable the size of the pupil to be altered so that the amount of light entering the eye can be varied. The lens is a transparent, crystalline biconvex structure that lies behind the iris and is supported by a suspensory ligament. The ciliary body incorporates a smooth muscle, the ciliary muscle, which is able, by contracting, to alter the shape of the lens so that light can be focused on the retina. The ciliary body is also the source of the aqueous humour which is secreted into the posterior chamber and passes through the pupil into the anterior chamber. From there, it passes out through the canal of Schlemm that lies in the angle between the cornea and the anterior surface of the iris. In the canal of Schlemm, the aqueous humour is absorbed into the venous system. The composition of aqueous humour is similar to that of plasma, with the exception of the protein content, which is about 15 mg per cent compared with approximately 7.0 gm per cent in plasma. Like CSF, it differs in composition in a number of respects from a protein free filtrate of plasma and is formed by a process of active secretion. As a circulating fluid, it carries nutrient materials to the avascular lens and cornea and it maintains the intraocular pressure at a level of between 10 and 20 mm Hg.

The retina consists of four layers of cells of which the outermost, that is the layer in contact with the choroid, is a layer of pigment epithelium. The next layer is the layer of receptor cells, which are of two types, namely rods and cones.

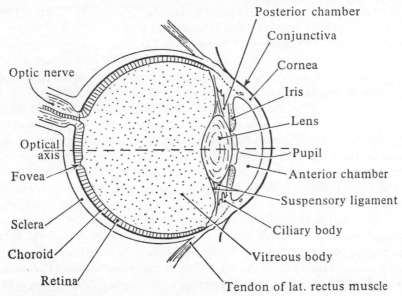

FIG. 8.1. The structure of the human eye.

These connect with the bipolar cells which are the first sensory neurone of the visual system. The layer nearest the inner surface of the retina is the ganglion cell layer, which contains the cell bodies of the second sensory neurone, the nerve fibres of which give rise to the optic nerve. Since the receptor cells lie closest to the choroid, light has to pass through all the other cell layers in order to activate the receptors.

The optic nerve leaves the eye at the optic disc, or nerve head, passing through the sclera to travel back through the orbit to enter the skull. After leaving the orbits, the two optic nerves cross at the chiasma and pass back as the optic tracts to the lateral geniculate bodies, or the superior colliculi. The third sensory neurone arises in the geniculate bodies to give rise to the optic radiations that pass back to the visual cortex. The optic nerve enters the eyeball through a lattice of scleral tissue which is known as the lamina cribrosa.

The vitreous body makes up the bulk of the content of the eyeball and consists of a network of fine collagen fibres in which is held fluid that is similar in composition to aqueous humour, but more viscous due to the presence in it of a mucopolysaccharide, hyaluronic acid.

The anterior surface of the cornea is protected by the eyelids which, when they are closed, shut off the entry of light into the eye. An additional protective function is served by the presence of tears, which are secreted by the lacrimal glands and irrigate the surface of the cornea.

The eyeball is moved within the orbit by the contraction of the extraocular muscles. These are the superior and inferior recti, the lateral and medial recti and the superior and inferior oblique muscles. They serve to turn the eye upwards, downwards, medially and laterally and also to rotate it clockwise and counterclockwise. The actions of the extraocular muscles are complex. Their coordinated action during conjugate gaze is an example of a highly organized arrangement of reciprocal innervation. Thus, in lateral gaze to the right, there is contraction of the right lateral rectus with relaxation of the right medial rectus and opposite changes in the corresponding muscles of the left eye. Weakness or paralysis of one or more of the external ocular muscles results in the two eyes no longer being correctly aligned on the same object, so that the images are no longer situated on the same point on the retina of each eye and double vision results.

The arrangement which has been described of a single eyeball with an aperture and a lens through which the image is focused on to the retina is one that is largely confined to vertebrates. Insects and crustaceans have what is known as a compound eye. The compound eye consists of many individual units known as ommatidia, each of which has a lens that focuses the light on to light sensitive retinula cells. Activation of the retinula cells leads to excitation of a centrally placed eccentric cell, which is the nerve fibre of the ommatidium. Microelectrode recording from the eccentric cell of Limulus or the horseshoe crab, has provided useful information regarding the genesis of the generator potential in sensory end organs (see also chapter 7).

THE RETINA

The retina contains not only the receptor cells, viz, the rods and cones, but also the nerve cells of the first and second sensory neurones of the visual pathway which are arranged vertically in the layers of the retina (Fig. 8.2). In the human eye, the rods are between 10 and 20 times as numerous as the cones, but there is much variation in the proportions of rods to cones in different forms of vertebrate life. In general, cones are associated with diurnal vision and are necessary for the appreciation of shape and colour. Rods are organized to be sensitive to small intensities of illumination and so are adapted to nocturnal vision. The cones tend to prevail in the retinae of vertebrates of predominantly diurnal habit, whereas rods are prevalent in the eyes of nocturnal animals. In the human eye the cones are concentrated in the central part of the retina, the fovea centralis, whereas the rods predominate in the periphery of the retina.

The central part of the retina is essential for the perception of colour and form, but it cannot perceive in poor lighting. The peripheral part of the retina

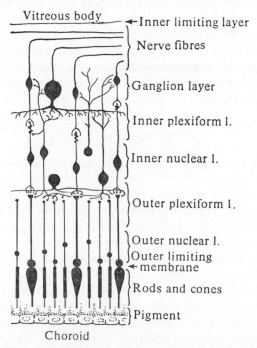

Fig. 8.2. The arrangement of cells in the human retina. After Walls, G. L. (1963). *The Vertebrate Eye and its Adaptive Radiation*. New York: Hafner. (Courtesy of Cranbrook Institute of Science, Michigan.)

where the rods are concentrated is essential for night vision. The rods are more slender than the cones, but each have a similar structure consisting of an outer segment that contains the light sensitive pigment and an inner synaptic body which connects with the bipolar cells. The bacillary layer of the retina, in which the rods and cones lie, consists of an outer nuclear layer that contains the cell bodies and an outer plexiform layer in which they form synaptic connection with the dendrites of the bipolar cells. The bipolar cells connect with the ganglion cells in the inner plexiform layer. Horizontal connection between the cells of the retina are provided by the horizontal and amacrine cells, which have their bodies in the inner nuclear layer.

The bipolar cells consist of three types (Boycott and Dowling, 1969), viz, midget bipolars which each connect with a single cone, flat bipolars that connect with small groups of the order of seven cones and diffuse bipolars which may connect with as many as 50 rods. In this way, many cones have a one to one relationship with bipolar and ganglion cells, whereas large numbers of rods may converge on a single bipolar cell. Although there are many horizontal connections between cones, and between cones and rods, the one to one relationship which provides a direct pathway between each cone and the intermediate cells, and hence to the individual optic nerve fibres, is important in terms of the resolving power of the eye, which is necessary to secure good visual acuity. The arrangement of the rods, by which perhaps hundreds of rods are connected to a single optic nerve fibre so that weak activation of single rods is magnified many times, has the effect that the part of the retina where rods predominate is highly sensitive to low intensities of illumination.

The Visual Pigments

In the vertebrate eye, the light sensitive mechanism involves the absorption of light energy on the photosensitive pigments that are situated in the outer segments of the visual receptor cells. Müller, in 1851, was the first to recognize that the rods contain a reddish pigment, which was later given the name of visual purple or rhodopsin. This is present in the outer segments of the rods and is bleached white when the retina is exposed to light.

Rhodopsin is a protein to each molecule of which is attached a chromophore group that has the property of absorbing light and it is responsible for the colour of the substance. When rhodopsin is exposed to light it undergoes a number of changes, the end result of which is that the chromophore group becomes separated from the protein or opsin. The chromophore group has been termed retinal and is in fact vitamin A aldehyde. Further exposure to light results in the alteration of this into vitamin A. If the eye is left in the dark, the changes are reversed and rhodopsin is reconstituted.

The pigment rhodopsin can be isolated from the eye by centrifugation in a detergent solution containing digitonin. If visual pigment is obtained in solution in this manner, it is possible to determine the proportion in which different wavelengths of visible light are absorbed by the solution by passing beams of light, of known wavelength and intensity, through the solution and recording the amount transmitted by means of a photocell. In the human eye, it is possible to measure the threshold sensitivity to light of different wavelengths. If this is done with the dark adapted eye, it is found that the curve representing spectral sensitivity of the eye matches very closely the absorption spectrum for rhodopsin.

Relatively little is known about the visual pigments that are present in the cones. One pigment that has been studied is a substance known as iodopsin, which has been extracted from the eye of chickens. This is of interest because the light sensitive cells in the eyes of the domestic fowls are predominantly cones (Wald, 1937). Cone pigments have not been extracted from the retinae of mammalian eyes (Brindley, 1970) but their presence has been demonstrated in the foveal region of the human retina by a process known as reflexion–densitometry (Rushton, 1959). In this method, if a light is shone into the eye the amount absorbed by the visual receptor cells can be determined from the intensity of energy at different wavelengths in the light reflected from the retina. By this means, two other pigments have been shown to exist in the foveal region of the eye and therefore, in the cones. One is a pigment which absorbs light in the red part of the spectrum and which has been called erythrolabe. The other is a pigment known as chlorolabe, which absorbs light in the green part of the spectrum.

Dark Adaptation

The sensitivity to light of the human eye is approximately 10,000 times greater after a period of $\frac{1}{2}$ hour in total darkness than it is when it has been exposed to

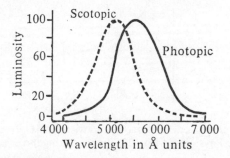

FIG. 8.3. Luminosity curves for scotopic and photopic vision. After Hecht, S. (1937), *Physiol. Rev.*, **17**, 239–290.

bright light. This process whereby the eye becomes more sensitive to light after a period in darkness is spoken of as dark adaptation. The visual process by which the dark adapted eye sees in conditions of poor illumination is spoken of as scotopic vision, as compared with vision in daylight, which is known as photopic vision. The dark adapted eye is not able to appreciate colour, but it does not respond equally to light of different wavelengths. Its maximum sensitivity is to a blue–green light having a wavelength of 500 nm. The curve for the spectral sensitivity of the dark adapted eye has the same shape as a curve which is plotted after exposure to daylight. However, the curve for daylight or photopic vision, shows a shift towards the higher frequency end of the spectrum with a maximum sensitivity at a wavelength of 560 nm (Fig. 8.3). This change in sensitivity was described originally by Purkinje in 1825 and has been called the Purkinje shift. These changes can be explained on the basis that scotopic and photopic vision depend on separate receptors, which is the principle of the duplicity theory of vision in which the rods are considered to form the receptors for scotopic vision in poor illumination and the cones the receptors for daylight vision and colour perception.

Since in the human eye the cones are concentrated in the fovea and the rods in the peripheral part of the retina, only the periphery of the retina is sensitive to light in the dark adapted eye. Dark adaptation, however, is not exclusively confined to the rods, although their change in sensitivity in darkness is very much greater than that of the cones. In animals with pure cone retinae, such as the grey squirrel, dark adaptation takes a relatively short time to develop, but the increase in sensitivity is not pronounced (Tansley, 1965). In the mixed retina

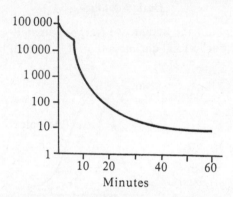

FIG. 8.4. Dark adaptation curve. After Kohlrausch, (1931), *Handbuch der normalen und pathologischen*. Physiologie Bd 122, Berlin: Springer-Verlag.

of the human eye, dark adaptation takes place in two stages. Initially there is a small increase in sensitivity that is complete in about seven minutes. This is followed by a much more marked increase in sensitivity which is complete after about an hour. This gives rise to a broken curve, the first part of which is probably due to the cones, and the second part to the rods (Fig. 8.4). Individuals with defective cone vision are known as rod monochromats and do not show a two stage dark adaptation curve.

The principal factor in dark adaptation is the regeneration of visual purple or rhodopsin which takes place in the dark. Dietary deficiency of vitamin A, an important constituent of rhodopsin, is one cause of night blindness. The maximum absorption of light by rhodopsin is in the blue–green part of the spectrum, and with wavelengths of greater than 640 nm very little bleaching will occur. For this reason, the wearing of red goggles enables people who have to work in dark surroundings to maintain dark adaptation if they are temporarily exposed to light. Regeneration of rhodopsin is not in itself sufficient to explain the marked increase in sensitivity of the retina which takes place during dark adaptation. There is evidence that changes in the neural organization of the retina are also important (Arden and Weale, 1954). Thus in the cat, the central portions of the receptive fields of the retina are surrounded by an inhibitory zone, which in the light adapted eye gives an off-response when the central zone is activated. In the dark adapted eye, this inhibitory effect of the peripheral portions of the receptive fields is lost (Barlow *et al.*, 1957). Dilatation of the pupil, which takes place in the dark, allows more light to fall on the retina, but this is a much less important factor in dark adaptation than the changes which take place in the retina.

Electrical Changes in the Retina

In an earlier section (see chapter 7) it was explained how the compound eye of the horse shoe crab Limulus had been used to study the development of the generator potential. This eye is composed of many separate units or ommatidia, each of which consists of light sensitive retinula cells that surround what appears to be the dendrite of a neurone known as an eccentric cell. Depolarization of the eccentric cell gives rise to a repetitive spike discharge in the nerve fibre at a frequency which increases with the intensity of illumination. The eye of Limulus is capable of dark adaptation, and in the dark adapted eye the frequency of discharge is greater for a given level of illumination. An interesting feature of the Limulus eye, which is paralleled in the vertebrate eye, is that the ommatidia are joined by a plexus of nerve fibres so that when one ommatidium is excited it gives rise to inhibition of its neighbours (Hartline, Wagner and Ratliff, 1956).

In the more complex retinae of vertebrates, it is possible to study the discharge either of individual optic nerve fibres or of individual retinal ganglion cells. This can either be done by recording from the optic nerve or by exposing the retina and recording from ganglion cells with a microelectrode. If the optic nerve fibres of the frog's retina are studied, three types of response can be recorded. One kind of fibre discharges when light falls on the retina and is known as an on-fibre. Another kind discharges only when the light goes off and is known as an off-fibre and the third and commonest variety, responds both when light reaches the retina and when it ceases, and is known as an on-off-fibre. Since the number of receptors in the retina is of the order of 150 times greater than the number of fibres of each optic nerve, many receptors must converge on each ganglion cell and therefore, a single optic nerve fibre connects with a wide receptive field, which may include many rods and cones. This convergence is more marked with rods than with cones, which in the human eye may have a one to one relationship with ganglion cells. If the receptive field is plotted by stimulating the retina with point sources of light and recording from a single nerve fibre it is found that the receptive field is circular in shape. In the frog it is about 1 mm in diameter. The convergence of fibres on the ganglion cell allows summation to take place, so that two spots of light falling on different parts of the field may together cause excitation, although either alone may be too weak to excite. In the frog's retina, the centre of the receptive field is many times more sensitive to light than the periphery. With some on-off ganglion cells, the threshold to off stimuli is lower at the periphery than the centre, so that a stimulus which produces an on response at the centre of the field will produce an off response at the periphery (Hartline, 1940; Barlow, 1953).

In the mammalian retina, it is also possible to distinguish between on and off elements, but the organization is more complex. The mammalian eye also shows a continuous background of discharge in the absence of light, so that the effects of stimulating on and off elements is to alter the rate of this background discharge. The receptive fields in the mammalian retina also show contrary types of response in the centre and periphery. Reference has already been made to the disappearance of the contrast between the effects of central and peripheral stimulation on the receptive field, which occurs during dark adaptation when the whole field becomes smaller in extent, but responds only to one type of stimulus (Barlow *et al.*, 1957; see also Brindley, 1970 and Davson, 1972).

The Electroretinogram

If an electrode is placed on the cornea and another on the head, a potential difference can be recorded between the two electrodes, the electrode on the cornea being positive. This potential difference is derived from the resting potential that exists between the cornea and the back of the eye, and was discovered by DuBois Reymond in 1849. The eye thus acts as a dipole orientated along its longitudinal axis. If electrodes are placed in the outer and inner canthi at right angles to this axis, they will record potential changes whenever the eye moves. This is the principle underlying electro-oculography, which is a procedure by which movements of the eyes can be recorded electrically. In 1865, Holmgren found that the standing potential alters if light is shone on the eye. The same observation was made soon afterwards and independently in Edinburgh by Dewar and McKendrick (1873).

The electrical changes which occur on exposure to light are known as the electroretinogram. They arise in the cells of the retina, and can be clearly demonstrated in an experimental preparation in which recordings are made between one electrode placed on the outer and another on the inner surface of the retina. The electroretinogram can be readily recorded in the human subject, and has been widely applied as a diagnostic technique in the clinical study of retinal disorders. In practice, it is usual to record from one electrode placed over the cornea and a second electrode on the forehead near the eye. When this is done, the changes are usually described in terms of the corneal potential change.

The first change which follows the application of a light stimulus is a brief negative potential known as the *a* wave. The *b* wave which follows it is a positive potential, and there is then a slow positive change, which is known as the *c* wave. The final effect occurs when the light is switched off when there is an abrupt positive change, which is the *d* wave or off effect. Much has been learned regarding the characteristics of these potential changes by studying the electro-retinogram in eyes in which the sensitive cells are predominantly cones or pre-dominantly rods. Thus, the course of the retinogram is different in the cat and the guinea pig where the retinae are dominated by rods, from the pigeon or the squirrel where the retinal cells are largely composed of cones. In predominantly cone retinae, the *a* wave and the off effect are most prominent, whereas the *b* wave tends to be prominent where rods are the principal receptors and the *b* wave is particularly large in the dark adapted eye. The *b* wave is of particular interest because within certain limits, its amplitude is proportional to the log of the intensity of the stimulating light and, therefore, the amplitude of the *b* wave is a measure of the sensitivity of the retina. This is useful in measuring sensitivity in conditions of good illumination and after dark adaptation, and it provides a method by which the sensitivity of the retina to light of different wavelengths can be measured.

Granit (1947) has considered that the electroretinogram represents the alge-braic sum of several different electrical events taking place nearly simultaneously. This can be demonstrated by studying the eye of a cat exposed to anaesthesia or asphyxia, so that different components of the retinogram are lost successively. In this way, Granit has derived three components. The first, or PI component, is a slowly developing positive deflection which disappears in light adaptation and accounts for the *c* wave. PII is also positive, but develops more rapidly and is associated with the *b* wave. The PIII component is a negative deflection which is particularly prominent in the light adapted eye and accounts for the *a* wave (Fig. 8.5). Subsequent studies, in which electrical changes haves been recorded directly from the retina with microelectrodes, suggest that the *a* wave is due to activity in the rod and cone receptors and that the *b* wave is derived from the bipolar cells. The *c* wave apparently is the result of changes taking place in the pigment epithelium. The capacity of the retinal cells to give rise to electrical changes, which can be recorded across the retina as a whole, is related to their orderly arrangement in layers of perpendicularly aligned cells.

In cone retinae the speed of reaction is faster than in rod retinae, so that the *b* wave runs a shorter course in cone than in rod retinae. One effect of this is that if the eye is exposed to flickering light the potentials fuse at a lower frequency in rod than in cone retinae. In the human eye, if the subject looks at a flickering light the light can be perceived as separate flashes up to a frequency of approxi-mately 70 Hz. Fusion of potentials with the electroretinogram, however, occurs at frequencies of about 25 Hz unless very strong intensities of light are used. This is related to the fact that in the human eye the rods are very much more numer-ous than cones.

The potentials recorded in electroretinography range in amplitude from about

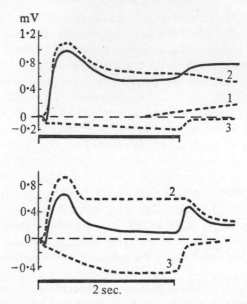

FIG. 8.5. The components of the electroretinogram in the dark adapted eye of the frog. Granit, R. and Liddell, L. A. (1934). *J. Physiol.* (*London*). **81,** 1–28.

0.10 to 1.0 mV. The latency of the *b* wave is shorter with strong stimuli than with weak, and with flashes used in clinical practice may be about 0.05 sec, the whole complex having a duration of the order of 1 sec. In clinical practice, a contact lens over the cornea may serve as the active electrode and the potential can be readily recorded after amplification on a direct writing pen recorder. Unless strong stimuli are used, the *a* wave is not conspicuous and the principle change observed is that due to the *b* wave. The electroretinogram ordinarily obtained in the human subject is the scotopic electroretinogram and is most satisfactorily recorded in the partially dark adapted eye. It is particularly valuable in the study of retinal disorders in children. Thus, in primary pigmentary degenerations of the retina, the retinal response may be markedly diminished, or even absent, and these changes may be present even when vision is apparently unaffected and the appearances of the fundus are normal. In detachment of the retina and arterial occulusion, the *b* wave may likewise be reduced, but in partial vascular lesions there may be an exaggerated *b* wave response.

The photopic electroretinogram is less easily studied, but may be obtained using high intensities of light. One method is to study the fusion frequency with high stimulus intensities when a diminished flicker fusion frequency may indicate defective function of the cones. A method of recording the retinogram, which avoids the use of a corneal electrode and is therefore less disturbing for children, makes use of an electrode on the bridge of the nose between the eyes and a vertex electrode as the reference point (Fig. 8.6). With this method, the signals are smaller and an averaging technique is necessary, but the procedure can be combined with the recording of cortical visual evoked responses (Tepas and Armington, 1962; Harden and Pampiglione, 1970).

Electro–oculography

Variations in the standing potential of the eyeball occur when the eye moves. The recording of these variations in potential with the electrodes on the canthal skin is the principle underlying electro–oculography. The technique is widely used for the recording of eye movements and forms the basis of electronystagmography. The relationship between the potential changes which take place in

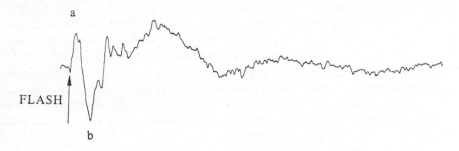

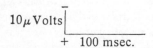

FIG. 8.6. Average of 128 responses to light flash recorded between electrode at nasion and at vertex. First large positive deflection is considered to represent the *b* wave of the electroretinogram.

the light adapted and the dark adapted eye depends on the condition of the pigmentary epithelium of the retina, and may provide useful information in the study of disorders of the retina.

The patient sits in front of a screen of diffuse lighting and directs his gaze alternately at two fixation lights 40° apart. After the subject has become accustomed to the procedure, it is carried out during a 12 min cycle of dark adaptation and then repeated during exposure to light. The sawtooth changes in potential produced by the eye movements are of higher amplitude during light adaptation than during dark adaptation, and the light peak/dark trough ratio is usually greater than 2.50. Low ratios occur particularly in primary pigmentary degenerations, but have also been recorded in a variety of retinal disorders. An abnormal electro–oculogram is not necessarily associated with an abnormal retinogram and the two techniques used together may be clinically useful.

Colour Vision

The human eye has the capacity to distinguish different wavelengths of the visible spectrum as separate hues. In the middle range of the spectrum it is possible to distinguish differences in hue of as little as 1 nm. Many more variations in colour arise from mixtures of hues. If a colour, or mixture of colours, includes white light it is known as a tint. Probably, there are more than 1500 different hues which can be distinguished in the visible spectrum. If the number of possible colour mixtures and tints is also considered, the enormous range of possibilities of colour perception can be considered.

The dark adapted eye which depends on rods for perception of light does not perceive colours in states of poor illumination, since colour vision is dependent on the spectral sensitivity of the cones, which are relatively insensitive to low levels of illumination. Colour vision in man is therefore best developed in the region of the fovea where the cones are concentrated. In animals, where only rods are present in the retina, colour vision is not possible. The converse is not necessarily true, since behavioural experiments have shown that many animals in which cones are present are devoid of colour vision, possibly because the central mechanisms for colour perception are absent. In general, colour vision is well developed in insects, birds and fish, but in mammals is only present to a marked extent in primates and man.

If different colours are mixed in different proportions, it is found that the three colours of red, green and blue, if mixed in appropriate proportions, can give rise to the sensation of white, or of any of the colours which occur in the spectrum. These three colours are therefore known as primary colours. For any colour there is another colour which, if mixed with it, will give rise to the sensation of white, and is known as its complementary colour. If one looks at a colour for a period of time and then stops looking at it, one may perceive for a short period of time an image of its complementary colour. In the trichromatic theory of colour vision, which was put forward originally by Thomas Young and developed by Helmholtz, it is argued that there are three varieties of cone, each of which is sensitive to one of the three primary colours. This view would seem to imply that there are three separate pigments, each corresponding to the spectral sensitivity of one of the three varieties of cone. Although less is known about cone pigments than is known about visual purple, which is found in the rods, more than one cone pigment has been shown to exist (see above). Spectral analyses of the cones have shown that different cones can be identified which have different spectral sensitivities.

If recordings are made from ganglion cells in the dark adapted eye, it is found that the discharge brought about by excitation of the retina with different wavelengths corresponds exactly to the absorption spectrum for rhodopsin. In the light adapted eye, however, different nerve fibres respond differently, according to the wavelength which is exciting the retina. Granit (1947) has found that optic nerve fibres can be divided into two varieties. One variety responds to a wide frequency band and these fibres he termed dominators. The other variety responds to a relatively narrow band of frequencies and these have been termed modulators. On this basis, the dominator response can be considered as the one which indicates the brightness of light applied to the light adapted eye. The cells that give rise to a dominator response may be connected with the three varieties of colour sensitive cone. The modulator response may arise, on the other hand, in cells which connect with one type of cone only. Further work on the retinae of many different species has shown that the same ganglion cell may give opposite responses to different modes of retinal stimulation. Thus, certain elements have been found to give an on response when the retina is activated by red and an off response when a green light is applied. Moreover, stimulation of the periphery and centre of a receptive field by different colours may give rise to opposite types of response (Daw, 1968).

The demonstration of different modulators for different wavelength bands is further evidence for specific receptors responsive to the primary colours. There are, however, features of colour vision which are not wholly explained by the trichromatic theory. One is the contrast between black and white. Although black is a sensation that occurs when light is withdrawn, it is different from the sensation experienced following stimulation in the region of the blind spot where nothing is perceived. One alternative to the trichromatic theory is the opponent colour theory originally put forward in 1875 by Hering. In this theory, six visual sensations are postulated, viz, black, white, blue, green, yellow and red, which can be divided into three opponent pairs white-black, yellow-blue and red-green. Hering postulated that there were three retinal substances, the synthesis of each of which produced the opposite effect to its breakdown. There are many difficulties in accepting this explanation, but the concept of opponent mechanisms does assist in explaining some of the phenomena of colour vision. Although there is no evidence for different effects resulting from synthesis and breakdown of retinal pigment, considerable evidence has accumulated that opposing effects may result from the opposite effects brought about by different modes of stimulation. Thus, it has been seen how microelectrode studies have identified neurones in the retina which give an on response with one wavelength of light and an off effect with the complementary colour.

Colour Blindness

Colour blindness is a relatively common disturbance of vision. It can occur as a hereditary disorder and the commonest variety is an inability to distinguish red from green which occurs in about 8 per cent of men and 0.45 per cent of women, being inherited as a sex linked recessive. It may also exist in an acquired form as a result of disease of the retina.

Colour blindness can be classified according to the trichromatic theory. The simplest and most complete form is known as monochromatism, in which colour is not appreciated at all and all colours appear as shades of grey. In the commonest form, it is the cones which are defective and the subject is known as a rod monochromat with poor central vision and low visual acuity. A much rarer form is known as cone monochromatism, in which visual acuity is unaffected so that the cones are presumably intact. It is not clear whether this disorder is due to defective colour appreciation by the cones or to some failure of the central mechanism. In dichromatism, all the colours that the subject is able to perceive can be matched with a mixture of two primary colours, so that it would appear that one of the three colour mechanisms is missing. In the protanope, the red mechanism is missing so that the subject is red blind. In the deuteranope, the subject cannot perceive green and in the much rarer variety, known as tritanopia, the mechanism for the perception of blue is not present. Protanopia and deuteranopia both give rise to inability to distinguish red from green. Defective colour vision can still occur even if all three mechanisms are present. In this situation, all three primary colours are necessary to match the colours of the spectrum, but not in the same proportions as in subjects with normal colour vision. This condition, which is relatively common, is known as anomalous trichromatism, and depending on which colour mechanism is weak may be termed protanomaly or deuteranomaly.

VISUAL ACUITY

Visual acuity, or the resolving power of the eye so that it is able to perceive fine detail, depends fundamentally on the fineness of grain of the retina. This depends on a number of different factors, including the size of the receptor cells and how densely they are packed, but particularly important is the number of cells which converge on a single optic nerve fibre. Since many rods may converge on a single neurone, whereas cones may have a one to one relationship with nerve cells, the ability to perceive fine detail depends very largely on the cones. In the human eye, visual acuity is very much greater in the macular region of the retina than in the peripheral parts and when viewing objects in bright illumination, rather than when the eye is dark adapted and rod vision predominates.

Accommodation

Good visual acuity depends not only on a properly functioning macula, but also on the ability of the lens of the eye to focus the image sharply on the retina. In the healthy eye, parallel rays of light from distant objects are focused on the retina. When a distant object is brought closer to the eye, its image is held in focus by the action of the ciliary muscle, which surrounds the lens and which by its contraction is able to increase the curvature of the lens. Eventually, a point is reached where the lens can alter its shape no further. This point that is at the shortest distance from the eye at which the object can be clearly seen is known as the near point. The process by which the lens alters its shape so that near objects can be held in focus is known as accommodation. When accommodation takes place, it is accompanied by convergence of the two eyes and constriction of the pupils. The constriction of the pupil which takes place in near vision increases the depth of focus and also enables the image to be seen with greater clarity by occluding the periphery of the lens where chromatic and spherical aberration may be particularly pronounced. The three effects of accommodation, vergance and pupillary constriction are mediated by the third cranial nerve through parasympathetic fibres, which originate in the Edinger–Westphal nucleus in the midbrain and relay through the ciliary ganglion. The excitatory stimulus for the near response is the perception that an image is out of focus. There is evidence that the reflexes concerned in the reaction are integrated in the temporo-occipital cortex (Jampel, 1959). In the Holmes–Adie, or myotonic, pupil, the reactions of the pupil both to light and accommodation may be abnormally slow, but on sustained convergence, a prolonged constriction may occur. A weak 2.5 per cent solution of mecholyl will have no effect on the normal eye, but in the Holmes–Adie syndrome causes a brisk constriction. There is evidence that the defect lies in the ciliary ganglion so that the pupil shows denervation hypersensitivity (Russell, 1956).

The ability of the lens to accommodate may approach 14 D in childhood but decreases to less than 2 D in old age. This failure to focus on near objects is known as presbyopia. An elderly subject may therefore require a convex lens in front of the eye if he is to read comfortably.

Errors of Refraction

Common defects in vision can arise from abnormalities in the shape of the eye or from abnormalities in the lens. In shortsighted, or myopic people, the eyeball is abnormally long. The effect of this is that parallel rays of light are focused in front of the retina and distant objects therefore appear blurred. Near objects, however, can still be focused on the retina. The condition can be corrected by wearing a concave lens. The reverse condition, or hypermetropia, occurs when the eyeball is abnormally short and parallel rays of light are therefore not properly in focus by the time they reach the retina. Distant objects can be focused by means of accommodation, but this is not possible with near objects, which can only be held in focus by means of convex spectacles (Fig. 8.7).

If the surface of the cornea and the lens are not completely spherical, images may be imperfectly focused on the retina since it is necessary for clear focusing to have a lens with equal curvatures along all the meridians. A defect of this kind is known as astigmatism, and can be corrected by using a lens which is made from cutting a cylindrical, instead of a spherical, piece of glass. A cylindrical

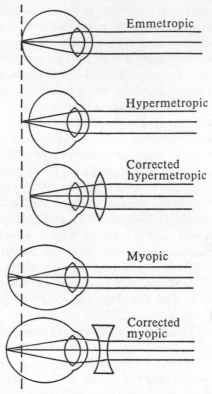

FIG. 8.7. Common refractive errors and their correction by lenses. After Bell,
G. H., Davidson, J. N. and Emslie-Smith, D. (1972). *Textbook of Physiology
and Biochemistry*. Edinburgh: Churchill Livingstone.

lens of this type will correct astigmatism provided the axis of the cylinder is
appropriately placed in relation to the defective meridian of the lens of the eye.

Measurement of Visual Acuity

The clinical measurement of visual acuity is carried out by determining the
distance apart at which separate images can be resolved when placed at a known
distance from the eye. One such test employs the Snellen test types, which embody
a set of letters, the details of which subtend a visual angle of 1 minute when held
6 m from the eye. If the subject is able to read this test type, his visual acuity is
said to be 6/6. With a visual acuity of half this value, he will only be able to read
the test type at 6 m distance if the details are large enough to subtend an arc of
1 minute at 12 m distance. At this level, the visual acuity is said to be 6/12.
The largest type on the standard chart has lettering where the details subtend

1 minute at 60 m distance, and the visual acuity of a person able to read this type at 6 m is said to be 6/60. Where defective visual acuity is the result of errors of refraction by the lens of the eye, it may generally be corrected by placing a suitable lens in front of the eye.

The Light Reflex

The amount of light that enters the eye is determined by the size of the pupil, which is the central aperture of the iris. The sphincter and dilator muscles of the iris enable it to act as a diaphragm. The pupil is constricted in bright light and dilates when the light is dim. The muscles of the iris are innervated by parasympathetic fibres from the third nerve, which cause constriction of the pupil and sympathetic fibres from the superior cervical ganglion, which bring about dilatation of the pupil. If a bright light is shone into the eye, both pupils will constrict. The constriction of the opposite pupil is known as the consensual light reflex. The afferent fibres are in the optic nerve, and they end in the pretectile nucleus in the midbrain where a further relay passes to the third nerve nucleus. In the Argyll Robertson pupil, both the direct and consensual reactions to light are lost, but the convergence reaction is retained. Unlike the Holmes–Adie pupil, which is characteristically large, the Argyll Robertson is generally constricted, which is difficult to explain if the lesion is in the efferent parasympathetic pathway. The site of the lesion remains unknown, but Lowenstein (1956) has reviewed the evidence in favour of a lesion in the final afferent neuron of the reflex arc close to the third nerve nucleus.

The function of the pupil in protecting the eye from bright illumination is particularly important in nocturnal animals which have highly sensitive retinae. In some animals, such as the cat, which are adapted to a nocturnal habit and like to bask in the sun during the day, the pupil is no longer circular in shape, but will contract to a vertical slit through which very little light can pass.

BINOCULAR VISION AND THE VISUAL FIELDS

Many clues are available which enable an individual with a single eye to judge distance. These include the apparent size of an object and the ability to appreciate perspective and also to assess the amount of accommodation required to see near objects in sharp focus. Precise judgment of distance, however, depends on the ability to use two eyes to obtain a stereoscopic perception of depth. Stereoscopic vision comes about because a very slightly different image is projected on to corresponding points of each retina. These images become subjectively fused so that they are seen in three dimensions. It will be appreciated that in binocular vision, although each eye has its own clearly defined field of vision, the fields of vision of the two eyes overlap over a considerable part of their extent.

In clinical practice, the study of the visual fields has considerable localizing value. This comes about through the particular anatomical arrangement of the visual pathway. In all vertebrates, the two optic nerves cross at the chiasma so that the visual field of one eye is perceived by the opposite half of the brain. In mammals, however, this decussation is incomplete and in the primates, including man, half the fibres in the optic nerve cross and the other half remain on the same side. The fibres that cross are those from the nasal half of the retina which subserve the temporal visual field. Those that are uncrossed are from the temporal half of the retina that subserve the nasal visual field. In this way, the whole

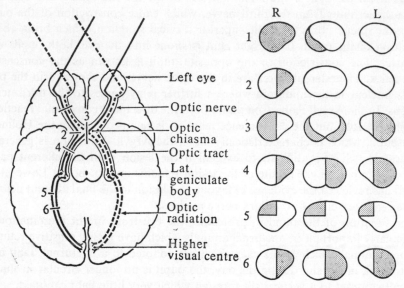

Left eye
Optic nerve
Optic chiasma
Optic tract
Lat. geniculate body
Optic radiation
Higher visual centre

FIG. 8.8. The visual pathway and the effect of lesions in various situations on the field of vision.

visual field, representing one half of space, is represented on one side of the brain and vice versa. Thus, injury to one optic nerve will produce a defect in the visual field of that eye, but injury to the visual pathway behind the chiasma will produce what is known as a homonymous field defect, in which the subject is unable to see in either the right or the left half of space (Fig. 8.8).

The visual field may be measured by means of a perimeter in which the subject fixates a point in the centre of an arc that is marked in degrees so that the fixation axis of the eye at any point on the arc can be identified. A test object is brought in from the periphery of the arc, and the visual angle at which it is perceived is recorded on a perimeter chart. The normal visual field measured in this way extends about 100° to the temporal side, 60° to the nasal side, 60° upwards and about 70° downwards. The blind spot lies slightly more than 15° to the nasal side of the fixation point. Disease of the optic nerve may be associated with abnormal blind spots or scotomata. These can be mapped out accurately if the central part of the visual field is projected on to a large black screen, known as a B,errum screen, generally placed 2 m away from the patient.

THE CENTRAL VISUAL PATHWAYS

The optic tracts are made up of the axons of the ganglion cells of the retina, half of which have crossed at the chiasma and come from the contralateral eye. They end in the thalamus in the lateral geniculate bodies, which contain six layers of cells that are separated by six layers of nerve fibres. The layers are arranged so that layers 1, 4 and 6 contain fibres from the opposite retina, whereas layers 2, 3 and 5 contain uncrossed fibres. The retina is projected on the lateral geniculate body, so that the representation of the macula lies between sectors derived from the upper and lower segments of the retina. Not all fibres in the optic tract end in the lateral geniculate body. Thus, those concerned with the light reflex pass instead through the superior colliculus to relay in the pretectal nucleus in the midbrain. The connections within the geniculate bodies are complex and each optic nerve axon gives off branches to connect with a number of geniculate cells. There is evidence also that the geniculate cells are influenced by fibres which come from the cortex. The receptive fields of the geniculate cells have been studied by stimulating the retina with point sources of light. They resemble the fields of the optic nerve fibres in that they are circular in shape and arranged in concentric rings, so that if stimulation of a central zone gives rise to an on response, the surrounding region will give rise to an off response and vice versa (Hubel and Wiesel, 1961).

The axons of the geniculate cells form the geniculo-striate bundle which passes as the optic radiation to end in the striate area of the occipital pole which corresponds to area 17 in Brodman's numeration. Close to it are two areas of different cytoarchitecture known as area 18 or the parastriate cortex and area 19 or the peristriate cortex and these have been considered to represent association areas for the visual cortex. The geniculo-striate fibres end by connecting with neurones in layer IV of the striate cortex and these in turn make connection with cells in the adjoining layers. In this part of the brain, the cells are grouped in vertical columns, and an electrode inserted at right angles to the surface may connect with numerous cells subserving the same receptive field.

The arrangement of receptive fields in the cortex is considerably more complex than in the retinal ganglion cells or the geniculate neurones. In general, the receptive fields of cortical neurones are arranged side by side and not concentrically. Thus, a strip of retina, which if stimulated gives rise to an on response in a cortical neurone, may lie parallel to a strip which gives rise to an off response.

Linear fields of this type may be derived from the combination of several circular fields belonging to a group of geniculate neurones. Cortical neurones with receptive fields of this type have been termed 'simple units' and these apparently converge on higher order neurones or 'complex units', which will only discharge when light crosses a receptive field in a particular direction and so respond to the orientation of the stimulus. 'Complex units' in turn may project on 'hypercomplex units'. The simple cortical units are perhaps particularly adapted to registering movement, but the complex units are necessary for the more elaborate processes of pattern recognition (Hubel and Wiesel, 1962 1968).

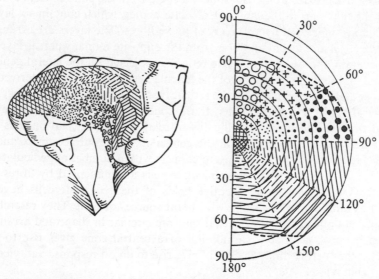

FIG. 8.9. Projection of visual fields on cortex. After Holmes, G. (1918). *Brit. J. Ophthal.*, **2**, 353–384.

The projection of the retina on the occipital pole has been mapped out in the human brain by studying the localization of blindness, which occurs if small portions of the visual cortex are damaged. Gordon Holmes (1918) made a systematic study of the effect of gunshot wounds on this part of the brain which has largely been confirmed by more recent studies. The results of this work show that the fibres from the upper part of the retina, which represent the lower part of the visual field, end on the superior lip of the calcarine fissure, whereas fibres from the lower segment of the retina end on the lower lip of the fissure. The macular fibres are situated posteriorly and end in an area of cortex which is disproportionately large in relation to the size of the macular area of the retina (Fig. 8.9). The point to point relationship between different parts of the retina and different parts of the cortex has been confirmed in experimental animals by applying stimuli to the retina with point sources of light, and recording evoked potentials from the cortex (Talbot and Marshall, 1941). It is of interest that this point to point relationship between retinal receptor cells and cortical neurones is maintained, in spite of the considerable interconnections which take place between the nerve cells of the visual pathway. The point to point representation of the cortex has also been demonstrated, in man, by stimulating the exposed occipital cortex at neurosurgical operation when the subject will see a small white point of light in a certain position of the visual field. This principle has been made us of by Brindley in developing a visual prosthesis to enable a blind person to see. This consists of a set of radio transmitters which are worn on a hat and transmit signals to a group of radio receivers implanted between the parietal bone and the pericranium that activate electrodes applied to the occipital pole. In the patient studied, stimuli applied to the electrodes appeared as point sources of light, and simultaneous stimuli applied to several electrodes gave rise to a coherent visual pattern (Brindley and Lewin, 1968).

Electrical recording from cortical neurones has shown that many are responsive to stimuli from both the right and the left visual fields. In some, the receptive fields are separated by a difference in projection of the order of about 1°. This sensitivity of certain cortical cells to slightly disparate binocular fields is probably a necessary factor in the fusion of images in binocular vision. It is of interest, that if kittens are deprived of binocular vision by occlusion of one eye or surgical production of a squint, the cortical cells become permanently insensitive to binocular stimulation. This does not occur in older animals, and it would appear that there is a phase in maturation when the central connections necessary for stereoscopic vision become defective if they are not used. In man, the critical period seems to be in the first four years of life when squint or congenital cataract may lead to permanent amblyopia (Hubel and Wiesel, 1963; 1970; Barlow *et al.*, 1967; Whitteridge, 1972).

MOVEMENTS OF THE EYES

Although not all vertebrates are able to move their eyes, nearly all have the same paired extraocular muscles that are present in the human subject, namely the superior and inferior recti, the internal and external recti and the two oblique muscles. Only mammals are capable of conjugate eye movement. All other vertebrates, if they have eye movements at all, are able to move their eyes independently. Birds are capable of very little movement of the eyes in the orbits, nearly all alterations in gaze being accomplished by movements of the head. The eye muscles are capable of rapid controlled movements and the motor units are small, generally containing less than 20 muscle fibres (Torre, 1953). The rate of motor unit discharge is considerably greater than in muscles elsewhere in the body, and may reach a rate of several hundred/sec (Björk and Kugelberg, 1953a). Electromyography has thrown considerable light on the contraction of the eye muscles during conjugate movement. Thus, it has been found that in the primary or resting position of the eye all the extraocular muscles are contracting continuously. However, when the eye moves from one to the other side, the electrical activity in the muscle bringing about the movement is increased, while that in its antagonist decreases. In a slow deviation, this relaxation may be incomplete, but in rapid movement, contraction of the active muscle may be accompanied by complete relaxation of its antagonist (Björk and Kugelberg, 1953b).

Eye movements can be classified as saccadic, or rapid movements, such as occur with sudden shifts of gaze and smooth following movements, such as occur when following a slowly moving object. Although common laboratory animals, such as the cat and dog, are without muscle spindles in the eye muscles, they are present in the human eye muscles and in those of certain other animals, such as the sheep and the goat. Both spindle afferents and γ efferents are present, and it would appear likely that, in mammals in which finely controlled eye movements are important, the spindles play an important part in proprioceptive control (Cooper, Daniel and Whitteridge, 1955). Animals which make use of only limited ocular movements largely employ movements of the head to control their gaze, and it is of interest that the muscles of the neck are particularly richly supplied with spindles.

The nervous elements which directly supply the extraocular muscles are the nuclei of the third, fourth and sixth cranial nerves, which lie in the midbrain and the pons. Since conjugate movement depends on the co-ordinated contraction and relaxation of opposing muscles, these nuclei are connected by interneurones which run in a structure known as the posterior longitudinal fasciculus. These structures constitute the lower motor neurone responsible for initiating co-ordinated movements of the eyes. Little is known regarding the higher centres in the brain responsible for controlling conjugate movement. It is clear that in simpler forms of life, centres in the upper part of the brain stem, in particular the superior colliculi, are particularly important in the control of eye movements. In man, eye movements have been obtained by stimulating the occipital cortex and it may be that this part of the brain is important particularly in connection with reflex movements of the eyes in response to visual stimuli. Certainly, damage to this part of the brain and the pathway between it and the ocular motor nuclei may seriously effect the fixation reflex. Stimulation of the frontal lobe, in particular the region close to the precentral gyrus, will give rise to movements of the eyes, especially lateral gaze towards the opposite side, and it is likely that voluntary control of eye movement is exercised through this part of the brain. Many structures, however, are concerned in the control of conjugate movement. These include not only cortical centres but also the labyrinths and vestibular system, and the cerebellum and its connections in the brain stem.

In disease of the nervous system, damage to the peripheral nervous pathway controlling the extraocular muscles, that is to the lower motor neurone, will give rise to paralysis of individual muscles, which will result in misalignment of the eyes to produce a visible squint and double vision. Disease affecting the higher centres concerned with eye movements or their pathways connecting them with the ocular motor nuclei, will give rise to paralysis of conjugate gaze, either in a vertical or lateral direction. Disease affecting the structures concerned in the fine control of conjugate movement will give rise to disturbances of gaze, of which one of the most important in clinical practice is nystagmus. This will be considered further in connection with the vestibular system.

REFERENCES

ARDEN, G. B. and WEALE, R. A. (1954). Nervous mechanisms and dark adaptation. *J. Physiol.* (*Lond.*), **125**, 417–426.

BARLOW, H. B. (1953). Summation and inhibition in the frog's retina. *J. Physiol.* (*Lond.*), **119**, 69–88.

BARLOW, H. B., FITZHUGH, R. and KUFFLER, S. W. (1957). Change of organization in the receptive fields of the cat's retina during dark adaptation. *J. Physiol.* (*Lond.*), **137**, 338–354.

BARLOW, H. B., BLAKEMORE, C. and PETTIGREW, J. D. (1967). The neural mechanism of binocular depth perception. *J. Physiol.* (*Lond.*), **193**, 327–342.

BJÖRK, A. and KUGELBERG, E. (1953a). Motor unit activity in the human extraocular muscles. *Electroenceph. clin. Neurophysiol.*, **5**, 271–278.

BJÖRK, A. and KUGELBERG, E. (1953b). The electrical activity of the muscles of the eye and eyelids in various positions and during movement. *Electroenceph. clin. Neurophysiol.*, **5**, 595–602.

BOYCOTT, B. B. and DOWLING, J. F. (1969). Organization of the primate retina: light microscopy. *Phil. Trans.*, **255**, 109–184.

BRINDLEY, G. S. and LEWIN, W. S. (1968). The sensations produced by electrical stimulation of the visual cortex. *J. Physiol.* (*Lond.*), **196**, 479–493.

BRINDLEY, G. S. (1970). *Physiology of the Retina and Visual Pathway*. London: Arnold.

COOPER, S., DANIEL, P. D. and WHITTERIDGE, D. (1955). Muscle spindles and other sensory endings in the extrinsic eye muscle. *Brain*, **78**, 564–583.

DAVSON, H. (1972). *The Physiology of the Eye*. 3rd Edn. Edinburgh: Livingstone.

DAW, N. W. (1968). Colour-coded ganglion cells in the goldfish retina: an extension of their receptive fields by means of new stimuli. *J. Physiol.* (*Lond.*), **197**, 567–592.

DEWAR, J. and McKENDRICK, J. G. (1873). On the physiological action of light. *J. anat. Physiol.*, **7**, 275–282, cited by Granit (1947).

GRANIT, R. (1947). *Sensory Mechanisms of the Retina*. London: Oxford University Press.

HARDEN, A. and PAMPIGLIONE, G. (1970). Neurophysiological approach to disorders of vision. *Lancet*, **1**, 805–808.

HARTLINE, H. K. (1940). The receptive fields of optic nerve fibres. *Amer. J. Physiol.*, **130**, 690–699.

HARTLINE, H. K., WAGNER, H. G. and RATLIFF, F. (1956). Inhibition in the eye of Limulus. *J. gen. Physiol.*, **39**, 651–673.

HOLMES, G. (1918). Disturbances of vision by cerebral lesions. *Brit. J. Ophthal.*, **2**, 353–384.

HUBEL, D. H. and WIESEL, T. N. (1961). Integrative action in the cat's lateral geniculate body. *J. Physiol.* (*Lond.*), **155**, 385–398.

HUBEL, D. H. and WIESEL, T. N. (1963). Receptive fields in striate cortex of very young visually inexperienced kittens. *J. Neurophysiol.*, **26**, 994–1002.

HUBEL, D. H. and WIESEL, T. N. (1962). Receptive fields, binocular interaction and functional architecture in the cat's visual cortex. *J. Physiol.* (*Lond.*), **160**, 106–154.

HUBEL, D. H. and WIESEL, T. N. (1968). Receptive fields and functional architecture of monkey striate cortex. *J. Physiol.* (*Lond.*), **195**, 215–243.

HUBEL, D. H. and WIESEL, T. N. (1970). The period of susceptibility to the physiological effects of eye closure in kittens. *J. Physiol.* (*Lond.*), **206**, 419–436.

JAMPEL, R. S. (1959). Representation of the near-response on the cerebral cortex of the macaque. *Am. J. Ophth.*, **48**, 573–581.

LOWENSTEIN, O. (1956). The Argyll Robertson pupillary syndrome: mechanism and localization. *Am. J. Ophth.*, **42**, 105–121.

RUSHTON, W. A. H. (1959). Visual pigments in man and animals and their relation to seeing. *Progr. Biophys.*, **9**, 239–283.

RUSSELL, G. F. M. (1956). Pupillary changes in the Holmes–Adie syndrome. *J. Neurol. Neurosurg. Psychiat.*, **19**, 289–296.

TALBOT, S. A. and MARSHALL, W. H. (1941). Physiological studies on neurol mechanisms of visual localization and discrimination. *Amer. J. Ophthal.*, **24**, 1255–1264.

TANSLEY, K. (1965). *Vision in Vertebrates*. London: Chapman and Hall Ltd.

TEPAS, D. I. and ARMINSTON, J. C. (1962). Electroretinograms from non-corneal electrodes. *Invest. Ophthal.*, **1**, 784–786.

TORRE, A. (1953). Nombre et dimensions des unites motrices dans les muscles extrinseques de l'oeil et, en general, dans les muscles squelettiques relies a des organes de sens. *Arch. Suisses Neurol. Psychiat.*, **72**, 362–376.

WALD, G. (1937). Photo-labile pigments of the chicken retina. *Nature*, **140**, 545–546.

WHITTERIDGE, D. (1972). Binocular vision and cortical function. *Proc. roy. Soc. Med.*, **65**, 947–952.

CHAPTER 9

Hearing and Balance

THE APPRECIATION OF SOUND

The organ of hearing is essentially a mechanical transducer that is sensitive to rapid changes in air pressure. In the human ear, it is able to resolve changes in air pressure occurring at a frequency of up to 20,000 Hz. In this respect, it is greatly more sensitive than receptors in the skin which may be sensitive to vibration, but only up to frequencies of between 500 and 1000 Hz. On the other hand, many animals can hear sound at considerably higher frequencies than the human ear can appreciate. Thus, cats can hear sounds with a frequency of up to 50,000 Hz and bats may hear notes of 100,000 Hz.

The human ear shows a considerable ability to distinguish between different frequencies, which are recognized as changes in pitch. Some individuals can appreciate as many as 2,000 different changes in pitch. A musical note consists of sound in which the vibrations are occurring regularly and non periodic vibrations can be recognized as noise. The loudness with which sound affects the human ear depends partly on its amplitude, and the quality, or timbre, of a note depends on the harmonics or overtones that are present, in addition to the dominant frequency. The sensitivity of the human ear is dependent on the frequencies of sounds to which it is exposed and is maximum at frequencies in the range of 1000 to 4000 Hz. This is a higher range of frequency than the frequencies that commonly occur in human speech, where the dominant frequencies are less than 500 Hz. The range of intensities of sound which can be heard, that is, the difference between the intensity of the minimal stimulus which is audible and the loudest noise that the subject will tolerate is considerable, the loudest tolerable sound having an intensity of approximately 10^{12} times the threshold. For this reason, the intensity of sound is generally expressed on a logarithmic scale and the decibel (dB) is the standard unit of notation.

A dB is 1/10 of a bel, which is the log of the ratio of two intensities of sound. Thus, a dB is 10 log $_{10}$ of the ratio of a particular sound intensity to the intensity

179

of sound at an arbitrarily selected intensity level. In practice, this reference level is taken as a sound which is at about the threshold of hearing for a 1000 Hz note, that in absolute terms, corresponds to a sound of r.m.s. p of 0.0002 dyn/cm^2. A note of 100 or 10^2 times threshold may be spoken of as 2 bels or $10 \times 2 = 20$ dB and a note of 10^{12} times threshold may be spoken of as 10×12 or 120 dB above threshold.

THE MECHANISMS OF HEARING

The Structure of The Ear

The transducer action of the ear depends on an arrangement which enables the pressure changes of sound in air to be transmitted to a fluid medium. The vibrations in the fluid medium are transmitted to the basilar membrane in the inner ear, the vibration of which sets up changes in sensitive hair cells that in turn activate the fibres of the auditory nerve. The external ear and the middle ear contain the mechanism which transmits the pressure changes from the air to the cochlear fluid. The inner ear, or cochlea, contains the mechanism for the excitation of nervous tissue.

The external ear consists of a closed tube through which pressure changes are transmitted to the tympanic membrane. The middle ear contains three small bones, the malleus, the incus and the stapes. The malleus is attached to the tympanic membrane and moves with it. This movement is transmitted to the incus, which rocks the stapes, the footplate of which is attached to the oval window that opens into the inner ear. The middle ear contains air, which is maintained at atmospheric pressure, since it communicates with the pharynx via the eustachian tube. Below the oval window is the round window, which is closed by a membrane that allows movement and recoil of fluid within the inner ear.

The internal ear is situated in the petrous temporal bone. It consists of a set of membranous chambers and passages known as the membranous labyrinth, which is enclosed within a cavity hollowed out of the bone, and known as the bony labyrinth. The anterior part of the membranous labyrinth includes the organ of hearing that is known as the duct of the cochlea. Behind this are the saccule and the utricle and further back the three semicircular ducts. The portions of bony labyrinth that surround these parts are known as the cochlea, the vestibule and the three semicircular canals. The lateral wall of the vestibule is directed towards the tympanic cavity and communicates with it through the oval and round windows. The membranous labyrinth is filled with fluid known as endolymph, which is similar in content to intracellular fluid with a high concentration of potassium. The fluid which surrounds the membranous labyrinth and fills the bony labyrinth is similar in content to cerebrospinal fluid, although it has a relatively high concentration of protein.

The cochlear portion of the inner ear consists of a tapering spiral cone or modiolus, round which a spiral tube is coiled. The spiral tube is divided longitudinally by the basilar membrane and the vestibular, or Reissner's membrane, to form three spiral canals. The centre of these canals is the cochlear duct, which communicates at its lower end with the saccule and contains endolymph. It is separated by the vestibular membrane from the scala vestibuli and by the basilar membrane from the scala tympani. Both these channels contain perilymph (Fig. 9.1.)

The organ of Corti lies on the basilar membrane and contains two sets of sensory cells, a single row of internal hair cells and three rows of external hair cells (Fig. 9.2). The hair cells are the receptor cells for hearing and are each

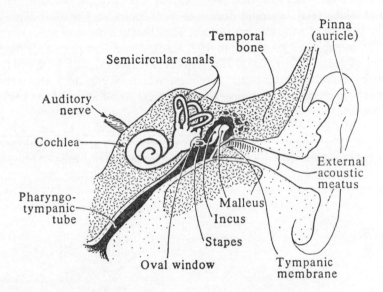

FIG. 9.1. Structure of the ear.

innervated by fibres derived from the bipolar nerve cells in the spiral ganglion, the axons of which form the acoustic part of the eighth nerve. Within the organ of Corti is the tunnel of Corti, which is situated between the internal and external hair cells, and contains perilymph. The endolymph in the scala media is separated from the interior of the organ of Corti by the reticular membrane, through which the hair cells pass to end in the gelatinous substance that constitutes the overlying tectorial membrane. When movements of the basilar membrane take place, the hairs, which are in contact with the reticular membrane, are exposed to shearing stresses, and it is these which bring about excitation.

The first stage in the sequence of events when sound reaches the external ear is that the vibration of the tympanic membrane sets up backward and forward movements of the ossicles in the middle ear. This enables the vibration to be transmitted to the fluid medium of the internal ear, which causes upward and downward movements of the basilar membrane. It is these which give rise to shearing of the hair cells and excitation of the nerve fibres.

Microphonic Effect of the Cochlea

In 1930 Wever and Bray found that if electrodes were placed on the auditory nerve of the cat, and the potentials amplified and played into a loudspeaker, this would give rise to reproduction of the sounds falling on the cat's ear. These changes are clearly not due to action potentials occurring at the same frequency as sound, since audible sound occurs at frequencies very much higher than a nerve is capable of transmitting signals. Thus, nerve fibres are generally refractory to frequencies of greater than 1000 Hz, but cochlear potentials have been recorded of greater than 50,000 Hz from certain species, such as the bat. It has since been established that the potentials which Wever and Bray recorded represent a microphonic response to mechanical stimulation of the cochlea by sound waves.

To record the cochlear microphonic, it is not necessary to record from the nerve itself. The potentials can be readily recorded by means of an electrode on the round window with an indifferent electrode on the face. Although this

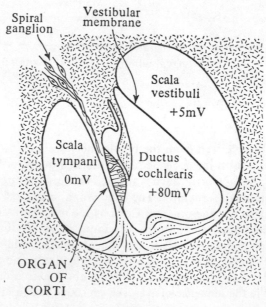

(A)

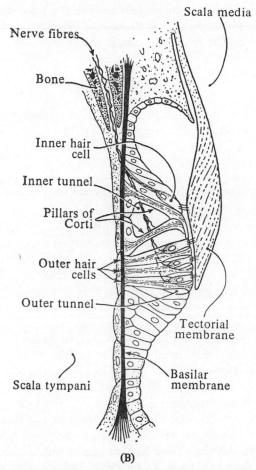

Scala media

Nerve fibres

Bone

Inner hair cell

Inner tunnel

Pillars of Corti

Outer hair cells

Outer tunnel

Tectorial membrane

Scala tympani

Basilar membrane

(B)

FIG. 9.2. (a) Cross section of the cochlea. (b) Detail of the organ of Corti.

microphonic potential is clearly distinct from the action potentials in the auditory nerve, which have been recorded with microelectrodes and found to have the characteristic properties of nerve action potentials, such as all-or-nothing effect and refractory period, there is evidence that the microphonic discharge of the cochlea may be the stimulus which excites the discharge in the sensory neurones.

The origin of the cochlear microphonic may be related to the potential difference that exists between the endolymph in the cochlear duct and the perilymph in the scala tympani and the scala vestibuli. The endolymph in the scala media is approximately 80 mV positive to the perilymph in the other two chambers. If the basilar membrane moves downwards, the endolymph becomes more positive, and if it moves upwards, it becomes less positive. This potential change which occurs with movement of the basilar membrane is probably related to shearing stresses that occur on the hair cells, and is the probable source of the micro-phonic potential.

Frequency Discrimination

In the human ear, frequency discrimination is most marked at medium and high intensities of sound. Helmholtz suggested that the mechanism of frequency discrimination was that hair cells in different parts of the basilar membrane responded preferentially to different frequencies of sound. This concept that receptors which correspond to a particular pitch are located on specific sites on the membrane has remained as the 'place theory' of frequency discrimination. Evidence in favour of this hypothesis is that injury to parts of the organ of Corti may cause selective loss of frequency perception. Moreover, it has been found that high notes activate preferentially the basal turn of the cochlea and low notes the apical end. This differential sensitivity may depend in part on the mechanical properties of the basilar membrane (von Bekesy, 1956).

It does not appear that particular nerve fibres respond exclusively to particular frequencies. Recordings from single fibres have shown that fibres in the apical part of the cochlea may respond only to the lower frequencies, whereas those in the basal turn may respond to higher frequencies also. Many single fibres respond to a fairly narrow frequency band at low intensities of stimulation, but to a wider frequency band at higher intensities. Frequently, fibres show a fairly sharp cut–off at an upper frequency limit (Tasaki, 1954). As the sensory neurones connect with neurones more centrally placed in the auditory pathway, it has been found that the cut–off occurs at a lower frequency so that the higher order neurones respond to a relatively restricted frequency band. Another mechanism for sharpening pitch discrimination has been described in the cochlear nucleus, where it has been found that a given tone may activate some units at the same time inhibiting others (Galambos, 1956). Neurones connected with different parts of the basilar membrane are spatially separated in the auditory pathways and in the auditory cortex, where there is a clearly defined tonotopic organiza-tion.

The Central Pathway of Hearing

The bipolar ganglion cells in the spiral ganglion that is situated in the cochlea in the spiral canal of the modiolus form the first sensory neurone for hearing. Their central axons enter the pons where they divide to enter the dorsal and ventral cochlear nuclei. There second order neurones arise and cross the pons to ascend in the lateral lemniscus to the inferior colliculus. From the inferior colliculus, fibres pass to the medial geniculate body, from which a final relay passes in the auditory radiations to the auditory cortex in the temporal lobe. A proportion of the fibres that cross in the pons form a layer of fibres known as the trapezoid body, and some relay in the nuclei of the trapezoid body or in the superior olivary nucleus. The auditory pathway differs from other sensory pathways in that the simple three neurone pathway from first sensory neurone to cortex is not a feature, and the neurones connecting the thalamus with the cortex may be fifth or higher order neurones. Only a proportion of the auditory neurones cross during their course, so that hearing is bilaterally represented in the cortex. Scarcely any loss of hearing occurs if the auditory cortex is destroyed on one side.

TESTS OF AUDITORY FUNCTION

Deafness

Although deafness can result from destruction of the central auditory pathways, the cause of deafness is more commonly peripheral and, in practice, deafness may be classified as either conductive deafness or perceptive deafness. Conductive deafness can occur as a result of obstruction of the external auditory meatus by wax, damage to the tympanic membrane or inflammation in the middle ear. In otosclerosis, the stapes becomes fixed in the oval window. Perceptive deafness may be due either to pathology affecting the sensory cells of the cochlea or to disease affecting the auditory nerve or its central connections.

Tuning Fork Tests

If a person has defective hearing, the simplest test to distinguish conductive from perceptive deafness is to compare the hearing conveyed by air conduction and by bone conduction, using a tuning fork of 256 Hz. In Rinné's test, a tuning fork is placed against the mastoid bone and when the patient can no longer hear it, it is then placed beside the external auditory meatus. In the normal subject, hearing is more acute by air conduction than by bone conduction, but in middle ear deafness bone conduction is more effective than air conduction. In Weber's test, the tuning fork is placed on the vertex of the skull and in the presence of normal hearing the sound is heard equally in both ears. In middle ear disease, the sound is heard better on the affected side, but in perceptive deafness the sound appears louder on the healthy side.

Audiometry

In audiometry, an electronic oscillator is used to test the sensitivity of the ear to different intensities of sound at different frequencies. Using pure tones, the threshold of hearing at selected frequencies is determined. The audiogram is constructed by plotting the hearing loss in dB for each frequency, using the

G

average threshold of hearing of a population of young adults as the reference level. If an earphone is placed over the ear and a vibrator applied to the mastoid process, the threshold values for both air and bone conduction can be plotted. In conductive deafness, air conduction is selectively impaired and the hearing loss includes the whole range of audible frequencies. In perceptive deafness, the hearing loss may affect particularly the higher frequencies of sound.

A number of refinements have been introduced into the audiometry tests to try and distinguish between end organ deafness due to cochlear lesions and nerve, or retrocochlear deafness. One approach depends on the observation that, whereas cochlear fatigue may give rise to a small decrease in the auditory response to a continuous tone, retrocochlear lesions may show excessive adaptation to pure tone stimuli (Johnson and House, 1964). In Bekesy audiometry, the audiogram is prepared using both a continuous and an interrupted tone as stimulus. With each stimulus, the patient gives a signal when a sound which is progressively increased becomes audible, or at the point when a decreasing sound disappears. In subjects with normal hearing or with conductive deafness, the curves obtained with continuous and interrupted stimuli are the same (type I). In cochlear deafness, at frequencies above about 1000 Hz, cochlear fatigue results in a small decrease in the sensitivity to continuous tones, so that two narrowly separated curves are obtained (type II). With nerve deafness there may be a relatively severe fall in the sensitivity to continuous tones either in the upper frequency range only (type III) or throughout the whole frequency spectrum (type IV) and the curves may be widely separated.

In the test for recruitment of loudness (Fig. 9.3) the subject is simultaneously presented with sound in each ear of different intensities, which are progressively increased in loudness. When recruitment is present, it is found that loud noises appear equally intense in the two ears, but soft noises are heard much less acutely in the affected ear. Recruitment is not present in conductive deafness or retrocochlear deafness and is only generally present in cochlear disease, such as that which may occur in Meniere's syndrome. It probably occurs because in cochlear disease the most sensitive receptors are affected first. Where recruitment of loudness exists, the subject may be able to appreciate small increments of loudness not perceptible by the normal ear. This is the basis of the short increment sensitivity index (sisi) in which the subject is exposed to a continuous tone, the intensity of which is increased by about 1 dB for periods of a few seconds. This test is valuable where recruitment of loudness cannot be clearly demonstrated, as may be the case in bilateral cochlear disease.

The above tests all depend on the co-operation of the subject, but it may also be important to recognize deafness in infants or in brain damaged individuals who are unable to co-operate. This can be done by monitoring the EEG changes that take place in response to auditory stimuli. A useful method is to record the cerebral evoked responses which occur in response to signals from a pure tone audiometer, a technique that can be carried out when the subject is asleep (see

a. AUDIOGRAMS

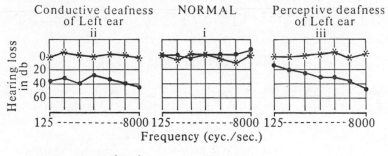

b. LOUDNESS BALANCE DIAGRAMS

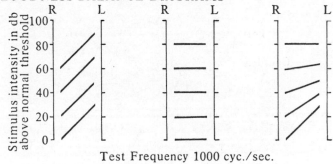

Test Frequency 1000 cyc./sec.

c.

FIG. 9.3. Diagram to show audiograms (a) and loudness balance diagrams (b and c) in (i) normal subject (ii) subject with conductive deafness in the left ear and (iii) subject with perceptive deafness in the left ear. (b) and (c) represent alternative methods of representing recruitment of loudness. Recruitment is particularly characteristic of perceptive deafness due to cochlear lesions. After Dix, M. R. (1956). *Brit. med. Bull.*, **12**, 119–124.

chapter 12). A less elaborate procedure is to condition the patient so that a galvanic skin response (see chapter 11) is evoked by an auditory stimulus.

THE VESTIBULAR SYSTEM

The vestibular apparatus forms the inner ear in association with the cochlea. It consists of the three semicircular ducts, which are situated within the semi-

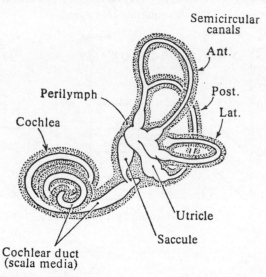

FIG. 9.4 Lateral view of the labyrinth.

circular canals at right angles to each other, and connect with the utricle and the saccule, which separate them from the cochlea. Each semicircular duct has a wide portion at one end known as the ampulla. This contains the sense organ or crista ampullaris, from which hair cells protrude and are embedded in a jelly like structure called the cupula. The utricle and saccule carry hair cells on the lining epithelium, which support gelatinous masses containing calcium carbonate, and are known as the otoliths. The cavities of the membranous labyrinths are filled with endolymph (Fig. 9.4).

In man, the utricle is the principal otolith organ and it appears to respond particularly to gravitational pull, although it may also respond to sudden linear acceleration of the head. By reacting to gravitational pull, it is able to respond to changes in the position of the head, a function which it shares with the proprioceptors in the neck muscles. In the semicircular ducts, the hair cells respond to movement of the endolymph, which may be brought about by angular acceleration of the head. The vestibular apparatus is innervated by the vestibular portion of the eighth nerve that passes into the medulla to end in the vestibular nuclei, but some fibres pass direct to the cerebellum. Fibres from the vestibular nuclei may pass down to the spinal cord in the vestibulospinal tract, which arises largely from the lateral vestibular (Deiter's) nucleus or ascend in the brain stem to the thalamus, from which fibres pass to the cortex of the temporal lobe. There are also important connecting pathways with other nuclei in the brain stem, in particular, the posterior longitudinal fasciculus that connects the vestibular nuclei with the external ocular muscles.

If action potentials are recorded from nerve fibres arising in the semicircular ducts, it is found that the fibres are normally discharging, even when the head is at rest. Angular acceleration of the head in one direction will result in an increase in the discharge rate from one horizontal canal, while at the same time that from the other is inhibited. When movement ceases, the movement of fluid in the canals is reversed, so that the previously excited afferent nerve is now inhibited and vice versa.

The information transmitted from the labyrinths, together with that obtained from proprioceptors in the body and from from the visual system, is extremely important in the maintenance of body posture (see chapter 10). If the labyrinths in man are destroyed, there is at first a marked disturbance of posture and gait, but with time, loss of the labyrinthine reflexes is compensated by reflexes from the eyes and proprioceptors. By means of its connections with the nuclei supplying the extraocular muscles, the labyrinths are able to exert a controlling influence on the visual axis during movements of the head. Disturbed function of the labyrinths is one factor in the production of nystagmus.

Tests of Vestibular Function

Tests of vestibular function in clinical use are directed principally to identifying abnormalities in the labyrinths and their central connections. Disordered function of the semicircular canals may give rise to a sensation of vertigo, which is a subjective feeling of abnormal movement in space that may be associated with nausea and vomiting. The patient may also have a disturbance of balance and gait and may misjudge the position of objects when he points to them, so that he past points. In addition, there is a disorder of ocular movement which takes the form of a repeated oscillating movement of the eyes from side to side that is known as nystagmus. Of these features, nystagmus is particularly amenable to analysis and the study of nystagmus following various manoeuvres has become the basis of many of the tests of vestibular function.

Rotational Nystagmus

If a subject is seated in a chair with his head bent forwards to bring his horizontal canals into the plane of rotation, and the chair is then rotated, the eyes go into a rotatory nystagmus as though they were attempting repeatedly to maintain fixation on an object in front. The nystagmus consists of a slow movement of the eyes in the direction opposite to the rotation, followed by a rapid movement in the reverse direction. By convention, the direction of the quick component is

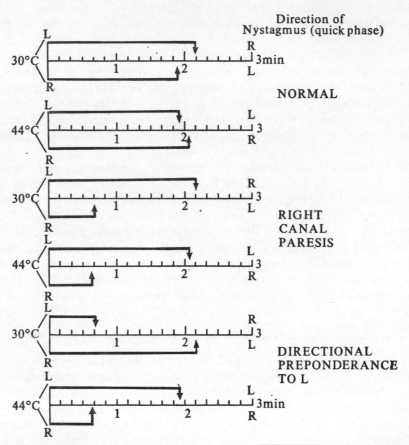

FIG. 9.5. Diagram to show duration and direction of nystagmus which follows irrigation of either ear with water at 30°C and 44°C for 40 secs. The lower two examples illustrate the caloric responses representing canal paresis and directional preponderance.

always taken as the direction of the nystagmus. However, the slow component is the one produced by action of the labyrinths and the quick component is due to a central correcting mechanism. If the rotation is maintained for longer than 20 or 30 sec the nystagmus will cease, but at the end of rotation the nystagmus will again occur and will last about 20 to 30 sec, but now the slow component will be in the direction of rotation. Rotational and postrotational nystagmus result from movement of the endolymphh in the semicircular canals.

The Caloric Test (*Fig.* 9.5)

Movement of endolymph in the canals can also be produced by passage of warm or cold water into the external auditory meatus and this provides a useful clinical test of labyrinthine function (Fitzgerald and Hallpike, 1942). In this test the subject lies with his head bent 30° forward so that the lateral canal lies in the vertical plane. If water at 7°C above body temperature (44°C) or 7° below (30°C) is passed into the external meatus movement of the fluid in the semicircular canal will give rise to nystagmus.Thus warm water causes an upward flow of endolymph towards the ampulla and nystagmus occurs with the quick component towards the side stimulated. Cold water produces a downward flow of endolymph and nystagmus occurs with the quick component towards the opposite side. The caloric test, by its relative simplicity and reproducibility, has become a frequently applied test of vestibular function. If the sensitivity of one semicircular canal is reduced or if one vestibular nerve is damaged, stimulation may fail to produce nystagmus or the nystagmus may be of shorter duration. A second type of abnormality is known as directional preponderance. This means that there is increase in nystagmus to one side with a corresponding reduction in nystagmus to the opposite side. Directional preponderance can result from a vestibular lesion at any level between the semicircular canals and the vestibular nuclei. Its clinical significance lies in the fact that it is directed to the contra-lateral side to the lesion which causes it. Hallpike (1965) has postulated that it results from imbalance between tonus elements that exist in the utricles and the vestibular nuclei and which have a function in the control of conjugate gaze. On this basis, the tonus of one vestibular apparatus may be regarded as tending to shift the gaze toward the opposite side.

Central and Peripheral Nystagmus

Nystagmus evoked by rotation or by caloric stimulation is similar in character to the nystagmus which results from disease of the labyrinth. Characteristically, this is a rapid, horizontal rotatory nystagmus and in disease of the labyrinths it is frequently transient. A highly characteristic feature is the direction of the quick component, which is determined by the direction of flow of the endolymph in the semicircular canals and is constant in direction and independent of the direction of gaze of the patient. Thus, warm water in the left external meatus will produce nystagmus with a quick phase to the left, regardless of the direction of gaze. A destructive lesion of the labyrinth or the vestibular nerve may give rise to nystagmus with the quick phase toward the healthy side. Nystagmus which arises from disease affecting central structures, such as the cerebellum or the brain stem, is less constant in direction than labyrinthine nystagmus and frequently the direction of the quick and slow components is dependent on the direction of gaze. If this is the case, the slow component is towards the fixation point and the quick component towards the midline, regardless of whether the patient is looking to the right or left. Central nystagmus is also not infrequently vertical. With lesions affecting the posterior longitudinal fasciculus, there may

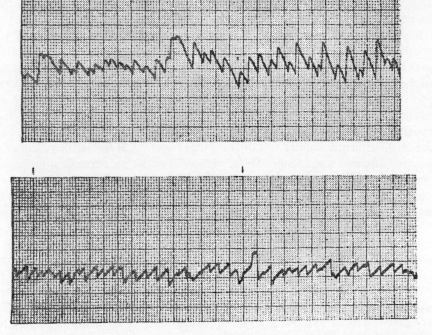

FIG. 9.6. Two examples of nystagmus recorded by electronystagmography. The upper record shows nystagmus to the right (direction of quick phase), the lower shows nystagmus to the left. The recording arrangements are such that an upward movement of the pen occurs when the eye moves to the right, a downward movement when the eye moves to the left. Maran, A. G. D. (1966), *Scot. med. J.*, **11**, 379–387.

occur a dissociated nystagmus known as internuclear ophthalmoplegia, in which there is paresis of the adducted eye with a course jerky nystagmus of the abducted eye. Positional nystagmus, occurring only after placing the head in a particular posture, may occur both in vestibular and central lesions, but the peripheral form is characteristically transient and may be associated with severe vertigo.

Electronystagmography (*Fig.* 9.6)

An important advance in the study of nystagmus has been the development of the technique of electronystagmography (Aschen, Bergstedt and Stahle, 1956).

In this method, the corneoretinal potential is recorded by electrodes placed close to the right and left outer canthi, with an indifferent electrode on the forehead. Eye movements give rise to potential changes which can be recorded on a pen recorder. The pens are conventially arranged so that an upward deflection refers to a deviation to the right and a downward deflection to a deviation of the eyes to the left. This method has the advantage that it has a definite end point, which is particularly useful in caloric testing, and one can be certain of the direction of the fast and slow components of the nystagmus. In addition, it is possible to record the nystagmus with the eyes closed in total darkness.

With this method, a number of criteria have been established which may help to distinguish central from peripheral nystagmus. Thus, nystagmus that is due to labyrinthine or other peripheral lesions may be particularly prominent when recorded in darkness and in general, the quick component is in one direction only. With central nystagmus, the nystagmus may be abolished both in darkness and by eye closure and the direction of the quick component may depend on the direction of gaze (Hood, 1967).

Optokinetic Nystagmus

Optokinetic nystagmus will occur in the healthy subject and may be seen, for example, when the subject looks out of a railway carriage when the train is moving or when the subject is standing still and looks at a moving part of the environment. It can be clinically tested by asking the subject to look at a rotating striped drum. The eyes respond by a slow movement in the direction of movement of the drum and a rapid movement in the opposite direction. Optokinetic nystagmus is of clinical interest because, although in animals it can be elicited in the absence of cerebral hemispheres, in man it requires the integrity of the parietal and temporal lobes. With lesions particularly affecting the parieto-temporal cortex, it may be absent or impaired or may show a directional preponderance so that it is only present when the drum is rotated in one direction but not in the other (Carmichael, Dix and Hallpike, 1954).

REFERENCES

ASCHAN, G., BERGSTEDT, M. and STAHLE, J. (1956). Nystagmography. Recording of nystagmus in clinical neuro-otological examinations. *Acta Oto. laryngologica. suppl.*, **129**, 1–103.
VON BEKESY, G. (1956). Current status of theories of hearing. *Science.* **123**, 779–783.
CARMICHAEL, E. A., DIX, M. R. and HALLPIKE, C. S. (1954). Lesions of the cerebral hemispheres and their effects upon optokinetic and caloric nystagmus. *Brain*, **77**, 345–372.

FITZGERALD, G. and HALLPIKE, C. S. (1942). Studies in human vestibular function 1. Observations on the directional preponderance ('nystagmusbereitschaft') of caloric nystagmus resulting from vestibular lesions. *Brain*, **65**, 115–137.

GALAMBOS, R. (1956). Suppression of auditory nerve activity by stimulation of afferent fibres to cochlea. *J. Neurophysiol.*, **19**, 424–437.

HALLPIKE, C. S. (1965). Clinical otoneurology and its contributions to theory and practice. *Proc. roy. Soc. Med.*, **58**, 185–196.

HOOD, J. D. (1967). Recent advances in the electronystagmographic investigation of vestibular and other disorders of ocular movement. In: *Myotatic, Kinaesthetic and Vestibular Mechanisms*. Ciba Foundation Symposium. Ed. de Reuck, A. V. S. and Knight, J. London: Churchill.

JOHNSON, E. W. and HOUSE, W. F. (1964). Auditory findings in 53 cases of acoustic neuromas. *Arch. Otolaryng.*, **80**, 667–677.

TASAKI, I. (1954). Nerve impulses in individual auditory nerve fibres of guinea-pig. *J. Neurophysiol.*, **17**, 92–122.

WEVER, E. G. and BRAY, C. W. (1930). The nature of acoustic response: the relation between sound frequency and frequency of impulses in the auditory nerve. *J. exp Psychol.*, **13**, 373–387.

CHAPTER 10

The Control of Posture and Movement

Some of the reflexes involved in postural mechanisms have been described in previous sections. In this chapter an account is given of the organization of postural reflexes. This is followed by an account of certain of the central structures and processes concerned with the control of movement.

POSTURAL REFLEXES

The standing posture of the body is maintained through a system of reflexes which are mediated largely through the spinal cord and brain stem and which require the higher centres in the brain for their integration.

The fundamental reflex necessary for standing is the extensor reflex, which opposes the action of gravity and which can be evoked by stretching the extensor muscles. If a muscle is stretched, the muscle spindles are activated so that afferent impulses arise that excite the anterior horn cells to bring about a reflex contraction which opposes the stretching force. If the spinal cord of an animal is divided, stretch reflexes can be demonstrated below the section, but they are not well maintained and the animal cannot maintain a standing posture. Normally the stretch reflexes are activated by centres in and above the brain stem and this activation is mediated in part through the γ efferent fibres which activate the spindles (see chapter 6).

If a lesion is made at a higher level so that in addition to the spinal cord, certain brain stem nuclei are left intact, the stretch reflexes are so well maintained that the antigravity muscles maintain a state of constant exaggerated contraction. This state of heightened extensor tonus is known as decerebrate rigidity. An animal in this state is able to stand if placed on its feet, although its posture is abnormal and it has no ability to right itself if it falls. Sherrington found that in order to obtain decerebrate rigidity it was necessary to divide the brain stem caudal to the red nucleus but rostral to the vestibular nucleus. It could be abolished by section of the dorsal nerve roots which carry afferent impulses into the spinal cord. Clearly it must be due to augmentation of the stretch reflexes by impulses arising at the level of the vestibular nucleus and which are released from inhibitory control by higher centres. It is now known that much of the regulatory influence on the excitability of the stretch reflexes is centred in the brain stem reticular formation which contains regions that have excitatory and inhibitory effects on the extensor stretch reflexes.

If the section is made through the brain at a higher level so that the midbrain and the thalamus are preserved, the animal is able to adopt a normal posture in which extensor tonus is preserved but is not exaggerated and flexor tone is no longer deficient. The thalamic animal is also able to right itself if it falls.

The detailed analysis of postural reflexes has been very largely carried out by Magnus and de Kleyn and the broad conclusions were summarized by Magnus in his Croonian lecture (Magnus, 1925). In general, postural reflexes can be classified as either static reflexes which are concerned with maintaining a particular attitude, stance or posture, and stato-kinetic reactions which occur in response to movement.

It has been seen that the maintenance of postural tone in the antigravity muscles depends largely on reflexes initiated by impulses from proprioceptors in the extensor muscles. The maintenance of a particular stance, which depends on the immediate performance of corrective movements in response to any deviation from the position held, depends on the receipt of information from a wide variety of sense organs that signal alterations in the position of the body. These include proprioceptive sense organs in muscles and joints, which in addition to signalling changes in the tonus of postural muscles, can indicate when the position of one part of the body has altered in relation to another, as for example when movement of the head activates proprioceptors in the neck. Touch and pressure receptors in the skin can set up reactions if part of the body is in contact with the ground and the labyrinths respond to changes in position of the head. Sense organs which respond to distant stimuli also play a part in postural adjustments. The eyes are particularly important in this respect. Postural reflexes can also be considered in terms of whether they are local reactions originating in or close to the muscles which are activated, or general reactions which are generated by signals arising from more distant receptors.

The Positive Supporting Reaction

The contraction of the extensor muscles, which is brought about by the stretch reflex, is not in itself adequate to maintain the standing posture. The limbs must be maintained as rigid props and for this there must be fixation of the joints, brought about by simultaneous contraction of the extensors and their antagonists. This occurs through an important local reflex which is known as the positive supporting reaction. The afferent stimulus for this comes from the sole of the foot. If pressure is applied to the sole of the foot or if the toes are separated so that the interosseus muscles are stretched, the muscles of the limb contract to convert it into a rigid pillar-like prop. Thus, whenever the foot is placed on the ground the positive supporting reaction will occur. Although pressure on the skin may initiate the reflex, it is not an essential part of the afferent stimulus since the reaction will still take place if the skin has been anaesthetized. If the digits are squeezed or flexed the reaction is overcome and the joints of the limb undergo flexion. This is known as the negative supporting reaction, and provides a mechanism whereby a flexion movement of the toes may free the limb for movement.

The Crossed Extensor Reflex

If an animal is standing on four legs and a painful stimulus is applied to one leg so that it is withdrawn, contraction takes place in the extensor muscles of the contralateral limb and the standing posture of the animal is maintained. Since this reflex is producing an effect on muscles lying in the same segment, it may be spoken of as a segmental reflex. In a four footed animal the crossed extensor response in the hind limbs may be accompanied by forelimb extension also and vice versa, and this is spoken of as an intersegmental reflex (see chapter 6).

The Influence of Head Posture

Information regarding the position of the head in space is derived from the labyrinths, and information regarding the position of the head in relation to the rest of the body from proprioceptors situated in the neck. These two sets of receptors set up reflexes which are important in maintaining the standing posture. These reflexes can be readily demonstrated in decerebrate animals. Under normal circumstances, the tonic neck reflexes and the labyrinthine reflexes act together, but the tonic neck reflexes have been studied in isolation in animals from which the labyrinths have been removed and the labyrinthine reactions in animals in which the position of the neck has been rigidly fixed.

The effect of the neck reflexes is that if the head is turned to one side, the limbs on the side to which the head is turned extend, whereas the extensor muscles on the opposite side relax. If the head is bent backwards the hindlimbs extend whereas the forelimbs relax; the opposite effect is observed if the head is bent forwards. The labyrinth reactions are mediated by the otolith organ that responds to the position of the head in space. They bring about an increase in extensor tonus when the animal is recumbant, a decrease when it is prone. The centres for these reflexes are situated in the lowest part of the medulla and the first two segments of the cervical cord.

Both the tonic neck and the tonic labyrinthine reactions also have an influence on the external ocular muscles, the effect of which is to maintain the direction of gaze, notwithstanding changes in the position of the head.

Righting Reflexes

A decerebrate animal cannot right itself if it falls. An animal with the midbrain intact, however, will not only maintain a standing posutre with a normal distribution of extensor and flexor tonus but is able reflexly to revert to its normal posture if it falls. The righting reflexes can be studied in a midbrain or thalamus animal, and include labyrinthine reflexes which will bring the head to its normal upright position, neck reflexes which align the body correctly with the head and reflexes from the skin which will right the body of a labyrinthectomized animal if it is placed on its side on a board so that the surface of the body is stimulated asymmetrically. The effect of these reflexes are illustrated very clearly by what happens to a cat if it falls when it always lands on its feet. Even if the cat falls with its feet upwards, the labyrinthine righting reflexes will cause its head to turn and become vertical and then the neck reflexes cause its body to turn and align itself with its head. This will take place even if the cat is unable to see, but in cats and dogs and higher mammals visual righting reflexes make it possible for the animal to right itself rapidly even after labyrinthectomy.

The centres of the brain necessary for the integrity of the righting reflexes include the pons, where the neck righting reflexes are integrated, and the midbrain, where the labyrinthine and body righting reflexes are centred. The visual reflexes are mediated through the cerebral cortex.

The wide variety of righting mechanisms provides an assurance against loss of this function and Magnus in 1925 wrote:

'The multiplicity of reflexes, causing and maintaining the correct position, makes it intelligible how labyrinthless deaf–mutes can stand and walk without apparent disturbance. Only if brought under water, where the optical impressions cannot be used and no body righting reflexes can be evoked, are they completely disorientated and will be drowned if they are not helped out of the water.'

Placing and Hopping Reactions

The postural mechanisms which have been described above, all, with the exception of those depending on vision, depend on reflexes which can take place in a decorticate preparation. More complex postural reactions are only possible if the cerebral cortex is intact. One of these is the hopping reaction that takes place to restore the centre of gravity when an animal is pushed off balance. This is a complex reaction which is also less efficiently performed if the cerebellum is damaged. The placing reactions can occur both in response to visual and tactile stimuli. Thus, if an animal is lowered on to a table it will, if able to see, place its limbs so that they will support the body without further adjustment. If the animal is blindfolded and the hindlegs are placed on the table it will rapidly adjust the position of the limbs so that they are correctly placed to support the body. These placing reactions are not present in a newborn baby and Roberts (1967) has suggested that they cannot be explained simply as inborn reflexes but must depend also on a learning process.

THE CEREBRAL CONTROL OF MOVEMENT

In the above section an account has been given of certain of the reflexes necessary for maintaining the standing posture. Many of these are basically spinal reflexes, but they require to be supplemented by reflexes centred in the brain and they are in varying degrees under the influence and control of centres in the brain stem and cerebral hemispheres. In the more complex forms of life the higher centres of the brain become increasingly important in the performance of organized movement. Thus, although some varieties of fish can swim if the cord is transected below the medulla, and spinal frogs may be able to jump and fish and amphibia in general show normal locomotion if the medulla is intact, a spinal mammal cannot stand, and birds and mammals are unable to move about unless the higher centres of the brain are intact. In the study of the cerebral control of movement, it is useful to designate as the motor system those structures which are concerned in the control of movement together with their connecting pathways.

Traditionally it has been customary to speak of the motor system as consisting of two divisions, viz, the pyramidal or corticospinal system and the extrapyramidal system. The corticospinal system may be regarded as a system of fibres which arise from neurones in the motor area of the brain in the precentral gyrus and pass without interruption to the motor neurones in the brain stem and spinal cord. Its function has been considered to be that of transmitting the impulses which initiate voluntary movement. The extrapyramidal system includes a complex system of fibres that pass from various parts of the cortex to end in subcortical nuclei, such as the basal ganglia, the reticular formation and brainstem nuclei, which in turn give off ascending, descending or interconnecting relays. This classification of the motor system is clinically useful, but there are difficulties in its application since not all fibres carried in the pyramidal tracts are derived from the motor cortex or pass directly, without synapse, to the anterior horn cells. A further structure, that is related to the motor system and which has powerful co-ordinating and regulatory functions in connection with the control of movement, is the cerebellum.

An important concept, which was introduced into neurology by Hughlings Jackson and which is of particular importance in connection with disorders affecting the motor system, is that of positive and negative signs. It depends on the idea that the nervous system has evolved into a system of functional levels, the more recently developed having a controlling influence on the more primitive. A negative sign represents loss of function due to destruction of the part of the system that is concerned with that function. A positive sign is one produced by an intact part of the nervous system which is released from control by another part that has suffered damage. On this basis, one would expect a lesion of the corticospinal or pyramidal system to produce negative signs, notably paralysis of the affected part, without any of the increase in reflex activity which occurs in spasticity. The extrapyramidal system is partly excitatory and partly inhibitory and lesions in it produce a wide variety of positive and negative signs. Lesions of the pyramidal tract are seldom confined to corticospinal fibres because throughout most of its course its fibres are intermingled with extrapyramidal fibres, many of which have an inhibitory action on reflexes at a spinal level. For this reason, damage to the pyramidal pathway generally produces the negative sign of paralysis together with the positive signs of hyperactive reflexes and varying degrees of spasticity.

THE CORTICOSPINAL OR PYRAMIDAL SYSTEM

The Motor Cortex

The earliest experiments which showed that movements of the opposite side of the body would result from electrical stimulation of the exposed cortex were carried out by Fritsch and Hitzig in 1870, who used galvanic current to stimulate the brain of the dog. These observations were confirmed and developed soon afterwards by Ferrier. The idea that movements are represented on the convolutions of the brain had been advanced a short time before by Hughlings Jackson on the basis of his observations on focal epileptic seizures. Later studies, notably those of Grünbaum and Sherrington (1903) on different animals, including the higher anthropoids, have made it possible to map out those areas of cortex which give rise to particular movements following electrical stimulation. Bartholow, in 1874, stimulated the cortex of a patient who had a skull defect resulting from a chronic abscess and produced contralateral movements as well as tingling sensations, and subsequently neurosurgeons, in particular Cushing and Foerster, showed that the cerebral cortex could be stimulated in conscious patients undergoing surgery under local anaesthesia to produce movements and sensations in particular parts of the body. By this means, Penfield and his colleagues were able to produce precise maps of the motor areas of the human cortex. (Penfield and Boldrey, 1937.)

The principal motor area of the cortex lies in the precentral gyrus and is the mirror image of the principal sensory area which lies in the adjacent postcentral gyrus. The cells of the motor cortex give rise to the fibres which comprise the pyramidal tracts and include the giant pyramidal cells of Betz, which lie in that part of the cortex which has been designated in Brodmann's histological classification as area 4. However, the Betz cells account for only a relatively small proportion of the fibres of the pyramidal tract, and the representation of the body over the motor cortex extends rostrally to include Brodmann's area 6. The size of the cortical areas is conditioned by the variety and complexity of the movements they subserve. Thus, the largest cortical areas are those representing the hand, especially the thumb, and the face, and particularly the tongue (Fig. 10.1). Hughlings Jackson regarded the motor cortex as the 'middle level' of cerebral organization and he envisaged that movements were represented at this

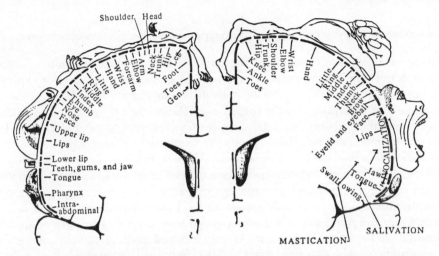

FIG. 10.1. Diagram to show projection of body on the contralateral postcentral gyrus (left) and representation of movements on the motor cortex (right). Motor and sensory homunculus obtained by direct stimulation of exposed cortex in patients operated on under local anesthesia. Penfield, W. and Rasmussen, T. (1950). *The Cerebral Cortex of Man.* New York: Macmillan.

level in overlapping fields of excitability. On the other hand, others have found evidence for a punctate representation of individual muscles (see Walshe 1943, Phillips 1973).

On the medial surface of the brain rostral to the precentral motor area is a smaller area of cortex which also will give rise to motor responses following stimulation. This is known as the supplementary motor area. Stimulation of the supplementary motor area produces slower movements of the contralateral side of the body than those that follow stimulation of the precentral motor area (Penfield and Welch, 1951). Excision of either the precentral motor area or the supplementary motor area, in man, will give rise to paralysis. In lesions of the supplementary motor area, however, spasticity may be a conspicuous feature.

Although the areas which will give rise to organized movement following electrical stimulation form a relatively small part of the cerebral cortex, experimental work has shown that the fibres of the pyramidal tract arise from relatively extensive areas of the cortex and that a substantial proportion arise from the postcentral regions. Two methods of study have provided useful information in tracing the source of pyramidal fibres. One is to study which areas of cortex need to be removed or destroyed to cause degeneration of pyramidal tract fibres (Russell and DeMeyer, 1961). Another is to determine the sites from which evoked potentials may be recorded on the cortex after antidromic impulses have been set up in the pyramidal tracts by stimulation of the medullary pyramids (Woolsey and Chang, 1947).

The Pyramidal Pathway

The somatotopic arrangement of the parts of the body on the motor cortex accounts not only for the effect of experimental stimulation, but also for clinical phenomena, such as the spread of convulsive movements in a focal epileptic seizure that is determined by the spread of excitation over the cortex. The representation of the body on the motor strip covers a relatively wide area. Lesions in this situation will not infrequently give rise to paralysis of only a portion of the contralateral half of the body, for example, a single limb. In the internal capsule the somatotopic representation occupies a smaller area, since the fibres from the cortex have converged and damage to this part is likely to cause a relatively complete hemiplegia. This also applies to the pyramidal pathway in the brain stem where the fibres are still more crowded together and where, in addition, somatotopic organization has been largely lost and fibres from areas of cortex representing widely differing parts of the body are situated close together (Barnard and Woolsey, 1956).

Although in the cat it appears that the pyramidal fibres end at synapses that connect with interneurones, in primates, many make direct connection with spinal motoneurones (Hoff and Hoff, 1934; Bernhard and Bohm, 1954). It is possible, by using weak anodal stimuli applied directly to the cortex, to bring about a highly localized excitation of cortical neurones and by recording with electrodes in the spinal cord to identify sites on the cortex which will excite particular spinal motoneurones. By this method, it has been shown that motoneurones can be excited by groups, or colonies of cortical neurones, and that the colonies concerned with distal muscles appear to be concentrated into a narrower area of cortex than those concerned with proximal muscles (Phillips, 1967).

Of particular interest, in connection with the cerebral control of movement, is the possibility that there exist tonic and phasic pyramidal tract neurones comparable to the tonic and phasic motoneurones which have been demonstrated in the spinal cord (see chapter 5). Evarts (1965) has provided evidence for this by stimulating cortical neurones antidromically from the medullary pyramids and showing that large neurones have fibres that have a rapid conduction velocity and discharge during active movement of the limb, whereas other fibres derived from smaller nerve cells are tonically active when the contralateral limbs are quiescent.

Weak antidromic stimulation of pyramidal tract fibres will produce inhibitory postsynaptic potentials in cortical neurones. This is likely to be due to excitation of recurrent collateral branches which have an inhibitory effect similar to that produced by the Renshaw loop in the spinal cord. The latency of the effect is sufficient to allow passage through a single inhibitory interneurone and in some instances, is long enough to include a polysynaptic inhibitory pathway. This recurrent inhibitory system seems likely to have an important stabilizing effect on cortical motoneurone discharges and is of possible clinical importance as a mechanism for preventing the uncontrolled spread of discharge that may occur in epilepsy (Phillips, 1959; Stefanis and Jasper, 1964; see Eccles, 1969 and Granit, 1970).

The monosynaptic connections which have been demonstrated between pyramidal tract neurones and spinal motoneurone, involve the α neurones in the spinal cord. Although stimulation of the motor cortex can activate the muscle spindles, it is not known how far excitation of the γ pathway may take place directly or must pass through subcortical connections in the brain stem and elsewhere.

Disease and Injury Affecting the Corticospinal System

If the motor cortex or the pyramidal tract suffers injury in man, as a result of trauma or invasion by a tumour or destruction by haemorrhage, the usual consequence is paralysis of the contralateral side of the body together with spasticity (see chapter 6). Whereas paralysis is a negative sign, spasticity is clearly a positive sign, or release phenomenon. The presence of both paralysis and spasticity in patients with pyramidal lesions would therefore imply that the corticospinal system has both excitatory and inhibitory effects on voluntary movement. However, it is only in a few localized situations, such as the decussation of pyramids, that the pyramidal tract can be shown to consist almost entirely of fibres derived from cortical pyramidal cells. Moreover, disease affecting the pyramidal tracts frequently involves other descending pathways at the same time.

Although lesions confined to the pyramidal pathway are rare in man, they can be produced in animals by section of the medullary pyramids. Tower (1940) carried out a detailed study of the effects of both unilateral and bilateral section of the pyramids in the rhesus monkey. Following unilateral section, there occurred paresis of the opposite side of the body which was associated with hypotonicity of the muscles, so that the limbs hung loosely from the body, with sluggish tendon reflexes and diminished or absent abdominal and cremasteric reflexes. In the rhesus monkey, it is not possible to obtain a consistant pathological extensor plantar response, but this is obtained following pyramidal section in the chimpanzee. The impairment of movement did not take the form of complete paralysis, but instead, there was difficulty in performing specific co-ordinated movements, such as fine movements of the fingers.

The effects of lesions of the motor area of the cortex in the monkey likewise include poverty of movement on the contralateral side, and spasticity is absent unless the supplementary motor area is also damaged. It is of interest that a lesion confined to one precentral motor area may result in contralateral impairment of movement, with hypotonia and diminished tendon reflexes, but is also associated with loss of abdominal reflexes and an abnormal plantar response. Travis found that removal of one supplementary motor area had little effect, but after bilateral ablation, there was marked flexor spasticity, yet the plantar responses remained flexor and the abdominal reflexes were preserved (Travis, 1955a and b). The position is not absolutely clear, however, for Denny-Brown (1966) has found little spasticity after removal of the supplementary area. He concludes that removal of the rostral part of the motor area leads to a general release of stretch reflexes and is associated with the hemiplegic posture.

There is a strong case for considering that the spasticity that is so generally a feature of clinical hemiplegia in man is not the direct consequence of damage to the pyramidal pathway, but is related to simultaneous injury to neighbouring descending fibre systems which exert a controlling influence on reflex activity in the spinal cord. Isolated lesions of the pyramidal pathway are probably rare in man. However, it is of interest that in an early or slight lesion affecting this system, clumsiness of fine movements of, for example, the hand may be a more conspicuous feature than weakness. If it is remembered that accurate movement requires not only activation of the musculature but also close correlation of movement with sensory information, it is reasonable to anticipate that the earliest effect of injury to the sensory-motor cortex is likely to be impairment of controlled voluntary movement.

Paralysis resulting from hemisphere lesions and damage to the descending pathways is frequently associated with muscular atrophy of the affected part. This is much less pronounced than the wasting which results, for example, from a peripheral nerve lesion, and it has generally been attributed to the effects of disuse which arises from the paralysis. The suggestion has been made, however, that it could result from the withdrawal of a trophic influence from cortical neurones on spinal motoneurones. There is some evidence that in hemiplegia there may be loss of nerve cells in the spinal cord (Botez, 1971; McComas *et al.*, 1971).

THE EXTRAPYRAMIDAL SYSTEM

It is convenient to include those parts of the motor system which are not included in the direct pathway between the cortex and the motor neurones, viz, the corticospinal or pyramidal system, under the general heading of extra-pyramidal system. Walshe (1947) has used the expression to include efferent cortical systems, other than pyramidal, as well as those subcortical systems of neurones which are concerned with movement. As such it is not a homogeneous system. It includes the system of fibres that pass between the cortex, the basal ganglia and the thalamus and brain stem nuclei on the one hand, the cortico strio reticular system, and the cerebellum on the other. Its role in the control of movement differs widely in different species and has been greatly modified in the course of evolution. In the higher mammals, the cortex of the fore-brain has assumed increasing importance in the control of movement. In simpler forms of life, movement is very largely controlled by subcortical centres. Thus, fish and amphibia can swim and move about with little impairment of control provided the brain stem is intact. In birds, which are capable of a highly complex variety of organized movement, the fore-brain is made up largely of corpus striatum. Elaborate behaviour patterns are possible in the absence of cortex, provided that the corpus striatum is intact. In man, the mode of action of the subcortical centres of the brain, and in particular the basal ganglia, remains poorly under-stood, but they are clearly of great importance in the control of movement and posture. Disease affecting these structures may be followed by many varieties of disordered movement.

The Basal Ganglia

The basal ganglia are a group of fore-brain nuclei and include the caudate nucleus, the putamen, the claustrum and the globus pallidus. These discharge into a group of brain stem nuclei, which include the subthalamic nucleus or corpus Luysii, the substantia nigra, the red nucleus and the reticular formation. The caudate nucleus, the claustrum and the putamen are together known as the corpus striatum. The putamen and the globus pallidus are sometimes referred to as the lentiform nucleus. However, it is usual to consider the structures forming the corpus striatum together, since they have a similar development and histo-logical structure, and are distinct from the globus pallidus, which is also spoken of as the pallidum. The structures comprising the striatum share a common development from the lateroventral wall of the telencephalic vesicle. They contain two distinct populations of neurones, viz, small to medium sized cells of 10–30μ diameter and large cells of about 55μ. The pallidum is derived from the diencephalon and is composed predominantly of larger cells of about 40–60μ which tend to be longer and narrower than the large cells of the striatum (Mettler, 1968).

The basal ganglia receive afferents from the cerebral cortex, from the thalamus and also from the brain stem nuclei, in particular the substantia nigra. The corpus striatum discharges into the globus pallidus and the outflow from the pallidum is principally to the brain stem nuclei, but fibres also pass between it and the thalamus. Many of the downgoing fibres from the globus pallidus end by connecting with cells of the reticular formation in the pons and medulla (Fig. 10.2).

There is much that is not understood regarding the functions of the basal ganglia. It has not been possible to ascribe clearly defined functions to the individual structures which comprise the system. One reason for this is that access to this part of the brain for experimental purposes is difficult. Another is that the basal nuclei interact with each other in a complex set of circuits which influence and are acted on by widely separated parts of the nervous system.

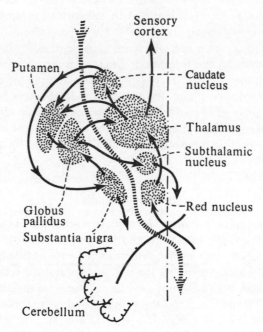

FIG. 10.2. Diagram to show basal ganglia and principal connections.

Lesions of the basal ganglia give rise both to negative signs, due to loss of function, and to positive signs, resulting from release of function. Although much has been learned from experimental studies in which particular structures have been stimulated or destroyed, a great deal of what is known arises from the study of disease of the basal ganglia, which results in important disturbances of posture and movement. The treatment of these disorders by the surgical production of discrete lesions in the basal nuclei has provided useful additional information. The pharmacological study of amines that may be active as chemical transmitters in this part of the brain has added to the knowledge derived from earlier clinical and experimental studies.

Experimental Lesions of the Basal Ganglia

The effect of stimulation of the caudate nucleus is to bring about the arrest of spontaneous movement. This was first demonstrated in the cat by Mettler (1942) and has subsequently been confirmed many times by different workers. Destruction of the caudate nucleus, on the other hand, is followed by hyperactivity and Denny-Brown, in his Croonian lectures (1960 and 1962), has described how bilateral ablation of the caudate nucleus in the monkey results in a continuous restless pacing of the animal up and down the cage. Stimulation of the putamen has likewise been found to result in inhibition of movement. Lesions of the putamen in monkeys have been followed by generalized rigidity of the limbs and walking has been handicapped by defective placing reactions (Denny-Brown, 1962).

Mettler observed no marked effects following stimulation of the globus pallidus, and unilateral lesions in animals also have little effect. Denny-Brown (1960) produced bilateral lesions of the globus pallidus in the monkey placed so as to interrupt the efferent pathway. Following this, the animals were at first unable to stand and lay in a flexed posture with limbs firmly flexed. Gradually, the animals learned to walk, but both visual and tactile placing reactions were defective. Labyrinthine and optic righting reflexes were lost so that if the animals were held upside down and allowed to fall, they failed to right themselves. These effects were not produced by lesions which spared the efferent outflow. The production of rigidity, poverty of movement and defective postural reastions by experimental lesions of the globus pallidus is of interest in connection with the clinical condition of Parkinson's disease, since bradykinesia, defective righting reflexes and rigidity may all be present in this disease. On the other hand, surgical lesions stereotactically placed in the globus pallidus are effective in relieving both the rigidity and tremor of Parkinson's disease (see below).

Considerable interest attaches to the substantia nigra, since cell loss in this region is an important pathological finding in many patients with Parkinson's disease. It is known also that many of the neurones, the axons of which end in the corpus striatum where they contain relatively high concentrations of dopamine, are situated in this part of the brain. Carpenter and McMasters (1964), however, found that unilateral lesions in monkeys had no observable effect and that the effects of stimulation were inconspicuous. Experimental lesions in this situation may, however, on occasion give rise to hypokinesia without rigidity or tremor (Sourkes and Poirier, 1966; Stern, 1966).

The Pharmacology of the Basal Ganglia

In an earlier section the distribution in the brain and the role as possible chemical transmitters of a number of biologically active substances has been discussed. the substances which are of particular interest as possible transmitters in the basal ganglia include acetylcholine and the amines noradrenaline, dopamine and 5-hydroxytryptamine (5-HT). Particular interest attaches to dopamine since the concentration of this substance in the basal ganglia is markedly reduced in Parkinson's disease. The administration to patients with this disease of its precursor L-DOPA has been followed by clinical improvement.

Gross analysis of cerebral tissue has shown that, whereas noradrenaline is present in high concentrations in the hypothalamus and the midbrain, dopamine has its highest concentration in the caudate nucleus. Histochemical studies (see chapter 4) have confirmed the gross analysis in that the hypothalamus shows dense accumulations of fibres containing noradrenaline and the caudate nucleus a dense fluorescence due to dopamine. Neurones containing 5-HT are present in the brain stem, where there are also neurones containing catecholamines. The monoamines present in neurones are found in highest concentration in the nerve terminals. The amines are mainly concentrated in varicosities that lie in close contact with cell bodies or dendrites and which are found along the whole length of the nerve terminals. They may be specialized structures in which monoamines are formed, stored and later released. The cell bodies of neurones which contain dopamine are found in the midbrain, in the zona compacta of the substantia nigra, and contain only small concentrations of dopamine. The axons arising from these cells have low concentrations of dopamine, but if they are divided, the concentrations of amine in the proximal portions increases sufficiently to allow ready identification. It would appear that there is a continuous transport of amine storage granules from the cell bodies to the terminals via the nerve fibres. These findings have made it possible to map out in detail the course of nerve pathways involved in the monoamine system and in particular, to demonstrate a system of neurones that contain dopamine, have their cell bodies in the substantia nigra and give rise to fibres which terminate in the striatum (see Fuxe and Anden, 1966).

A number of possible transmitter substances have been applied by microelectrophoresis to the cells of the caudate nucleus. If acetylcholine is applied in this way, it is found to give rise to an increased discharge of caudate neurones. Noradrenaline and dopamine, on the other hand, each reduce spontaneous activity, dopamine having the more marked effect. They also reduce activity which has been induced by application of acetylcholine (Bloom *et al.*, 1965). If the substantia nigra is stimulated, the neurones of the striatum undergo inhibition (Connor, 1968).

Another method of study has been to adminster drugs which modify the action of transmitter substances in the brain. One approach has been to administer reserpine, which causes depletion of amines, and then restore the amine concentration by administering their precursors, the active substances do not readily penetrate the blood brain barrier. (Carlsson, 1966). If reserpine is given to rats, this results not only in depletion of brain and tissue 5-HT and noradrenaline, but also of dopamine. This depletion of dopamine can be restored by giving its precursor L-DOPA. If drugs such as reserpine or chlorpromazine are given to man or animals, a parkinsonian syndrome is induced. Whereas reserpine causes a marked depletion both of dopamine and its metabolite methoxytyramine, after chlorpromazine there is no alteration in brain dopamine, but a marked increase occurs in its metabolites, in particular homovanillic acid. A possible explanation of the effects of chlorpromazine and other phenothiazine drugs is that it causes a competitive blockade of dopamine receptors.

It is of interest that effects similar to those which result from dopamine depletion can be produced by the administration to laboratory animals of substances which have a cholinergic effect. Two substances which have been studied are tremorine (1,4-Dipyrrolidino-2-butyne) and its metabolite oxytremorine. These are muscarinic agents comparable in potency to acetylcholine and lacking either nicotinic or anticholinesterase properties. Administration to laboratory animals produces a syndrome characterized by tremor, rigidity, lack of spontaneous movement and marked parasympathetic stimulation. Monkeys take on the appearance of parkinsonism. The effects are reversed by atropine and other drugs which are of value in Parkinson's disease (Jenden, 1966).

The Clinical Symptoms of Basal Ganglia Disease

Martin and his colleagues (1962) have characterized disorders of voluntary movement as giving rise to positive and negative symptoms. The positive symptoms include rigidity, tremor and a variety of complex involuntary movements. The negative symptoms include a generalized impoverishment of movement or bradykinesia and a number of disturbances of postural control. In Parkinson's disease, both positive and negative symptoms occur, but in other disorders of the basal ganglia, such as Huntington's chorea, the torsion dystonias and Wilson's disease, involuntary movements may predominate. Marsden and Parkes (1973) have classified involuntary movements into five main clinical categories, viz., tremor, chorea, myoclonus, tic and torsion dystonia, or athetosis. Of these tremor, chorea and torsion dystonia are clearly recognized as dyskinesias related to basal ganglia disease. Myoclonus and tics, on the other hand, have a less clearly defined relationship to the extrapyramidal system, but both can give rise to movements which closely resemble those of other dyskinesias in particular those of chorea. Although myoclonus is frequently associated with epilepsy, it occurs in many patients who do not have fits. Halliday (1967) has described a form in which the jerks are relatively slow and prolonged as 'extrapyramidal myoclonus'. The disorders of movement considered in the present section are listed below.

(1) Rigidity—plastic or cogwheel

(2) Tremor
    a. Static
    b. Postural
    c. Intention
(3) Chorea
    a. Generalized
    b. Hemichorea
(4) Athetosis
(5) Torsion Dystonia
(6) Bradykinesia

Rigidity

The rigidity which occurs in Parkinson's disease is sometimes referred to as plastic or lead pipe in quality since it represents a relatively unchanging resistance throughout the whole range of a passive movement. It differs from the hypertonus of spasticity where the resistance to passive stretch gradually increases to a maximum and then gives way. Sometimes the resistance to passive movement in Parkinson's disease has an irregular intermittent character when it is termed cogwheel rigidity. This has been assumed to be due to its modulation by a superimposed tremor. However, in Parkinson's disease, cogwheel rigidity is not infrequently present before tremor is evident. Lance *et al.* (1963) have suggested that, in some instances, the cogwheel effect is related to an exaggeration of physiological tremor (see below). Rigidity may be first noted in the flexors of the fingers and wrist and although it generally affects both flexors and extensors, it tends to be more pronounced in the flexor muscles.

Rigidity can be markedly diminished by section of the dorsal roots (Pollock and Davis, 1930) and intramuscular procaine can also reduce rigidity without causing loss of muscle power (Walshe, 1924; Rushworth, 1960). It would appear that rigidity must, in some measure, depend on the integrity of the stretch reflex arc and possibly the γ efferent system. It has been suggested that the principal factor in rigidity is hyperactivity of the γ efferent system. However, there is increasing evidence that rigidity is largely influenced by an increased discharge of α neurones. If a rat has a lesion placed in the substantia nigra, the dopamine content of the neostriatum is lowered, but there are no marked motor effects until the animal is given reserpine. The animal then develops a unilateral akinetic syndrome with tremor and predominantly flexor rigidity on the affected side. Administration of L-DOPA leads to marked hyperactivity on the unaffected side. Steg (1964, 1966) has recorded the activity of α and γ fibres in single fibres in the ventral roots and found that after reserpine, the discharge of γ fibres ceases and α discharge is increased. This effect was reversed by administration of L-DOPA, which also abolished the rigidity and akinesia. The effect of reserpine could be mimicked by cholinergic drugs such as physostigmine. These experiments suggest that one function of the nigrostriatal dopaminergic system is to regulate the balance between γ efferent and α motoneurone activity, and that dopamine and acetylcholine exert opposing actions in this connection.

The recovery of the amplitude of the H reflex (see chapter 6) after a conditioning stimulus has been studied as a measure of the excitability of the α motoneurones pool. It has been found that in patients with parkinsonian rigidity, the H reflex recovers more rapidly after a conditioning stimulus than in normal controls, and this may be reversed by thalamotomy (Olson and Diamantopoulos, 1967) and by treatment with L-DOPA (McLeod and Walsh, 1972). This is also consistent with an increased excitability of the α motoneurone pool in patients with rigidity.

It is not known which centres in the basal ganglia bring about the changes that give rise to rigidity, but experimental lesion of the putamen may be followed by marked rigidity. Surgical lesions in the globus pallidus and its outflow to the thalamus and in the ventrolateral nucleus of the thalamus will abolish ridigity, so it would appear that the disturbance lies in a lack of balance between different portions of a circuit which includes these structures.

Tremor

The tremor of Parkinson's disease is unique in that, characteristically, it is present when the limb is at rest and as such, it must be distinguished from postural tremors, which are only present when a limb is maintaining a posture, and from intention tremor which develops when a voluntary movement is carried out. Characteristically, it is a slow tremor with a frequency of 5–6 Hz and consists of regular alternating contractions of agonists and antagonists. Often it is most evident at the fingers, the regular adduction and abduction movements of the thumb in relation to the flexed fingers giving rise to the classical 'pill-rolling' movement. Eventually, it may be present in both upper and lower limbs, affecting the tongue, the jaw and in some cases, the whole head. Frequently it is present in the eyelids when the eyes are lightly but not firmly closed. It disappears during sleep but may be brought on or enhanced by anxiety or sometimes by mental concentration. When it is severe, it may no longer be completely abolished by the maintenance of a posture or by voluntary movement. In some cases of Parkinson's disease, the tremor is not conspicuous at rest but becomes obvious during movement. Denny-Brown (1962) has maintained that the association of movement with tremor is of limited value in determining its nature. He suggests that parkinsonian tremor, athetosis and chorea are all related disorders of posture. On this basis, the action tremor of Parkinson's disease may represent a variant of the same process. Others have maintained that it is a separate entity, possibly related to physiological tremor (Lance *et al.*, 1963; Marshall, 1968).

The physiological mechanisms underlying parkinsonian tremor are unknown and there is no certain information regarding the location of the lesions responsible for its production. It is of interest that unlike rigidity, it is not abolished by infiltration of an affected muscle with local anaesthetic (Walshe, 1924). It is abolished, however, by stereotactic lesions in the same part of the brain as are effective in relieving rigidity, viz, the globus pallidus, its outflow to the thalamus and the ventrolateral nucleus of the thalamus. When electrodes have been implanted into several different situations in the thalamus during stereotactic surgery for the relief of tremor, regular spike discharges have been recorded which occur at the same rate as the tremor (Albe-Fessard *et al.*, 1967). It may be, therefore, that tremor arises from a disturbance arising in a circuit which includes the thalamus and possibly the pallidum and the cerebral cortex, and which is normally under inhibitory control from other parts of the basal ganglia system. Since treatment with L-DOPA is capable of relieving parkinsonian tremor, it is possible that the nigrostriatal pathway has an inhibitory function in this respect.

Postural tremor can arise from a variety of conditions and one of the most widely studied varieties is physiological tremor, which is present in nearly all healthy individuals. This is absent at rest, but is present whenever a limb maintains a posture and persists throughout a voluntary movement. It involves all muscle groups, but cannot normally be seen with the naked eye, requiring special transducers to record it. In adult life it has a frequency of the order of about 10/sec but is slower in childhood and in old age. It can be recorded from the lower limbs in complete paraplegia and may be absent in patients with tabes, so its mechanism would appear to depend on the integrity of the spinal reflex arc. It has been suggested that its mechanism may therefore arise from oscillation around a servoloop which includes the muscle, the efferent and afferent neurones and possibly the γ efferent system. A number of individuals have a tremor which may be severe enough to provoke attention, but which in other respects, has the characteristics of physiological tremor. This has been given the name of essential tremor, or familial tremor, since it may be inherited as a Mendelian dominant. Usually no treatment is necessary for this condition, but it is of interest that in severe cases it can be relieved by stereotactic thalamotomy. If it is inherently the same as physiological tremor and depends on oscillation in a servo loop at spinal level, it is evident that this oscillation must normally be exposed to damping from centres in the brain and that the thalamus is included in this system (Marshall, 1968). Other forms of postural tremor such as those associated with anxiety, thyrotoxicosis and fatigue may also be exaggerations of physiological tremor but the tremor of cerebellar disease is unrelated and more probably the result of hypotonia. Intention tremor (see below) is only present during a voluntary movement and occurs in disease of the cerebellum generally when it affects the pathway leading from the cerebellum to the red nucleus. It is the result of breakdown of the servo mechanism whereby the cerebellum acts as an error detector in carrying out a voluntary movement.

Dystonia, Athetosis and Chorea

Denny-Brown (1962) has defined dystonia as a fixed attitude of the body which is associated with other extrapyramidal disorders of movement. Many localized dystonias may occur and were a conspicuous feature of postencephalitic parkinsonism. In the later stages of Parkinson's disease, the body assumes a posture of generalized flexion, which has been referred to as generalized flexion dystonia. Torsion dystonia occurs in its most severe form as dystonia musculorum deformans which may occur as a hereditary disorder with either a dominant or recessive inheritance. The relatively common disorder of spasmodic torticollis is probably a mild form of torsion dystonia. In dystonia musculorum deformans the most conspicuous pathological change is dense bilateral scarring of the putamen. It is of interest that some cases of Wilson's disease, where there is deposition of copper in the basal ganglia, progress to a terminal hemiplegic state which Denny-Brown has termed hemiplegic dystonia. These patients may show severe scarring with cavitation of the putamen on one side.

Athetosis is a disorder of movement and posture in which the body moves slowly from one dystonic posture to another. It may involve the upper and lower limbs, the face and tongue. Its most severe form is the condition known as double athetosis, in which the pathology resembles that of dystonia musculorum deformans with severe scarring of the putamen on either side. Athetosis can develop in adult life as a complication of cerebral vascular disease, but more commonly it presents in childhood in association with cerebral palsy.

In chorea, the movements are more rapid and affect the face, tongue, and distal portions of upper and lower limbs. They show no evident relationship to posture and occur seemingly at random without achieving any evident purpose. Transient grimacing movements of the face are common and may closely resemble tics or habit spasms. If choreiform movements become slow and increase in amplitude, they may gradually come to take on the character of athetosis and one may speak of choreoathetosis. In Huntington's chorea, which is inherited as an autosomal dominant, the pathological changes affect predominantly the putamen, the caudate nucleus and the frontal cortex. In Sydenham's or rheumatic chorea, no definite changes have been noted in the basal ganglia. Unilateral chorea, which is known as hemiballismus, may sometimes develop following a vascular lesion affecting the contralateral subthalamic nucleus and is also an occasional complication of stereotactic thalamotomy.

It is of interest that a variety of forms of dystonia may occur as a complication of drug therapy. Occasionally, patients who have been on treatment over an extended period with phenothiazines may develop an orofacial dyskinesia which persists even after withdrawal of the drug. Dyskinesia may also develop in the course of treatment with L-DOPA in Parkinson's disease. This may take various forms including torticollis, inward rotation of the foot and grimacing movements of the face. The changes are reversible in that they cease on withdrawal of the drug and they do not occur in healthy volunteers who take L-DOPA (Barbeau, 1970). The movements resemble those which may occur in Huntington's chorea and it is interesting that in this condition the movements may be reduced by administration of either reserpine or tetrabenazine, which deplete the brain of catecholamines. If we regard the globus pallidus as having a facilitatory effect on movement that is inhibited by the striatum, this is consistant with the association of pathological damage to the striatum with involuntary movement. Some of the actions of L-DOPA might be explained on the basis of an inhibitory effect on neurones in the striatum.

Bradykinesia and Disturbances of Posture

Generalized slowness of movement with loss of associated movements is one of the cardinal features of Parkinson's disease and is almost invariably present in some degree. There is poverty of facial expression with infrequent blinking, the arms cease to swing during walking and when the patient sits he appears to sit unnaturally still with a complete absence of fidgeting movements. Fine voluntary movements such as fastening and unfastening buttons become slow and difficult and the handwriting becomes irregular and small. As time goes on, all movement becomes progressively slowed and the patient finds that everyday tasks take progressively longer to carry out. It becomes increasingly difficult for the patient to initiate a voluntary movement. Here it is of interest that even severely disabled patients retain the ability to move quickly in an emergency situation or under the influence of strong emotion, a feature which has been termed 'kinesia paradoxa'.

Bradykinesia is not, as a rule, benefited by stereotaxic surgery, but may diminish markedly after administration of L-DOPA, an effect which can perhaps be interpreted as related to re-establishment of the inhibitory action of dopamine on the cells of the striatum. If the pallidum contains neurones which have a facilitatory effect on movement, depression of the inhibitory action of the striatum may lead to a restoration of natural movement. Experimental lesions of the globus pallidus in monkeys result in profound akinesia and it is possible that in a number of conditions where bradykinesia is a feature, such as carbon monoxide poisoning, the disturbance may result directly from the effect of damage to the pallidum.

Martin and his colleagues (1962) have drawn attention to the marked disturbances of posture which occur particularly in postencephalitis Parkinson's disease. Thus, there may be failure of postural fixation of the head or even the trunk which may be flexed to nearly 90°. The reflexes which maintain equilibrium may be lost so that the patient may topple over if pushed and the ability to rise from the supine to standing posture may be gravely impaired. Experimental lesions of the globus pallidus result in loss or severe impairment of the righting reflexes. It is likely that this part of the brain is implicated in the disturbances of postural control which occur in Parkinson's disease. Denny-Brown (1960) has emphasized the importance of the globus pallidus in the integration of movement and has referred to it as the 'head ganglion' of the motor system in primates.

The Reticular Formation

The brain stem contains in addition to the long ascending and descending tracts of white matter that pass through it, and the nuclei of the cranial nerves that emerge from it, a number of important centres of grey matter which are concerned in the control of posture and movement. These include the substantia nigra, the subthalamic nucleus, the vestibular nuclei and the red nucleus. In addition, the brain stem contains a central network of neurones that extend rostrally from the medulla to the thalamus and which is known as the reticular formation. This is an important interconnecting centre receiving ascending fibres from the spinal cord and also many connections from the cerebral cortex, basal ganglia, cerebellum and the sensory nuclei in the brain stem. The nerve cells in the reticular system give rise to ascending fibres which pass to the cerebral cortex through the thalamus and probably also by independent pathways. These ascending pathways from the reticular formation have given rise to the name ascending reticular activating system (see chapter 12). Descending fibres from the reticular formation pass to the spinal cord in the reticulospinal tract. The descending reticular system has been shown to exert important effects on the control of movement.

Magoun and his colleagues (see Magoun, 1950) have shown that stimulation of the caudal part of the reticular formation in the medulla gives rise to depression of spinal reflexes and motor activity induced by cortical stimulation, and will also abolish decerebrate rigidity. Stimulation of the rostral and lateral parts of the formation gave rise to facilitation of motor activity and enhancement of reflexes. These observations were made on anaesthetized animals. It is of interest that stimulation of the reticular formation with implanted electrodes in the conscious animal has been followed by co-ordinated stepping movements and changes in posture (Sprague and Chambers, 1954).

The Cerebellum

The cerebellum arises embryologically as an outgrowth of the roof of the fourth ventricle. In simpler forms of life, the cerebellum is an outfolding of the fourth ventricle with vestibular connections. This forms the major part of the cerebellum in fish and amphibia and the flocculonodular lobe or archicerebellum in mammals. In birds and mammals, the cerebellum is highly developed and the anterior and lateral lobes have extensive connections with the spinal cord and the cerebral hemispheres.

The cerebellum has no direct connections through a descending pathway with the motor neurones in the spinal cord and removal of the cerebellum is not followed by any loss of voluntary movement. Damage to the cerebellum is, however, followed by difficulty in performing co-ordinated movement and it is evident that its function lies in the control and regulation rather than in the initiation of movement. This control is possible because the cerebellum receives information from the vestibular apparatus, from proprioceptors in the limbs and from the cerebral cortex. Through its outflow it is able to influence both the cortex and subcortical nuclei in the brain stem. Sherrington emphasized its importance in the control of postural reactions and termed it the 'head-ganglion of the proprioceptive system' (Sherrington, 1906). Eccles has likened the cerebellum to a computer which controls movement by integrating sensory information to act as an error detector. It is of interest that it appears to exert its control, to a large extent, through inhibitory mechanisms, since the cells of the cerebellar cortex exert an inhibitory action on the outflow from the cerebellum through the cerebellar nuclei. They are exposed to varying degrees of inhibition through the afferent fibres which act on the cells of the cerebellar cortex (Eccles, 1969).

Anatomical Structure

The anatomy of the cerebellum is complex and more than one terminology has been applied to it, but it has been found convenient to distinguish the earliest portion of the cerebellum to evolve, viz, the flocculonodular lobe, from the remainder of the cerebellum that forms the corpus cerebelli. The corpus cerebelli is separated from the flocculonodular lobe by the posterolateral fissure and is itself divided into an anterior and a posterior lobe by the fissura prima. The flocculonodular lobe has been termed the archicerebellum, the anterior lobe and certain midline structures of the posterior lobe, the paleocerebellum, and the lateral lobes of the cerebellum, the neocerebellum. The medially situated portion of the cerebellum is termed the vermis, in contrast to the hemispheric portions. The cerebellar hemispheres have an outer layer of gray matter, the cerebellar cortex, and a deeper layer of white matter. In this lie three pairs of nuclei which are close to the roof of the fourth ventricle. These nuclei include the most medially situated nucleus fastigii, the nuclei globosus and emboliformis and the laterally placed dentate nuclei.

The efferent outflow from the cerebellar cortex is to the deeply situated nuclei. Thus, the medial portion of the cerebellum, or the vermis, sends fibres to the fastigial nuclei, the intermediate portions to the nuclei globosus and emboliformis and the more laterally placed parts to the dentate nuclei. The output from the flocculonodular lobe is to the vestibular nuclei. The efferent fibres from the fastigial nuclei pass to the vestibular nuclei and the reticular formation, the efferents from the laterally placed nuclei go to the red nucleus and to the thalamus. Afferent impulses to the cerebellum pass to the cerebellar cortex and enter the cerebellum through the inferior, middle and superior cerebellar peduncles, and are derived from both the spinal cord and the cerebral cortex.

Histologically, the cerebellar cortex consists of three layers, viz, an outer or molecular layer, a layer of Purkinje cells and an inner layer of granule cells. The Purkinje cells provide the sole efferent outflow from the cerebellar cortex and they project to the vestibular nuclei and to the deep nuclei of the cerebellum.

Two types of fibre enter the cerebellum and project on to the Purkinje cells. The first are the climbing fibres, which arise in the cells of the superior and inferior olivary nuclei. They end by connecting with the dendrites of the Purkinje cells which ramify in the molecular layer of the cortex. In general, each Purkinje cell does not receive more than one climbing fibre afferent, although it is possible that one climbing fibre may activate more than a single Purkinje cell. Climbing fibres pass to all areas of the cerebellar cortex and they relay impulses, both from the muscles and skin, and from the cerebral cortex. A more complex input arrangement is provided by the mossy fibres, which do not connect directly with the Purkinje cells, but form synapses with the cells of the granular layer. The axons of the granule cells pass perpendicularly into the molecular layer where they bifurcate to become the parallel fibres, which travel parallel to the surface of the cerebellum and form excitatory synapses with the dendrites of Purkinje cells. In addition, they connect with other cells that have been shown to act as inhibitory interneurones. The first of these is the basket cell, the axon of which forms inhibitory synapses with the Purkinje cells. A second is the golgi cell, that sends fibres to connect with the granule cells. The mossy fibre input thus differs in a number of respects from that of the climbing fibres. Firstly, the one to one relationship of climbing fibre to Purkinje cell is not present, since each mossy fibre can connect with hundreds of Purkinje cells through the parallel fibres. Secondly, although the parallel fibres provide an excitatory connection by direct contact with the Purkinje cells, this effect is modified by the inhibitory loops provided by the interneurones, which are also activated by the parallel fibres.

The input to the cerebellum from the olivary nuclei passes via the climbing fibres to all parts of the cerebellar cortex. Other structures project via the mossy fibres and tend to be concentrated in particular regions of the cortex according to their source. Thus, the vestibular input ends principally in the flocculonodular lobe and the midline vermis of the anterior lobe. The spinocerebellar connections pass to both the posterior and anterior lobes but are concentrated in the medial portion of the anterior lobe. The corticopontine input passes to all portions of the cerebellum except the flocculonodular lobe, but the largest number of fibres ends in the lateral portions of the anterior and posterior lobes, that is in the cerebellar hemispheres.

Somatatopic Organization

The above anatomical description makes it possible to attach some functional significance to the different anatomical regions of the cerebellum. Thus, the flocculonodular lobe, which is connected predominantly with the vestibular

H

system is clearly concerned with posture and equilibrium. The anterior lobe and the medial part of the posterior lobe, which receive afferents from the spino cerebellar tracts and communicate with descending spinal pathways through the reticular formation and other brain stem nuclei, are concerned, perhaps predominantly, with stretch reflexes and postural tone. The lateral lobes of the

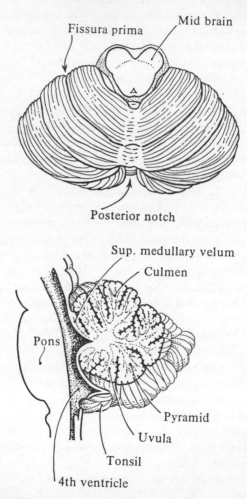

Fissura prima

Mid brain

Posterior notch

Sup. medullary velum

Culmen

Pons

Pyramid

Uvula

Tonsil

4th ventricle

Fig. 10.3. General morphology of cerebellum.

cerebellum have important connections with the cerebral cortex so that there is good reason to associate them with the control of voluntary movement. Electrophysiological studies in which it has been shown that evoked potentials can be obtained from particular points on the cerebellar cortex following stimulation of different portions of the body, have illustrated a different aspect of functional localization. Two separate representations have been recorded. In the anterior lobe, the body is represented with the hind limbs situated rostrally, the head caudally and each half of the body on the ipsilateral cortex. In the posterior lobe there is a separate representation with each half of the body represented bilaterally (Fig. 10.3), (Adrian, 1943; Snider and Stowell, 1944).

These areas of the cerebellar cortex, which are concerned with particular parts of the body, communicate with corresponding parts of the cerebral cortex. Thus, stimulation of the cerebellar cortex will give rise to evoked potentials in corresponding portions of the cerebral cortex and if the sensory-motor cortex of the cerebral hemispheres is stimulated, evoked potentials can be obtained from corresponding parts of the cerebellar cortex.

Ablation and Stimulation Experiments

The effect of removal of the cerebellum varies greatly in different forms of life. Thus, fish and amphibia may retain the ability to swim, but in birds, standing and flying may be grossly impaired. In dogs and cats, there may be opisthotonus and extensor rigidity immediately after cerebellectomy, with difficulty in standing and walking as compensation develops. In monkeys, this marked extensor rigidity is not seen, but there is disturbance of equilibrium, particularly after removal of the midline structures and impaired co-ordination after lesions affecting the hemispheres. In the decerebrate animal, removal of the cerebellum increases decerebrate rigidity, but this is associated with a decreased outflow along the γ pathway (Granit *et al.*, 1955). In cats that have had the cerebellum removed, extensor hypertonus develops, but this is accompanied by a decrease in the frequency of spindle afferent discharges and the rigidity is not blocked by section of the dorsal roots. Ligation of the arterial supply to the brain results in extensor rigidity that is due to necrosis of the anterior lobe of the cerebellum (Pollock and Davis, 1927). On the other hand, stimulation of the anterior lobe of the cerebellum may abolish decerebrate rigidity. This is apparently the result of inhibition of fusimotor activity. Granit (1970) has suggested that the cerebellum, and the Purkinje cells in particular, plays an important part in regulating the activity of the fusimotor system (see chapter 6).

Mode of Action of the Cerebellum

Much has been learned regarding the mechanisms of cerebellar action by studies carried out using techniques of microelectrode recording to study the responses of the Purkinje cells and their connections. This work has been largely developed by Eccles and his colleagues. If a microelectrode is inserted into the molecular layer of the cerebellar cortex, it is possible to record potentials from Purkinje cells which can be identified by stimulating the deep cerebellar nuclei and recording antidromic responses. If an electrode is inserted into the inferior olive, it can be used to activate climbing fibres and exert a powerful depolarizing effect on the Purkinje cells, which is all-or-nothing in character. Stimulation of the mossy fibre input can be carried out by stimulating a peripheral nerve, by applying stimuli directly to the mossy fibres or by activating the parallel fibres that are readily accessible to cortical stimulation and serve to connect the mossy fibre input to the Purkinje cells since they form the axons of the granule cells. Stimulation of the parallel fibres results in excitation of the Purkinje cells followed by

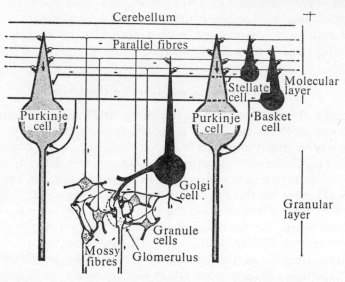

FIG. 10.4. Diagram showing the principal features that have been postulated for the mossy fibre input and the cerebellar glomerulus. The Golgi, stellate and basket cells are all inhibitory in action and are shown by convention in black. The broken line represents the glial lamella that ensheaths a glomerulus. The diagram is drawn as for a section along the folium and the main distribution of the basket and stellate cells should be perpendicular to the plane of the diagram, but they are also distributed as shown to a band of several Purkinje cells along the folium. The arrows indicate the direction of impulse propagation. Eccles, J. C. (1969). *The Inhibitory Pathways of the Central Nervous System.* Liverpool University Press.

hyperpolarization. It is clear therefore that the mossy fibres exert both an excitatory and an inhibitory effect on the Purkinje cells. The excitatory effect is due to the direct action of the parallel fibres on the Purkinje cells. The inhibitory effect comes about through the action of interneurones, in particular the basket cells, which are activated by the parallel fibres but which exert an inhibitory effect on the Purkinje cells, an effect which Eccles has termed 'feed-forward' inhibition. At the same time, a feedback inhibition takes place through a second set of inhibitory interneurones, the Golgi cells, which make inhibitory connection with the granule cells. It is of interest that the output of the Purkinje cells to the cerebellar nuclei is inhibitory in character, so that any effect of the afferent input on the Purkinje cells serves to vary their inhibitory output. Eccles has likened the process whereby the cerebellum achieves control on movement as one that is akin to sculpturing, where form is achieved by taking away from an amorphous mass (Eccles, 1966), (Fig. 10.4).

The functional role of the climbing and mossy fibre systems has been subject to much discussion. One hypothesis assumes that the Purkinje cells are under the excitatory and inhibitory influences of the mossy fibre system continuously and that the climbing system provides a 'read out' mechanism which can test the excitability of a Purkinje cell at any instant (Eccles *et al.*, 1967). Another hypothesis postulates that the mossy fibre input exerts a tonic effect on large numbers of Purkinje cells to establish the background level of inhibition on the cerebellar nuclei. The climbing fibres, on the other hand, activate small groups of Purkinje cells and are able thus to produce short periods of inhibition on the target cells of the Purkinje axons. The climbing fibres thus provide a phasic system which can modulate the tonic effects derived from the mossy fibreparallel fibre input (Llinas *et al.*, 1970).

Symptoms of Cerebellar Deficiency

The clinical disturbances of function which occur in patients with disease affecting the cerebellum were very fully described by Gordon Holmes in his Croonian lectures (1962) and later in the Hughlings Jackson lecture (1939). Later work has added little to his clinical descriptions. On the whole, the clinical effects of disease affecting particular parts of the cerebellum correlate well with what is known regarding the anatomical connections and functions of particular portions of the cerebellum. An interesting feature of cerebellar disease in man, is the ability of the brain to compensate for cerebellar damage. This is particularly evident after acute lesions when the immediate effects may be severe, but where compensation may eventually be nearly complete.

In disease affecting the flocculonodular lobe there is a profound disturbance of posture and balance that is sometimes referred to as trunk ataxia, in which the patient may walk unsteadily on a broad base and may tend to fall backwards. The difficulty in maintaining a vertical posture may be evident also when the patient attempts to sit upright in bed. Nystagmus may be present, but it may be difficult to demonstrate either hypotonia or ataxia of the limbs. If the midline and intermediate structures of the anterior lobe are affected, trunk ataxia is less marked, nystagmus may be absent but there is a marked disturbance of gait which is associated with ataxia that affects predominantly the lower limbs. The flocculonodular lobe may be affected by midline tumours of the cerebellum, in particular medulloblastomas, which most commonly occur in childhood. Asbury *et al.* (1959) have described changes which occur in the midline structures of the anterior lobe of the cerebellum in alcoholics. In disease affecting the posterior lobe and the cerebellar hemispheres, the disturbance of voluntary movement affects predominantly the upper limbs. The cerebellar hemispheres are particularly well developed in man. This part of the cerebellum is richly endowed with connections to and from the cerebral cortex receiving afferents from the corticopontine fibres and sending efferents via the red nucleus and the thalamus. Disease of this part of the cerebellum characteristically presents as defective modulation of voluntary movement.

In disease of one cerebellar hemisphere, disturbances of movement occur on the same side of the body as the lesion. The disturbance of voluntary movement is frequently accompanied by hypotonia, in the sense of a diminished resistance to passive movement. This hypotonia makes it difficult for the patient to maintain the posture of the outstretched limbs and may account for the postural tremor which is sometimes observed. It also accounts for the pendulous character of the tendon reflexes. Holmes (1922) has ascribed the nystagmus of cerebellar disease, which is essentially a fixation nystagmus in which the eyes drift slowly from the fixation point towards the midline and jerk toward the periphery, as due to a defect of postural tone in the muscles that maintain the posture of the eyes in the position to which they have been brought by voluntary movement. Disturbances of voluntary movement include dysmetria, in which the range of voluntary movements is disturbed so that, for example, a patient who tries to touch something may overshoot the mark, and decomposition of movements, in which a complex movement is broken into its component parts and carried out out of sequence. Intention tremor is an excellent example of the cerebellum failing to act as an error detector, so that the limb strays from its path during a voluntary movement and correcting movements give rise to course oscillations.

REFERENCES

ADRIAN, E. D. (1943). Afferent areas in the cerebellum connected with the limbs. *Brain*, **66**, 289–315.

ALBE-FESSARD, D., ARFEL, G., GUIOT, G., DEROME, P. and GUILBAUD, G. (1967). Thalamic unit activity in man. *Electroenceph. clin. Neurophysiol.*, suppl. **25**, 132–142.

ASBURY, A. K., VICTOR, M. and ADAMS, R. D. (1963). Uremic polyneuropathy. *Arch. Neurol. (Chicago)*, **8**, 413–428.

BARNARD, J. W. and WOOLSEY, C. W. (1956). A study of localization in the corticospinal tracts of monkey and rat. *J. comp. Neurol.*, **105**, 25–50.

BARBEAU, A. (1970). Rationale for the use of L-dopa in the torsion dystonias. *Neurology (Minneap.)*, **20**, 96–102.

BERNHARD, C. G. and BOHM, E. (1954). Cortical representation and functional significance of the corticomotoneuronal system. *Arch. Neurol. Psychiat. (Chicago)*, **72**, 473–502.

BLOOM, F. E., COSTA, E. and SALMOIRAGHI, G. C. (1965). Anaesthesia and the responsiveness of individual neurons of the caudate nucleus of the cat to acetylcholine, norepinephrine and dopamine administered by microelectrophoresis. *J. Pharmacol. exp. Ther.*, **150**, 244–252.

BOTEZ, M. I. (1971). Some clinical findings concerning muscular atrophy of central origin. *Europ. Neurol.*, **5**, 25–33.

CARLSSON, A. (1966). Morphologic and dynamic aspects of dopamine in the central nervous system. In: *Biochemistry and Pharmacology of the Basal Ganglia*. Ed. Costa, E., Coté, L. J. and Yahr, M. D. New York: Raven Press.

CARPENTER, M. B. and McMASTERS, R. E. (1964). Lesions of the substantia nigra in the Rhesus monkey. *Amer. J. Anat.*, **114**, 293–319.

CONNOR, J. D. (1968). Caudate unit responses to nigral stimuli: evidence for a possible nigro-neostriatal pathway. *Science*, **160**, 899–900.

DENNY-BROWN, D. (1960). Diseases of the basal ganglia, their relation to disorders of movement. *Lancet*, **ii**, 1099–1105 and 1155–1162.

DENNY-BROWN, D. (1962). *The Basal Ganglia and their Relation to Disorders of Movement*. London: Oxford University Press.

DENNY-BROWN, D. (1966). *The Cerebral Control of Movement*. Liverpool: Liverpool University Press.

ECCLES, J. C. (1966). Functional organisation of the cerebellum in relation to its role in motor control. In: *Muscular Afferents and Motor Control*. Ed. Granit, R. New York: John Wiley & Sons.

ECCLES, J. C. (1969). *The Inhibitory Pathways of the Central Nervous System*. Liverpool: Liverpool University Press.

ECCLES, J. C., ITO, M. and SZENTAGOTHAI, S. (1967). *The Cerebellum as a Neuronal Machine*. Berlin: Springer-Verlag.

EVARTS, E. V. (1965). Relation of discharge frequency to conduction velocity in pyramidal tract neurones. *J. Neurophysiol.*, **28**, 216–228.

FUXE, K. and ANDEN, N.-E. (1966). Studies on central monoamine neurons with special reference to the nigro-striatal dopamine neurone system. In: *Biochemistry and Pharmacology of the Basal Ganglia*. Ed. Costa, E., Coté, L. J. and Yahr, M. D. New York: Raven Press.

GRANIT, R. (1970). *The Basis of Motor Control*. London: Academic Press.

GRANIT, R., HOLMGREN, B. and MERTON, P. A. (1955). The two routes of excitation of muscle and their subservience to the cerebellum. *J. Physiol. (Lond.)*, **130**, 213–224.

GRÜNBAUM, A. S. F. and SHERRINGTON, C. S. (1904). Observations on the physiology of the cerebral cortex of the anthropoid ape. *Proc. roy. Soc. (Lond.)*, **72**, 152–155.

HALLIDAY, A. M. (1967). *The Clinical Incidence of Myoclonus in Modern Trends in Neurology*. 4. Ed. William, D. London: Butterworths.

HOFF, E. C. and HOFF, H. E. (1934). Spinal terminations of the projection fibres from the motor cortex of primates. *Brain*, **57**, 454–474.

HOLMES, G. (1956). *Selected Papers of*. Compiled and edited by Walshe, F. M. R. London: Macmillan.

JACKSON, H. (1932). *Selected Writings of*. Ed. Taylor, J. Vols. I and II. London: Hodder and Stoughton.

JENDEN, D. (1966). Studies on tremorine antagonism by structurally related compounds. In: *Biochemistry and Pharmacology of the Basal Ganglia*. Ed. E. Costa, Coté, L. J. and Yahr, M. D. New York: Raven Press.

LANCE, J. W., SCHWABM, R. S. and PETERSON, E. A. (1963). Action tremor and the cogwheel phenomenon in Parkinson's disease. *Brain*, **86**, 95–110.

LLINAS, R. R., HILLMAN, D. E. and PRECHT, W. (1970). Functional aspects of cerebellar evolution. In: *The Cerebellum in Health and Disease*. Ed. Fields, W. S. and Willis, W. D. London: Hilger.

McCOMAS, A. J., SICA, R. E. P., UPTON, A. R. M., AGUILERA, N. and CURRIE, S. (1971). Motoneurone dysfunction in patients with hemiplegic atrophy. *Nature*, **233**, 21–23.

McLEOD, J. G. and WALSH, J. C. (1972). H reflex studies in patients with Parkinson's disease. *J. Neurol. Neurosurg. Psychiat.*, **35**, 77–80.

MAGNUS, R. (1925). Croonian Lecture—Animal Posture. *Proc. roy. Soc. B.*, **98**, 339–353.

MAGOUN, H. W. (1950). Caudal and cephalic influences of the brainstem reticular formation. *Physiol. Rev.*, **30**, 459–474.

MARSDEN, C. D. and PARKES, J. D. (1973). Abnormal movement disorders. *Hospital Medicine*, **10**, 428–450.

MARTIN, J. P., HURWITZ, L. J. and FINLAYSON, M. H. (1962). The negative symptoms of basal ganglia disease. A survey of 130 postencephalitic cases. *Lancet* **ii**, 1-6 and 62–66.

METTLER, F. A. (1942). Relation between pyramidal and extrapyramidal function. *Res. Publ. Ass. nerv. ment. Dis.*, **21**, 150–227.

METTLER, F. A. (1968). Anatomy of the basal ganglia. In: *Diseases of the Basal Ganglia*. Vol. 6. Ed. Vinken P. J. and Bruyn, G. W. Amsterdam: North-Holland Publishing Co., pp. 1–55.

OLSEN, P. Z. and DIAMANTOPOULOS, E. (1967). Excitability of spinal motor neurones in normal subjects and patients with spasticity, Parkinsonian rigidity and cerebellar hypotonia. *J. Neurol. Neurosurg. Psychiat.*, **30**, 325–331.

PENFIELD, W. and BOLDREY, E. (1937). Somatic motor and sensory representation in the cerebral cortex of man as studied by electrical stimulation. *Brain*, **60**, 389–443.

PENFIELD, W. and WELCH, K. (1951). The supplementary motor area of the cerebral cortex. *Arch. Neurol. Psychiat.* (*Chicago*), **66**, 289–317.

PHILLIPS, C. G. (1959). Actions of antidromic pyramidal volleys on single Betz cells in the cat. *Quart. J. exp. Physiol.*, **44**, 1–25.

PHILLIPS, C. G. (1967). Corticomotoneural organization. *Arch. Neurol.* (*Chicago*), **17**, 188–195.

PHILLIPS, C. G. (1973). Cortical localization and 'sensorimotor processes' at the 'middle level' in primates. *Proc. roy. Soc. Med.*, **66**, 987–1002.

POLLOCK, L. J. and DAVIS, L. (1927). The influence of the cerebellum upon the reflex activities of the decerebrate animal. *Brain*, **50**, 277–312.

ROBERTS, T. D. M. (1967). Neurophysiology of postural mechanisms. London: Butterworths.

RUSHWORTH, G. (1960). Spasticity and rigidity: an experimental study and review. *J. Neurol. Neurosurg. Psychiat.*, **23**, 99–118.

RUSSELL, J. R. and DEMEYER, W. (1961). The quantitative cortical origin of pyramidal axons of Macaca rhesus. *Neurology*, **11**, 96–108.

SHERRINGTON, C. S. (1906). The integrative action of the nervous system. New York, reprinted 1947 Cambridge: University Press.

SNIDER, R. S. and STOWELL, A. (1944). Receiving areas of the tactile, auditory and visual systems in the cerebellum. *J. Neurophysiol.*, **7**, 331–357.

SOURKES, T. L. and POIRIER, L. J. (1966). Amines of the striatum: relation to experimental tremor in the monkey. In: *Biochemistry and Pharmacology of the Basal Ganglia*. Ed. Coste, E., Coté, L. J. and Yahr, M. D. New York: Raven Press.

SPRAGUE, J. M. and CHAMBERS, W. W. (1954). Control of posture by reticular formation and cerebellum in the intact, anaesthetized and unanaesthetized and in the decerebrated cat. *Amer. J. Physiol.*, **176**, 52–64.

STEFANIS, C. and JASPER, H. (1964). Recurrent collateral inhibition in pyramidal tract neurons. *J. Neurophysiol.*, **27**, 855–877.

STEG, G. (1964). Efferent muscle innervation and rigidity. *Acta physiol. scand.*, **61**, suppl. 225.

STEG, G. (1966). Effects on α- and γ-efferents of drugs influencing neostriatal mono-aminergic and acetylcholinergic transmission. In: *Control and Innervation of Skeletal Muscle*. Ed. Andrew, B. L. Edinburgh: Livingstone.

STERN, G. (1966). The effects of lesions in the substantia nigra. *Brain*, **89**, 449 478.

TOWER, S. S. (1940). Pyramidal lesion in the monkey. *Brain*, **63**, 36–90.

TRAVIS, A. M. (1955a). Neurological deficiencies after ablation of the precentral motor motor area in Macaca Mulatta. *Brain*, **78**, 155–173.

TRAVIS, A. M. (1955b). Neurological deficiences following supplementary motor area lesions in Macaca Mulatta. *Brain*, **78**, 174–198.

WALSHE, F. M. R. (1924). Observations on the nature of the muscular rigidity of paralysis agitans, and on its relationship to tremor. *Brain*, **47**, 159–177.

WALSHE, F. M. R. (1943). On the mode of representation of movements in the motor cortex with special reference to 'convulsions beginning unilaterally' (Jackson). *Brain*, **66**, 104–139.

WALSHE, F. M. R. (1947). On the role of the pyramidal tract in willed movement *Brain*, **70**, 329–354.

WOOLSEY, C. N. and CHANG, H.-T. (1947). Activation of the cerebral cortex by anti-dromic volleys in the pyramidal tract. *Res. Publ. Ass. nerv. ment. Dis.*, **27**, 146–161.

CHAPTER 11

The Autonomic System

The major part of the nervous system, which is concerned with the activation of skeletal muscle, that is to a large extent under voluntary control, has been termed the somatic nervous system and reflexes concerned with voluntary muscle are known as somatic reflexes. A separate division of the nervous system controls the action of smooth muscle, cardiac muscle and the secretion of the glands and is known as the autonomic nervous system. The autonomic system consists of two anatomically separate divisions, the sympathetic and the parasympathetic and these in general have opposing actions.

Anatomically autonomic efferent nerves differ from somatic motor nerves in that the efferent neurones lie outside the nervous system in peripheral autonomic ganglia. The nerve cells in the spinal cord, unlike somatic motor neurones, are not the final common pathway, and their nerve fibres which travel to the ganglia are known as preganglionic fibres. These are small myelinated B fibres, and because the myelin sheath gives them a white appearance, the bundles of fibres that they form are known as white rami communicantes. The postganglionic fibres are unmyelinated C fibres and arise from nerve cells in the autonomic ganglia. Afferent fibres arise in the viscera (see chapter 7) but although they may pass through the autonomic ganglia, they enter the cord through the dorsal roots where the first sensory neurone is situated. Since they follow the same course as somatic sensory nerves, it is generally held that the autonomic system is essentially a motor system. Another important difference between the autonomic and somatic systems is that although somatic motor nerves all have an excitatory function, inhibitory processes taking place centrally, autonomic nerves have an excitatory action on the heart, whereas in this situation parasympathetic nerves have an inhibitory effect.

Important actions of the sympathetic include dilatation of the pupils, acceleration of the heart, vasoconstriction, vasodilatation, dilatation of the bronchi, inhibition of intestinal motility and secretory activity and closure of the sphincters. Glucose is liberated from glycogen in the liver and the adrenal medulla is stimulated to secrete adrenaline, which leads also to dilatation of the blood vessels in skeletal muscle. These actions are all ones which take place before and during physical exertion. This led Cannon to say that the sympathetic prepares the body for fight or flight. The actions of the parasympathetic are, in general, opposite. Thus, it causes constriction of the pupils, slowing of the heart and increased motility of the intestines with outpouring of secretions. However, not every organ receives both parasympathetic and sympathetic innervation and in those that do, the two divisions are not necessarily equally important. Thus the arterioles, with certain important exceptions such as the salivary glands and the genitalia, have virtually no parasympathetic innervation and the action of the parasympathetic is considerably more important than the sympathetic in controlling the heart rate and the emptying of the bladder.

In all autonomic ganglia the chemical transmitter is acetylcholine, which is also liberated by postganglionic parasympathetic nerve fibres. Postganglionic sympathetic nerves on the other hand act by liberating noradrenaline, although there are a few exceptions, such as the sympathetic nerves which innervate the sweat glands and sympathetic vasodilator nerves to skeletal muscle, which liberate acetylcholine. In the central nervous system, the principal activating centres for the autonomic system are in the hypothalamus.

ORGANIZATION OF THE AUTONOMIC SYSTEM

The Sympathetic

The sympathetic outflow arises from nerve cells in the grey matter of the thoracic and upper lumbar segments of the spinal cord. These give rise to preganglionic nerve fibres, which end either in the ganglia of the sympathetic chain or in one of the peripheral ganglia that lie in the abdominal cavity. In general, the sympathetic ganglia, in contrast to the parasympathetic ganglia, are situated some distance from the organs which the sympathetic innervates, so that postganglionic fibres tend to be long and preganglionic fibres comparatively short.

The sympathetic chain consists of bundles of nerve fibres connecting a series of ganglia which lie on each side of the vertebral column. In the thoracic, lumbar and sacral regions there is one ganglion for each spinal nerve root but in the cervical region, these have fused into three, the superior, middle and inferior cervical ganglia. The inferior cervical ganglion is sometimes fused with the first thoracic to form the stellate ganglion.

Preganglionic fibres emerge from thoracic and upper lumbar segments and pass to the sympathetic chain in white rami communicantes. In the sympathetic chain, some connect with nerve cells in the corresponding ganglion, others pass up or down the chain to connect with neurones at other levels. A number pass out of the sympathetic chain without synapse to end in ganglia which lie in relation to abdominal viscera. These ganglia include the coeliac ganglion, the superior and inferior mesenteric ganglia, and the hypogastric ganglia. They are found in a complex series of nerve plexuses that lie in front of the aorta close to the origins of the large abdominal vessels. The nerves to these ganglia travel

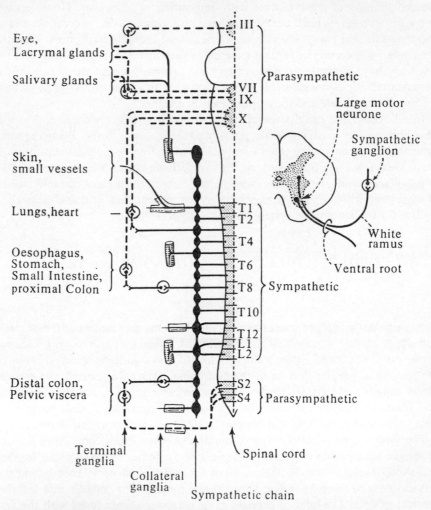

FIG. 11.1. Diagram to show main features of autonomic system.

in the splanchnic nerves and a few pass through the coeliac ganglion without synapse to end in the adrenal medulla.

Postganglionic fibres pass from the sympathetic ganglia to their destinations, either in association with spinal nerves or by travelling along with small arteries.

Those that are to travel with spinal nerves pass back from the sympathetic chain to the spinal nerve roots as grey rami communicantes. Although only the thoracic and upper two or three lumbar segments give off a white ramus, grey rami pass to all the spinal nerve roots. Sympathetic fibres are ultimately distributed to the skin, sweat glands, blood vessels, dilator pupillae muscle, thoracic organs and the abdominal viscera (Fig. 11.1).

The Parasympathetic

Preganglionic parasympathetic nerve fibres travel either in association with cranial nerves or in the pelvic nerves which arise from the second and third sacral segments. The preganglionic fibres are relatively long, the terminal ganglia lying close to the organ supplied. The third cranial nerve carries preganglionic fibres, which end in the ciliary ganglion whence postganglionic fibres pass to the constrictor pupillae and the ciliary muscle. The seventh cranial nerve carries fibres which end in the sphenopalatine ganglion which supplies the lachrymal gland. Other fibres in the seventh and ninth nerves pass to ganglia which supply the salivary glands. The tenth cranial nerve carries the parasympathetic supply to the thoracic and all the abdominal viscera except those supplied by the pelvic nerves.

Chemical Transmission in the Autonomic System

Chemical transmission at the neuromuscular junction and in the central nervous system has been discussed eleswhere (see chapter 4, 5 and 9). In the autonomic system, chemical transmission is of particular interest in that the concept of humoral transmission first developed in the study of this part of the nervous system. It is here also that the pharmacology of chemical transmission has been most thoroughly established. Furthermore, the therapeutic possibilities of modifying the chemical transmission of nerve impulses by drugs have been particularly prominent in connection with the autonomic nervous system.

Sympathetic Transmitters

The first suggestion that nerves might act by liberating a chemical transmitter was made by Elliott in 1904 who suggested that this might be the explanation for the previously noted (Langley, 1901) similarity between the effects of adrenaline and sympathetic stimulation. Later, in 1921, Loewi showed that stimulation of the vagus led to the liberation of a substance in the perfused heart of the frog that could cause slowing or arrest in a second heart. This action was abolished by atropine and if the sympathetic supply to the atropinized heart was stimulated, acceleration of the heart occurred. He called the substance which slowed the hear 'vagusstoff' and the substance liberated by the sympathetic fibres 'acceleranstoff'. Vagusstoff was later identified as acetylcholine. At about the same time, Cannon and Uridil (1921) showed that stimulation of the splanchnic nerves to the liver resulted in an increase in heart rate even if the adrenal gland was removed. This substance liberated by the hepatic nerves came to be known as sympathin. Sympathin produced in this way resembled adrenaline in certain respects. For example, it accelerated the heart and produced contractions of the nictitating membrane of the cat, after it had been rendered hypersensitive by denervation and treatment with cocaine. These are both strong effects of adrenaline, but its action in dilating the pupil or relaxing the uterus was weaker than that of adrenaline. Cannon and Rosenbleuth (1933) postulated that there must be two sympathins which they termed sympathin I (inhibitory) and sympathin E (excitatory). The matter was resolved in 1946 when von Euler showed that an extract of the splenic nerves had the characteristics of noradrenaline. It is now established that noradrenaline is the principle postganglionic sympathetic transmitter, adrenaline being liberated from sympathetic nerve endings in much smaller amounts. The reason why stimulation of the hepatic nerves has little effect on the uterus is that the uterus is less sensitive to noradrenaline than it is to adrenaline. Although adrenaline is the principal substance in the adrenal medulla, noradrenaline is also present in appreciable quantities.

Certain effects of adrenaline are blocked by substances such as ergotoxine or ergotamine. These include vasoconstriction and elevation of blood pressure, but not acceleration of the heart or relaxation of the uterus. Ahlquist (1948) suggested that adrenaline acted on two separate types of receptor which he termed α and β receptors. Activation of α receptors produced effects which were blocked by ergotamine. The effects of α activation included vasoconstriction, contraction of the uterus and dilatation of the pupil; those of β activation acceleration of the heart, vasodilatation and relaxation of the bronchi. When adrenaline and noradrenaline are compared, adrenaline is seen to act more or less equally on α and β receptors whereas noradrenaline acts almost exclusively on α receptors. Considerable interest has attached to the concept of α and β receptors since the identification of substances which block the action of adrenaline on the β receptors, such as propranalol, which has been found to be therapeutically useful in the control of cardiac arrhythmias.

The method by which adrenaline and noradrenaline are inactivated after release is unknown. It was originally considered that they were destroyed by the enzyme amine oxidase but it is doubtful if this is an important effect, although there is no doubt that other monoamines are destroyed by this enzyme.

A number of drugs have a marked effect on the liberation of noradrenaline. Alphamethyldopa interferes with the synthesis of noradrenaline by giving rise to the production of alphamethyl noradrenaline in its place, which is a relatively inactive substance and is therefore sometimes referred to as a false transmitter. Guanethidine and a number of other substances prevent the liberation of noradrenaline. Both αmethyldopa and guanethidine, by reducing vasoconstrictor tone, have been found to be useful in the treatment of hypertension. Reserpine also has an effect in lowering the blood pressure, which is secondary to its general effect in preventing the storage of catecholamines including noradrenaline.

Acetylcholine

The crucial experiment which showed that a substance, later identified as acetylcholine, was liberated in the body as a humoral transmitter was that of Loewi in 1921 when he showed that 'vagusstoff' would slow the isolated heart of the frog (see above). However, in 1914, Dale had shown that acetylcholine in low dosage could mimic the actions of muscarine and in higher dosage the actions of nicotine. Muscarine and nicotine are both alkaloids which have powerful pharmacological actions on the nervous system. Muscarine produces effects which closely resemble those resulting from parasympathetic stimulation, and the effects are blocked by atropine. Nicotine in small dosage stimulates the neuromuscular junction and autonomic ganglia and in higher dosage produces depression of conduction at both sites. The actions of nicotine are blocked by curare. Dale suggested that the actions of acetylcholine could be classified into nicotine- and muscarine-like actions. This has been a generally useful concept implying that in different situations there are specific receptors sensitive to muscarine or nicotine and that acetylcholine may react appropriately with either. This is now known to apply to the central nervous system also where both nicotine and muscarine actions of acetylcholine have been identified.

It was not definitely established that acetylcholine was present in the body until 1929 when it was isolated by Dale and Dudley. In 1933 Feldberg and Gaddum were able to show that if an autonomic ganglion was perfused with modified Ringer solution, acetylcholine could be isolated from the perfusate following preganglionic stimulation. It is now firmly established that acetylcholine is the chemical transmitter at parasympathetic nerve endings and at all autonomic ganglia. The actions of acetylcholine at the neuromuscular junction and in the central nervous system are discussed elsewhere where its synthesis, storage and fate are also reviewed (see chapters 4 and 5).

Transmission in Autonomic Ganglia

The evidence that acetylcholine is the chemical transmitter in autonomic ganglia is broadly similar to that in connection with its role in neuromuscular transmission (see chapter 4). The nature of the transmission process is clearly different in a number of respects. Firstly, the localization of cholinesterase is different since it is present in the preganglionic endings and not in the ganglion cells, so it is clearly not hydrolyzed after the nerve impulse as it is in muscle. Secondly the postsynaptic potential at the ganglion is more complex than the partial depolarization which constitutes the end–plate potential. Although the main effect of acetylcholine on the ganglion is on nicotine receptors, the effect of blocking agents on later phases of the postsynaptic potential suggests that the ganglion cell may, in addition, embody muscarine receptors and also adrenaline α receptors (Eccles and Libet, 1961).

A number of substances will produce transmission block at autonomic ganglia. Nicotine and tetramethylammonium produce a depolarization block, but their action at autonomic ganglia differs from that of depolarizing agents at the neuromuscular junction in that doses insufficient to produce block will produce effective stimulation. Substances which prevent the synthesis or release of acetylcholine, such as hemicholinium or botulinus toxin, will also produce ganglionic blockade. Curare will produce a competitive type block and a number of competitive blocking agents have been found clinically useful. Since ganglion block will block the sympathetic, the overall effect includes a reduction in vasoconstrictor tone and a fall in blood pressure. Ganglionic blocking agents, such as hexamethonium, pentolinium, mecamylamine and pempidine have been used as agents for the treatment of hypertension. Since ganglionic block affects the parasympathetic as well as the sympathetic, treatment with these agents is limited by side effects. They have been used less since the introduction of drugs which selectively block the release of noradrenaline from sympathetic endings. Since acetylcholine is not hydrolyzed in the autonomic ganglia by cholinesterase, as it is at the neuromuscular junction, anticholinesterases, such as neostigmine, are of little value in relieving competitive block in autonomic ganglia.

Denervation Hypersensitivity

Denervated skeletal muscle becomes hypersensitive to acetycholine, a change which is associated with the whole cell membrane and not merely the end–plate zone becoming excitable (see chapter 5). In the autonomic system denervation hypersensitivity is most marked after section of postganglionic fibres (Cannon and Rosenblueth, 1949), but the autonomic ganglia can also show denervation hypersensitivity. A similar hypersensitivity to adrenaline and noradrenaline may occur in organs which have been depleted of catechol amines by reserpine. The explanation of denervation hypersensitivity is unknown. With denervated skeletal muscle the hypersensitivity of the fibre membrane may be due to loss of some trophic factor from the motor neurone. Another factor at cholinergic endings may be the disappearance of cholinesterase following denervation. With adrenergic endings the mechanism is probably complex. Removal of noradrenaline from the site of action by enzymatic hydrolysis does not seem to be an important mechanism. There is evidence that after release from the granules in which it is stored, adrenaline is again taken up by the nerve ending and returned to the storage granules. Failure of this mechanism could account for denervation hypersensitivity (Hertting *et al.*, 1961). It is of interest that reserpine may cause depletion of noradrenaline in the nerve fibre by preventing its re-entry into the granules (Carlsson, 1964).

Denervation hypersensitivity is of clinical importance since the operation of sympathectomy rapidly loses its effect unless the preganglionic nerve fibres are divided. Russell (1956) has suggested that the impaired reaction of the Holmes–Adie pupil is due to parasympathetic denervation and that the tonic contraction and delayed relaxation are the result of supersensitization of the denervated sphincter pupillae to acetylcholine, liberated by intact parasympathetic nerves. There is pathological evidence that the lesion affecting the pupil lies in the ciliary ganglion (Harriman and Garland, 1968).

THE HYPOTHALAMUS AND AUTONOMIC INTEGRATION

Autonomic reflexes are organized at various levels in the nervous system. Thus, many autonomic reflexes are subserved at spinal level and will persist, after recovery from spinal shock, in the isolated cord. Under normal circumstances, however, they are subject to regulating influences from higher centres in the brain. Thus, reflex vasoconstriction and sweating may occur below the level of a spinal cord transection. Although they are not normally under voluntary control, sweating and vasoconstriction in the intact preparation are subject to changes in the body temperature and so come under the influence of the hypothalamus. The bladder reflexes are autonomic reflexes that are normally subject to voluntary control, but after cord transection may sometimes return as independent spinal reflexes.

In the brain stem there are also reflex centres which subserve autonomic reflexes but subject again to varying degrees of modification. The reflexes concerned with the contraction of the heart are mediated in the medulla. Although they are preserved after transection at the midbrain, emotional influences arising at a higher level under normal circumstances have important effects on the cardiovascular system.

Stimulation of the cerebral cortex will bring about autonomic discharges. Probably the most important cortical centres for the control of autonomic reflexes lie in the so-called visceral brain, or limbic lobe, which is particularly important in connection with emotional reactions. The principal subcortical integrating centre is the hypothalamus, which has widespread connections with other parts of the brain and with the autonomic outflow.

Connections of the Hypothalmus

The hypothalamus is a collection of nuclei that lie in the floor and walls of the third ventricle and extend backwards from the chiasma to the upper border of the pons. It lies above the pituitary to which it is connected by the pituitary stalk. The nuclei include anterior, middle and posterior groups. The supraoptic and paraventricular nuclei lie in the anterior group, the nuclei of the tuber cinereum comprise the middle group, and the posterior group include the posterior hypothalamic nuclei and the mamillary bodies (Fig. 11.2).

The hypothalamus receives afferents from the cerebral cortex and from the spinal cord, some of the latter afferents reaching it via the thalamus, others direct. Important afferent pathways include the medial fore-brain bundle which carries impulses from the cortex to the hypothalamus, the fornix that passes from the hippocampus to the mamillary bodies and the stria terminalis which connects the amygdala with the anterior nuclei. Efferents pass to the thalamus, which is probably the principal route to the cerebral cortex. Descending fibres pass initially to the reticular formation in the brain stem where fresh relays lead to autonomic neurones in the brain stem and the intermediolateral cell column of the spinal cord. The hypothalamicohypophysial tract passes from the supra-optic nucleus to the posterior lobe of the pituitary.

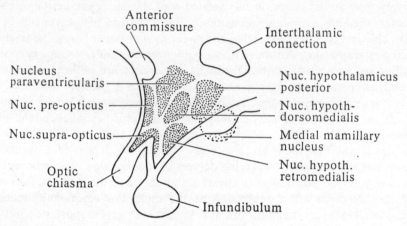

Fig. 11.2. The principal nuclei of the hypothalamus.

The experimental study of the hypothalamus has been carried out very largely by the application of localized stimuli through stereotactically placed electrodes (Hess, 1957). In this way, it has been shown that stimuli applied to particular sites will produce a wide range of visceral responses, including changes in blood pressure, micturition, salivation and pupillary responses. In addition, stimulation of the anterior hypothalamus in the cat gives rise to an aggressive reaction akin to rage. Another method of study has been by ablation experiments. Thus, lesions of the ventromedial nuclei in the tuber cinereum will give rise to obesity, suggesting that this part of the brain is important in connection with appetite and satiety. In addition to its other functions in relation to the autonomic system, the hypothalamus is an important integrating centre for the control of body temperature. Through its connection with the posterior pituitary it has an important role in the regulation of water balance. It also has an intimate connection with the anterior lobe of the pituitary. Since this gland has a controlling action on the endocrine system as a whole, it is able in this way also, to exert a regulating effect on the internal environment of the body.

Temperature Regulation

The maintenance of a constant body temperature depends on an appropriate balance between heat loss and heat production in response to changes in environmental temperature. In general, the mechanisms determining heat exchange depend on reactions such as vasodilatation, vasoconstriction and sweating which are mediated through the autonomic system, although reactions such as panting and shivering are mediated through somatic nerves. There is evidence that the control of body temperature is, to a large extent, integrated in the hypothalamus, the mechanisms of heat retention and heat production, viz, shivering and cutaneous vasoconstriction, being activated through the posterior hypothalamus. Moreover, the anterior hypothalamus appears to be sensitive to changes in temperature and so can respond to cooling or warming of the blood circulating through it (Hardy *et al.*, 1964). Likewise, pyrogens may also act on the hypothalamus, although there is no certain knowledge regarding their site of action. However, although the hypothalamus is undoubtedly sensitive to changes in internal temperature, there is no doubt that vasodilatation, vasoconstriction, shivering and possibly sweating may also occur as a result of peripheral reflexes resulting from changes in skin temperature. Thus, peripheral vasodilatation in response to warming the body and vasoconstriction after cooling can both occur abruptly, before any warming of the brain has taken place. The reflex pathway is not known, but it apparently passes through the brain as it is lost in patients with cervical cord transection. Shivering also will occur if the skin is cold, even if there is a rise in central temperature. This reflex is also lost if there is a lesion of the cervical cord (Johnson, 1966).

Water Balance

The amount of water which is reabsorbed by the distal tubules of the kidney is controlled by the antidiuretic hormone of the posterior pituitary. This substance is formed in the cells of the supra–optic nucleus of the hypothalamus, the axons of which form the hypothalamico hypophysial tract and it passes along the nerve fibres to be liberated in the posterior pituitary gland. Verney (1947) has shown that in the supra–optic nucleus there are cells which he has called 'osmoreceptors', which react to the osmotic pressure of the blood. A rise in the blood osmotic pressure, due for example to an increase in Na concentration, leads to an outpouring of hormone so that more water is reabsorbed from the kidneys. If the osmotic pressure falls, less hormone is secreted so that more water is lost.

Damage to the supra–optic nucleus leads to diabetes insipidus in which the patient drinks enormous quantities of water. Nicotine will stimulate the supra–optic nucleus to release antidiuretic hormone and so reduce the output of urine.

Endocrine Control

The capillaries in the vicinity of certain of the hypothalamic nuclei open into a set of portal channels that pass down the pituitary stalk and drain into the capillaries of the anterior lobe of the pituitary. Neurones in the hypothalamus liberate 'releasing factors' which act on the secretory cells of the pituitary to promote the secretion of hormone. Since the anterior lobe of the pituitary, in addition to secreting the growth hormone, liberates trophic hormones such as corticotrophin, thyrotrophin and the gonadotrophic hormones that promote the secretion of endocrine glands elsewhere in the body, the hypothalamus exerts a very wide influence on endocrine function throughout the body. In certain instances it participates in a delicate feedback controlling mechanism in that hormones liberated by the target glands exert an effect on the hypothalamic neurones to reduce the output of trophic hormone.

Control of Appetite

Damage to the ventromedial nucleus leads to obesity in animals due to an increase in food intake. Lesions in other areas will cause failure to eat. Drinking may also be affected by lesions and by the application of stimuli to other centres. The hypothalamus thus has an important role in the regulation both of eating and drinking (see reviews by Kennedy, 1966 and Fitzsimmons, 1966). The clinical significance of these observations is difficult to evaluate since pathological obesity and abnormalities of fluid intake may also be associated with disturbances of pituitary function. The physiological mechanisms both of hunger and thirst are complex and incompletely understood. The syndrome of anorexia nervosa has features resembling that of the effects that may be produced by hypothalamic lesions in rats, but Russell (1969) has pointed out that patients with this condition may experience normal hunger drives and has stressed the importance of psychological factors.

THE CLINICAL STUDY OF AUTONOMIC FUNCTION

In general, the function of the autonomic system is that of maintaining a constant internal environment in the body by means of circulatory and visceral reflexes. Paralysis of the autonomic system can be produced by the administration of ganglion blocking drugs. One of the effects of these is to produce a marked fall in blood pressure. However, severe damage to the autonomic system is compatible with life and removal of the entire sympathetic chain in the cat is not necessarily fatal, but the animal may be unable to adapt to physical exertion or changes in external temperature (Cannon *et al.*, 1929). In mice, a nerve growth factor can be isolated from the salivary glands which will promote growth of autonomic ganglia and an antiserum can be prepared to this which will produce an immunological destruction of the sympathetic system. If rats are made to undergo immunological sympathectomy in this way, they survive quite well, but a marked fall in blood pressure occurs if the adrenal medulla is also removed (Zaimis, 1967).

In man, disease of the nervous system may give rise to disturbances of autonomic function and, of these, effects on the circulatory reflexes are perhaps particularly important, but abnormalities in visceral responses and temperature regulation also occur. Physiological tests of autonomic function have proved useful in the recognition and understanding of these disorders. Since sympathetic postganglionic fibres are in many instances carried to their terminations in association with spinal nerves, tests of autonomic function are sometimes also useful in assessing the integrity of peripheral nerves.

Methods of Study

Autonomic reflexes which are accessible for clinical study include those regulating the calibre of the blood vessels, the pupillary responses, sweating, gastric secretion and micturition. Of these, the circulatory reflexes are of particular clinical importance and have provided a useful means of assessing the integrity of the autonomic system. The study of sweating and changes in skin resistance are useful in determining the integrity and area of innervation of peripheral nerves which carry sympathetic components, and also in distinguishing between lesions of the efferent and afferent pathways. Of the circulatory reflexes, Valsalva's manoeuvre is particularly useful. Helpful information has also been obtained from studying the effects of changes of posture on the arterial blood pressure.

Valsalva's Manoeuvre

In this procedure, the subject expires against a closed glottis immediately after taking a deep breath. A useful method of carrying this out is to blow against a column of mercury for a period of several seconds. The rise in intrathoracic pressure produced in this way decreases the venous return to the heart, so that the cardiac output falls and there is a decrease in blood pressure. This is immediately corrected by reflex vasoconstriction due to an autonomic reflex initiated by afferent stimuli arising from the baroreceptors. Return of the intrathoracic pressure to normal is followed by a rise in blood pressure to above the initial level. During the transient fall in blood pressure which occurs, there may be a brief increase in the heart rate that slows when the blood pressure rises again. If the autonomic reflexes are defective, the fall in blood pressure is no longer immediately corrected but, instead, the blood pressure continues to fall and at the same time the heart rate becomes more rapid. The blood pressure may take several minutes to regain its normal level and there is no overshoot (Fig. 11.3). To record these changes it is advantageous to have a continuous record of arterial blood pressure (Sharpey-Schafer, 1956; Spalding, 1966) but in the absence of this useful information can be obtained by a continuous ECG recording of the heart rate (Nathanielsz and Ross, 1967).

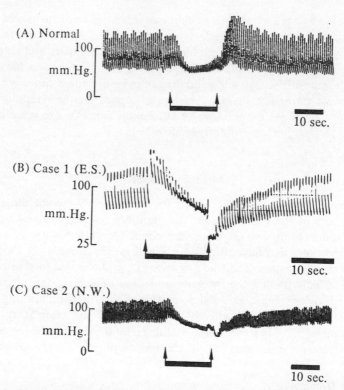

Fig. 11.3. Changes in blood pressure accompanying Valsalva's manoeuvre in A a normal subject and B and C 2 patients with postural hypotension due to autonomic failure (see Fig. 11.4). Johnson, R. H., Lee, G. de J., Oppenheimer, D. R. and Spalding, J. M. K. (1966), *Quart. J. Med.*, **35**, 276–292.

Effect of Postural Change

This can be studied by changing the posture of the subject or patient from the horizontal to vertical by means of a tilting table. This is normally associated with little alteration in blood pressure, but if the autonomic reflexes are impaired, there may be a marked fall in blood pressure (Fig. 11.4). Tilting table tests need to be carried out with caution in patients subject to postural hypotension, since in these subjects, the fall in blood pressure can be precipitous.

The adaptation of the body to a rise in blood pressure can be studied by observing the changes resulting from adopting the squatting posture. This has the effect of producing a rise in blood pressure, since the blood which is squeezed out of the leg veins increases the venous return to the heart and therefore the cardiac output. The blood pressure, however, soon falls in response to vasodilatation which occurs as a result of baroreceptor reflexes.

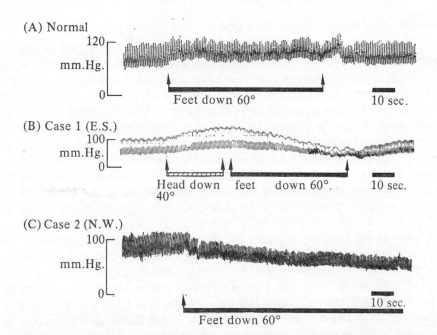

FIG. 11.4. Effect of change in posture on blood pressure in A a normal subject B and C 2 patients with orthostatic hypotension associated with autonomic failure due to a preganglionic sympathetic lesion in the nervous system. Johnson, R. H., Lee, G. de J., Oppenheimer, D. R. and Spalding, J. M. K. (1966), *Quart. J. Med.*, **35**, 276–292.

Changes in Peripheral Blood Flow

The calibre of both the arterioles and the veins is under sympathetic control and sometimes the innervation of the one may be affected independently of the other. The arterioles account for the peripheral resistance, whereas the tone of the venous system is an important factor in determining how much blood is pooled and how much is available to provide a venous return to the heart. The tone of both sets of vessels can be studied by venous occlusion plethysmography. If blood flow through the hand is measured at the same time as changes in blood pressure are produced by procedures such as the valsalva manoeuvre or alterations in posture, the changes in peripheral blood flow that occur provide a measure of the integrity of the autonomic reflexes in so far as they affect the peripheral resistance. The tone of the venous system, or capacity vessels, can be estimated by measuring the pressure in the veins of the hand as they become distended following venous occlusion. In healthy individuals, the distensibility of the veins alters with changes in intrathoracic pressure, but this reflex may be lost in patients with disturbed autonomic function.

Sweating, Skin Resistance and the Galvanic Skin Response

Since the sweat glands are supplied by sympathetic fibres, the ability to sweat over a given area of skin is a sign that the sympathetic outflow to that part of the body is intact. Since the sympathetic nerves to the sweat glands are carried along the peripheral nerves, a peripheral nerve lesion may be accompanied by loss of sweating over the region supplied by that nerve. Likewise, with a root lesion, sweating may be lost in a segmental distribution. Localized loss of sweating may occur in lesions affecting particular parts of the sympathetic system, as in Horner's syndrome, when a lesion affecting the superior cervical ganglion gives rise to loss of sweating over the face along with ptosis and constriction of the pupil. Following transection of the spinal cord, provided the transection is above a sufficient proportion of the thoracolumbar outflow, sweating may be lost during the phase of spinal shock, but later recovers so that stimuli, such as distension of the bladder, may give rise to intense sweating (see chapter 6).

To test the integrity of the innervation of the sweat glands the subject may be warmed under a heat cage. In the healthy individual, sweating will occur as the central temperature rises. The area of sweating can be mapped by dusting the patient with Quinezarine, which is a blue powder that turns purple in contact with water. Sweating also has a marked effect on the electrical resistance of the skin, which falls as sweating takes place. Measurements of skin resistance using an instrument known as a dermometer, have been used to map regions of denervated or sympathectomized skin (Richter, 1946). If a subject is exposed to a sudden unexpected stimulus, the autonomic discharge that occurs can be recorded as an abrupt fall in skin resistance which has been termed the galvanic skin response (GSR). The galvanic skin response has been widely studied by psychologists as a method of recording emotional responses, and its latency has been used to measure the conduction velocity in sympathetic fibres. Young children can be conditioned by an electrical stimulus so that a GSR occurs in response to a sound. This can be used as a test for deafness. It has been recorded in the presence of anhydrosis due to absence of sweat glands (Gilchrist, 1927) and after atropinization (Richter, 1927). It appears to be due, in part, to vasomotor changes in the skin (Carmichael *et al.*, 1941a and b). The fall in skin resistance which occurs in the GSR is accompanied by a small change in potential that can be recorded with suitable amplification. This may be seen as an artefact when recording the electroencephalogram. The underlying mechanism is not understood.

Lesions Affecting Afferent and Efferent Portions of the Reflex Arc

Autonomic reflexes can be affected by disease in either the afferent, central or efferent portions of the reflex arc. Thus, tabes dorsalis, where the disease affects the dorsal roots, affects the afferent pathway, cerebrovascular disease and centrally acting drugs may affect the central pathway and the efferent pathway may be damaged in lesions of the spinal cord and peripheral nerves. In clinical testing, the efferent arc is more readily tested than the central or afferent pathways. Lesions in these situations are generally only postulated if careful testing fails to demonstrate a lesion in the efferent pathway. If the lesion is found to lie in the efferent pathway, it may be possible to distinguish whether it is situated in the preganglionic or postganglionic nerves.

The integrity of the efferent pathway is tested by applying stimuli which excite the autonomic outflow by activating the cerebral centres and not the afferent pathways. Thus, a sudden noise or concentration on mental arithmetic will produce a measurable rise in blood pressure in many, but not all, normal subjects. Another method is to study the effects of indirect heating on the body, which by raising the temperature of the blood passing through temperature sensitive structures in the brain will cause both sweating and an increase in limb blood flow that can be recorded by venous occlusion plethysmography. A similar mechanism operates in the cold pressor test when immersion of the hand in cold water brings about a rise in blood pressure. Failure to elicit autonomic axon reflexes such as the sweating and piloerection produced by an alternating current or intradermal acetylcholine (see chapter 6) is evidence that the lesion lies in the postganglionic pathway (Bárány and Cooper, 1956).

Orthostatic Hypotension

Although disturbed autonomic function may occur in many different clinical syndromes and gives rise to a wide variety of symptoms, orthostatic or postural hypotension is a common manifestation of autonomic impairment and one which is of immediate clinical importance.

The maintenance of a normal blood pressure depends on many complex factors in which humoral as well as nervous mechanisms are involved. Important reflexes are activated by stimulation of baroreceptors in the aortic arch and carotid sinus. These connect with vasomotor centres in the medulla, so that if there is a rise in blood pressure the baroreceptors discharge and set up reflexes that slow the heart and relax the arterioles. The opposite effect follows a fall in blood pressure which is compensated by an increase in peripheral resistance and in cardiac output. The increase in cardiac output is due, in part, to a direct stimulating effect of the sympathetic system on the heart and possibly, also to an increase in the tone of the capacity vessels of the venous system. A further reaction to a fall in blood pressure comes about through an increased rate of secretion by the suprarenal cortex. This has the effect of causing retention of Na by the kidney so that the blood volume increases. The factors bringing about secretion of aldosterone are complex, but one that is important is the liberation of renin by the kidney. Renin is liberated following pressure changes in the juxta-glomerular vessels. In the normal subject, renin may be liberated if there is a fall in blood pressure or of blood volume or if the subject assumes the erect posture. Renin reacts with constituents of the plasma so that angiotensin II is formed, which activates the suprarenal to liberate aldosterone. There is evidence that the sympathetic system and circulating catecholamines play a part in renin release. Renin release has been found to be defective in certain patients with disturbed autonomic function (Chokroverty *et al.*, 1969; Bannister, 1971).

Postural hypotension may result from disease affecting the afferent, central or efferent segments of the autonomic reflex arcs. In the majority of cases, it arises as a secondary manifestation of a generalized disorder and is spoken of as secondary orthostatic hypotension. In primary orthostatic hypotension, the symptom is a prominent feature of a rare but important group of conditions in which disturbed autonomic function is the dominant characteristic.

Secondary orthostatic hypotension is a common condition in the elderly where loss of vasomotor reflexes may be the result of central changes in the brain, perhaps as a consequence of associated cerebrovascular disease (Johnson *et al.*, 1965). Other important causes include tabes dorsalis where the afferent segment of the autonomic reflexes are affected. In diabetic and other forms of peripheral neuritis, the lesion may affect both the afferent and the efferent pathways. In transection of the cord, the descending sympathetic pathway may be interrupted and postural hypotension is a particular hazard when the cord is damaged at or above the middorsal level.

Primary or idiopathic orthostatic hypotension has been considered to be part of a widespread degeneration of neurones in the central nervous system (Shy and Drager, 1960). In this syndrome, symptoms commonly develop in adult life. Disturbed bladder control is an early symptom, postural hypotension may be progressive and disabling, and as the disease advances parkinsonian features develop, sometimes with cerebellar ataxia. The pathological changes may be widespread, but the autonomic disorder may be related to loss of nerve cells in the intermediolateral cell column of the spinal cord (Johnson *et al.*, 1966). Postural hypotension may also be a feature of familial dysautonomia (Riley *et al.*, 1949). In this condition the cardinal features include defective lacrimation, excessive sweating, gastric hypermotility, insensitivity to pain and absent reflexes. A striking feature may be hypersensitivity to acetycholine. The nature of the underlying defect is unknown, but it has been suggested that one factor may be failure of production of a neurohumoral transmitter (Mahloudji *et al.*, 1970).

REFERENCES

AHLQUIST, R. P. (1948). A study of adrenotropic receptors. *Amer. J. Physiol.*, **153**, 586–600.

BANNISTER, R. (1971). Degeneration of the autonomic nervous system. *Lancet*, **ii**, 175–179.

BÁRÁNY, F. R. and COOPER, E. H. (1956). Pilomotor and sudomotor innervation in diabetes. *Clin. Sci.*, **15**, 533–540.

CANNON, W. B., NEWTON, H. F., BRIGHT, E. M., MENKIN, V. and MOORE, R. M. (1929). Some aspects of the physiology of animals surviving complete exclusion of sympathetic nerve impulses. *Amer. J. Physiol.*, **89**, 84–107.

CANNON, W. B. and ROSENBLUETH, A. (1933). Studies on conditions of activity in endocrine organs. XXIX. Sympathin E and Sympathin I. *Amer. J. Physiol.*, **104**, 557–574.

CANNON, W. B. and ROSENBLUETH, A. (1949). *The Supersensitivity of Denervated Structures*. New York: Macmillan.

CANNON, W. B. and URIDIL, J. E. (1921). Studies on the conditions of activity in endocrine glands. VIII. Some effects on the denervated heart of stimulating the nerves of the liver. *Amer. J. Physiol.*, **54**, 353–364.

CARLSSON, A. (1964). Functional significance of drug-induced changes in brain monoamine levels. *Progr. Brain. Res.*, **8**, 9–27.

CARMICHAEL, E. A., HONEYMAN, W. M., KOLB, L. C. and STEWART, W. K. (1941a). A physiological study of the skin resistance response in man. *J. Physiol. (Lond.)*, **99**, 329–337.

CARMICHAEL, E. A., HONEYMAN, W. M., KOLB, L. C. and STEWART, W. K. (1941b). Peripheral conduction rate in the sympathetic nervous system of man. *J. Physiol. (Lond.)*, **99**, 338–343.

CHOKROVERTY, S., BARRON, K. D., KATZ, F. H., DEL GRECO, F. and SHARP, J. T. (1969). The syndrome of primary orthostatic hypotension. *Brain*, **92**, 743–768.

DALE, H. H. (1914). The action of certain esters and ethers of choline and their relation to muscarine. *J. Pharmacol.*, **6**, 147–190.

DALE, H. H. and DUDLEY, H. W. (1929). The presence of histamine and acetylcholine in the spleen of the ox and the horse. *J. Physiol. (Lond.)*, **68**, 97–123.

ECCLES, R. M. and LIBET, B. (1961). Origin and blockade of the synaptic responses of curarized sympathetic ganglia. *J. Physiol. (Lond.)*, **157**, 484–503.

ELLIOTT, T. R. (1904). On the action of adrenaline. *J. Physiol. (Lond.)*, **31**, 20–21.

VON EULER, U. S. (1946). A specific sympatho-mimetic ergone in adrenergic nerve fibres (Sympathin) and its relations to adrenaline and nor-adrenaline. *Acta physiol. scand.*, **12**, 73–97.

FELDBERG, W. and GADDUM, J. H. (1934). The chemical transmitter at synapses in a sympathetic ganglion. *J. Physiol. (Lond.)*, **81**, 305–319.

FITZSIMONS, J. T. (1966). The hypothalamus and drinking. *Br. med. Bull.*, **22**, 232–237.

GILCHRIST (1927), cited by Richter, C. P. (1927), *Brain*, 216–235.

HARDY, J. D., HELLON, R. F. and SUTHERLAND, K. (1964). Temperature-sensitive neurones in the dog's hypothalamus. *J. Physiol. (Lond.)*, **175**, 242–253.

HARRIMAN, D. G. F. and GARLAND, H. (1968). The pathology of Adie's syndrome. *Brain*, **91**, 401–418.

HERTTING, G., AXELROD, J., KOPIN, I. S. and WHITBY, L. G. (1961). Lack of uptake of catecholamines after chronic denervation of sympathetic nerves. *Nature*, **189**, 66.

HESS, W. R. (1957). *The functional organisation of the diencephalon.* New York: Grune and Stratton.

JOHNSON, R. H. (1966). The autonomic nervous system and body temperature. *Proc. roy. Soc. Med.,* **59,** 463–466.

JOHNSON, R. H., LEE, G. DE J., OPPENHEIMER, D. R. and SPALDING, J. M. K. (1966). Autonomic failure with orthostatic hypotension due to intermedio-lateral column degeneration. *Quart. J. Med.,* **35,** 276–292.

JOHNSON, R. H., SMITH, A. C., SPALDING, J. M. K. and WOLLANER, L. (1945). Effect of posture on blood-pressure in elderly patients. *Lancet,* **I,** 731–733.

KENNEDY, G. C. (1966). Food intake, energy balance and growth. *Br. med. Bull.,* **22,** 216–220.

LANGLEY, J. N. (1901). Observations on the physiological action of extracts of the suprarenal bodies. *J. Physiol. (Lond.),* **27,** 237–256.

LOEWI, O. (1921). Über humerale Übertragbarkeit der Herznervenwirkung. I. Mitteilung. *Pflüg. Arch.,* **189,** 239–242.

MAHLOUDJI, M., BRUNT, P. W. and McKUSICK, V. A. (1970). Clinical neurological aspects of familial dysautonomia. *J. neurol. Sci.,* **11,** 383–395.

NATHANIELSZ, P. W. and ROSS, E. J. (1967). Abnormal responses to Valsalva Manoeuver in diabetics—Relation to autonomic neuropathy. *Diabetes,* **16,** 462–465.

RICHTER, C. P. (1927). A study of the electrical skin resistance and the psychogalvanic reflex in a case of unilateral sweating. *Brain,* **51,** 216–235.

RICHTER, C. P. (1946). Instructions for using the cutaneous resistance recorder or dermometer on peripheral nerve injuries, etc. *J. Neurosurg.,* **3,** 181–191.

RILEY, C. M., DAY, R. L., GREELEY, D. McL. and LANGFORD, W. S. (1949). Central autonomic dysfunction with defective lachrymation. 1. Report of five cases. *Pediatrics,* **3,** 468–478.

RUSSELL, G. F. M. (1956). Pupillary changes in Holmes–Adie syndrome. *J. Neurol. Neurosurg. Psychiat.,* **19,** 289–296.

RUSSELL, G. F. M. (1969). Metabolic, endocrine and psychiatric aspects of anorexia nervosa. *Scientific Basis of Medicine Annual Reviews* 1969. London: Athlone Press. 236–255.

SHARPEY-SCHAFER, E. P. (1956). Circulatory reflexes in chronic disease of the afferent nervous system. *J. Physiol. (Lond.),* **134,** 1–10.

SHARPEY-SCHAFER, E. P. and TAYLOR, P. J. (1960). Absent circulatory reflexes in diabetic neuritis. *Lancet,* **i,** 559–562.

SHY, G. M. and DRAGER, G. A. (1960). A neurological syndrome associated with orthostatic hypotension. *Arch. Neurol. (Chicago),* **2,** 511–527.

SPALDING, J. M. K. (1966). The autonomic nervous system and the circulation. *Proc. roy. Soc. Med.,* **59,** 461–463.

SPALDING, J. M. K. (1967). Some disorders of the circulation due to neurological disease. In: *Modern Trends in Neurology.* Ed. Williams, D. New York: Appleton, Series 4, **4,** pp. 193–208.

VERNEY, E. B. (1947). The antidiuretic hormone and the factors which determine its release. *Proc. roy. Soc. B.,* **135,** 25–106.

WALL, P. D. and CRONLY-DILLON, J. R. (1960). Pain, itch and vibration. *Arch. Neurol. (Chicago),* **2,** 365–375.

ZAIMIS, E. (1967). Immunological Sympathectomy. *Scientific Basis of Medicine Annual Reviews* 1967. London: Athlone Press. 59–73.

CHAPTER 12

The Cerebral Cortex

The cerebral hemispheres form the larger part of the brain in man and they are the seat of the most complex and highly developed forms of cerebral function. In the more primitive vertebrates, the fore-brain is closely related to the olfactory nerves. The relatively simple structure of the cortex of the primitive brain persists in the so-called archipallium that is found in mammals. Only mammals have, in addition to this, a multilayered folded cortex which is particularly well developed in the higher primates and in man. Deep to the cortex are the corpus striatum and basal nuclei, which are present in fish, and form the major part of the brain in birds. In man, the multilayered neocortex contains, in addition to extensive association areas, the function of which remains imperfectly understood, important centres that are concerned with recognition and interpretation of sensation and the initiation of voluntary movement. Although the archipallium in higher mammals is still concerned with the sense of smell, it has also become important in connection with autonomic regulation and probably also with emotional responses.

METHODS OF STUDY

Anatomical methods have been important in the study of the cerebral hemispheres. Identification of nervous pathways has been carried out by dividing nerve fibres and tracing the degenerated columns by means of staining techniques, which can distinguish normal myelinated fibres from fibres that have undergone degeneration with breakdown of the myelin sheath. Histological studies, particularly using the silver impregnation methods developed by Ramon y Cajal (1894), which will distinguish the different portions of the neurone and its processes, have clarified the cellular structure of the cerebral cortex.

An important physiological method has been to study the effect in experimental animals of stimulation of the cerebral cortex, either with electrical pulses or following the local application of substances, such as strychnine. In man, it has been possible to observe the effects of stimulating the exposed cerebral cortex at surgical operation. Both in animals and man, evoked potentials have been recorded from the brain following stimulation of sense organs or of afferent pathways. A valuable technique has been to record from microelectrodes inserted at different depths in the brain. The study of the effects of experimental removal of parts of the cerebral cortex in animals has been supplemented by information gained from the clinical study of patients with disease affecting particular parts of the brain or who have sustained brain damage. A great deal of information concerning higher cognitive functions, such as speech, can only be obtained from the human subject. Here, studies of the psychological aspects of nervous function have supplemented information gained from the examination of patients with disease of the brain.

THE STRUCTURE OF THE CEREBRAL CORTEX

The greater part of the cerebral cortex has a thin outer layer of grey matter, the thickness of which is maximal in the region of the precentral gyrus where it is about 3 mm thick. If the cerebral cortex is examined histologically, six layers can be identified. This laminated cortex is known as isocortex or neocortex. About one-twelfth of the cerebral cortex has a less clearly defined laminar structure comprising three layers of cells and is known as allocortex. This part of the cortex includes the cortex overlying the phylogenetically primitive archipallium, which because of its early association with the sense of smell, is also known as the rhinencephalon. The allocortex and the structures over which it lies are situated in the form of a ring that surrounds the upper part of the brain stem and for this reason, is sometimes given the name of the limbic lobe.

If the isocortex is looked at by the naked eye, differences can be seen between the cortex in different parts of the brain. In most parts of the brain, two layers of white matter can be seen in the cortex, which are known as the inner and outer lines of Baillarger and consist of fibres that run parallel to the surface. In the occipital cortex, however, only the outer line can be seen. Here it is thicker than elsewhere and has been called the white line of Gennari.

Histologically, the cerebral cortex contains two principal types of cell. These are firstly pyramidal cells, which have a pyramid shaped body from which apical dendrites extend towards the surface of the brain to make synaptic contact with the axons of cortical neurones. The axons of many of the pyramidal cells leave the cortex and pass into the white matter of the brain. The second type of cell is the stellate cell and the axons of these generally connect with other neurones in the cerebral cortex. Of the six layers of the cortex, the outer or molecular layer consists mainly of dendrites from the cells in the deeper layers and axons connecting different neurones within the cortex. One type of cell that is seen here is the horizontal cell, which sends fibres parallel to the surface to connect neigh-bouring parts of the cortex. The second and third layers are layers of pyramidal cells, and the fourth layer contains star pyramids and stellate cells. The stellate cells of the fourth layer connect with specific afferents from the thalamus. These specific afferents are derived from nuclei which form part of the main sensory pathway and send fibres to localized areas of cortex. Non-specific afferents from the thalamus are distributed to wide areas of cortex and connect with cells in all the cortical layers. The outer line of Baillarger lies at the level of the fourth layer. The fifth and sixth layers form the inner lamina of the cortex. The fifth is a layer which contains pyramidal cells and in the motor area of the cortex, it is in the

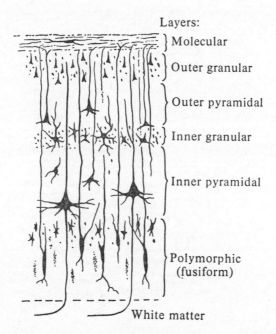

Layers:

Molecular

Outer granular

Outer pyramidal

Inner granular

Inner pyramidal

Polymorphic (fusiform)

White matter

FIG. 12.1. A simplified diagram to show histological layers of cerebral cortex.

fifth layer that the large pyramidal or Betz cells are found. The inner line of Baillarger lies at the deeper part of the fifth layer. The innermost layer is the fusiform cell layer and contains cells similar to the stellate cells, but which send their axons into the white matter. The afferent fibres that enter the cortex branch and ramify so that each afferent neurone is able to influence many thousands of cortical cells (Fig. 12.1).

Histological examination of the cerebral cortex shows differences in structure in different regions. This has led Brodmann and others to prepare maps of the cortex in which different cortical locations are marked by numbers according to the histological pattern. Histological differences are in general small, with the exception of a few regions, such as area 4 in the precentral gyrus where the giant pyramidal cells of Betz are a conspicuous feature. The functional significance of

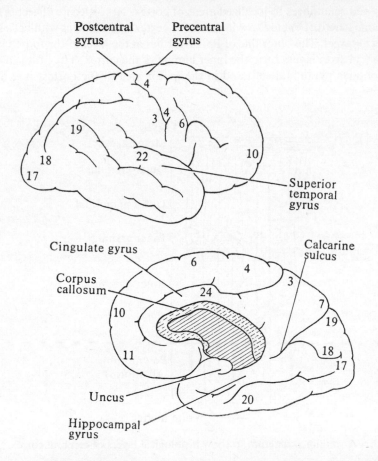

FIG. 12.2. Morphology of cerebral hemispheres to show lateral and medial aspects with main sensory and motor areas. The numbers are derived from Brodmann's cytoarchitectural classification.

the differences in histological structure in the different regions is not known. Nevertheless, the numerical maps which have been prepared have been a useful means of identifying areas of the cortex that have been exposed to histological study (Fig. 12.2).

GENERAL TOPOGRAPHY OF THE CEREBRAL HEMISPHERES

The general arrangement of the motor pathways out of the brain and the organization of the sensory input has been considered in earlier sections. The localization of the main sensory areas of the brain and the motor outflow can be fairly readily defined, but the organization of the brain as a whole, particularly in respect of mental function and emotional responses, is far less clearly established. Although damage to a particular part of the brain may lead to impairment or loss of a particular function, such as speech, it does not mean that the function concerned is necessarily localized specifically in that part of the brain, since it may be dependent on complex interactions from widely separate areas. In chapter 10, reference was made to Hughlings Jackson's concept of the nervous system as organized in terms of a hierarchy of functional levels. According to this conception, the first level comprised the brain stem and spinal cord and included the lower motor centres for movement; the second or middle level consisted of the motor area on the precentral gyrus and the third or highest level, where complex activity is organized, was made up of the prefrontal lobes. Jackson was also aware of the differentiation of function that exists between the right and left cerebral hemispheres particularly as regards speech. Penfield, on the other hand, has developed the concept that the highest level of the nervous system is not in the cortex of the hemispheres but in the central structures of the diencephalon. This part of the brain is necessary to maintain consciousness, and Penfield has defined this area as the centrencephalic integrating system.

Luria (1973) has considered that the brain should be thought of in terms of interdependent functioning systems or units. The first of these is defined as 'a unit for regulating tone or waking'. He regards the principal part of this as the reticular activating system in the diencephalon, which is necessary to maintain the state of alertness required for waking activity. In addition to receiving an afferent input from the environment, this part of the brain has an important role in maintaining homeostasis and has complex connections with the cerebral cortex. A second unit is 'the unit for receiving, analysing and storing information' and comprises the main sensory association areas that are situated on the cerebral convexity posterior to the central sulcus. The third unit is 'the unit for programming, regulating and verifying mental activity' and it is located in the hemisphere anterior to the central sulcus. The participation of all these units can be regarded as necessary for the carrying out of mental processes. Luria considers each of the units as hierarchical in structure, consisting of a primary or projection area which is under the influence of secondary and tertiary association areas of cortex. Thus, in the third unit, the motor area of the cortex is the primary projection zone corresponding to Jackson's middle level. The premotor cortex is conceived of as a secondary zone which gives rise to organized movements. The remainder of the frontal lobes that has wide connections not only with the brain stem but

J

with all other parts of the cortex, forms the tertiary zone concerned with the formation of programmes for the more complex forms of human activity.

Cerebral Dominance

The human brain and that of other mammals is a paired organ, the right cerebral hemisphere the mirror image of the left, each cerebral hemisphere controlling the sensory and motor functions of the opposite half of the body. The two cerebral hemispheres act in very close association. Information is transferred from one to the other by means of a large band of nerve fibres, which forms the great cerebral commisure or corpus callosum. Structurally, the two cerebral hemispheres are symmetrical. In animals other than man, the two cerebral hemispheres are of virtually equal functional importance. In man, there has developed specialization of function between the two hemispheres, so that certain capacities are predominantly under the control of one half of the brain. In most individuals, there is a strong preference for the right hand for the carrying out of skilled and complex movements. In these individuals one may speak of the left cerebral hemisphere as the dominant hemisphere as regards motor control. A smaller number of people, probably between 5 and 10 per cent, are left-handed and in these, the right hemisphere is dominant in this respect.

An important difference between the two hemispheres, in the human subject, is that in adults the left cerebral hemisphere is particularly important for speech, so that damage to the left hemisphere may result both in loss of the ability to understand speech and the ability to express oneself in words. There is some correlation between handedness and lateralization for speech in that in the majority of right-handed individuals, the left hemisphere is the dominant hemisphere for speech. In a proportion of left-handed individuals, the right hemisphere is the more important for speech, but this group appears to be a minority. Probably more than half of left-handed individuals will develop defects in language function if the left hemisphere is damaged. In young children, cerebral dominance for speech is less firmly established than in adults. In left-handed individuals, localization of language function in one side of the brain may be less complete than in right-handed subjects. If hemiplegia develops in early childhood as a result of damage to the left hemisphere, the operation of hemispherectomy can be performed with little adverse affect on speech or motor function, but operation on an adult with, for example, a glioma of the left hemisphere may be followed by severe disability.

Clinical studies have shown that there is specialization of function in the right and left hemispheres for other capacities in addition to language function. Thus, damage to the posterior parietal lobe may result in loss of the capacity to carry out voluntary purposive movements in the absence of any muscular paralysis. This disturbance is known as apraxia and may involve the inability to perform even a simple movement to command, ideomotor apraxia, or to perform an organized sequence of movements, ideational apraxia. Both these varieties of apraxia may result from a lesion of the left parietal lobe, in which case both sides of the body may be affected. A lesion of the corpus callosum separating the right from the left posterior parietal lobe may give rise to apraxia affecting the left side of the body only. On the other hand, actions which depend in some degree on the subject's awareness of space, such as dressing or arranging objects in a pattern, may be particularly affected by lesions of the right hemisphere. Thus, dressing apraxia is nearly always the result of a right sided lesion. Constructional apraxia, although it occurs with lesions of either hemisphere, is more likely to develop and is more severe when the right side of the brain is affected. Functions which do not depend on language formulation may be selectively affected by right-sided lesions. It appears that, in particular, the ability to form a mental image of the body and the spatial world is better developed in the right hemisphere than in the left. Thus, lesions of the right parietal lobe are particularly liable to give rise to loss of awareness or neglect of the left side of the body or of the left half of space (Hecaen, 1962).

Other differences between the right and left cerebral hemispheres have become evident from studies of patients who have had operations to remove portions of either the right or the left temporal lobe. Following left temporal lobectomy, patients perform relatively poorly in tests which involve the handling of verbal material. Following right temporal lobectomy, there may be difficulty in recognizing and interpreting visual patterns and in the recall and recognition of musical sequences. These deficits that result from unilateral hemisphere lesions are, in general, a feature of the human brain, since in animals it is usually necessary to produce bilateral lesions before any defect of discrimination or learning ability not wholly dependent on a sensory deficit can be demonstrated. One instance in man where the higher cerebral functions appear to be bilaterally represented is the ability to establish and recall short term memories. Thus, damage to both hippocampal areas results in loss of the ability to retain new information, although the patient can still recall the remote past. Unilateral lesions, on the other hand, have little effect (Scoville and Milner, 1957; Milner, 1962; Piercy, 1967). A full account of the interrelationships between the hemispheres has been given by Dimond (1972).

The Corpus Callosum

A further method which has been developed to study the independent functions of the two cerebral hemispheres is to analyse the changes that take place following lesions of the corpus callosum. The condition which results is one variety of what has been termed the disconnection syndrome. In animals, the corpus callosum has been divided as an experimental procedure. In man, it has been sectioned in the treatment of intractable epilepsy. Studies have also been carried out on patients with agenesis or tumours of the corpus callosum. Superficially, an individual with a lesion of the corpus callosum shows little abnormality, but he is not able to name objects which he feels with the left hand, although sensation in the left hand is intact and he can match objects identified by touch. He cannot, however, match objects held in the left hand with objects held in the right.

In animals, if both the corpus callosum and the optic chiasma are divided, it is possible to stimulate the visual system of the right and left sides independently so that tests of learning and discrimination can be applied to either hemisphere in isolation. When this is done, it is found that material learned by one half of the brain is not transferred to the other in the absence of an intact corpus callosum. Similarly, in the human subject, the ability of either hemisphere to respond to visual stimuli or perform certain functions can be tested following section of the corpus callosum. These studies confirm that the capacity for language expression is concentrated in the left hemisphere, but it is clear also that, at least in some individuals, some capacity for comprehension of verbal material exists in the minor hemisphere. Patients have been able to spell simple words with the left hand if given a pile of letters to handle. The relative absence of language function makes it difficult to fully assess the abilities of the minor hemisphere, but it has been found that in spite of the better motor control of the right hand, patients with callosal lesions may be better able to draw three dimensional figures with the left hand than with the right (Sperry, 1964; Gazzaniga and Sperry, 1967; Geschwind, 1970).

The Frontal Lobes

The motor functions of the frontal lobe and, in particular, the precentral motor cortex, have already been referred to in chapter 10. Although the portions of the frontal lobes that are anterior to the precentral area form a considerable mass of cerebral tissue, localization of function has not been so clearly established in this region as in other parts of the brain. Thus, performance in intelligence tests, memory, emotional responses, autonomic function and the control of movement are apparently unaltered following frontal lobectomy. As long ago as 1876, Ferrier showed that removal of the anterior part of the frontal lobes in monkeys gave rise to no motor loss or sensory deficit and the animals appeared capable of normal emotional responses. They did, however, lose all apparent active interest in their surroundings and became dull and apathetic. In a later series of experiments, Jacobsen (1936) found that if both frontal lobes were removed from monkeys, the animals eventually recovered to a stage where they could carry out problem solving tasks, such as tests which involve the use of sticks to reach and obtain food, with very little impairment compared with their performance before operation. He found, however, that when given what he described as a delayed response task, in which the animals had to remember under which of two cups food had been placed in order to gain a reward, the animal would fail in the test even when the interval between test and response was as short as a few seconds. Following unilateral frontal lobectomy there was no impairment of performance in any test. These observations might suggest that the frontal lobes are necessary for short term memory and recall. Subsequent work has shown that the defect in the performance of this task is primarily one of defective attention or concentration, so that the animal fails to register the information presented in the first part of the test. Thus, the monkeys with frontal lobe lesions can readily perform the delayed response test if their appetites are first stimulated by cold or drugs (Pribram, 1966).

In man, the effect of damage to the frontal lobes is, in general, one of apathy with a tendency to euphoria, defective attention and failure to appreciate the seriousness of a given situation. The well known case of Phineas Gage, which was described by Harlow in 1868, was that of a foreman who was struck during blasting operations by an iron bar that entered his skull and damaged the frontal lobe on each side. Although he remained able to work with apparently unaffected memory and intelligence, there was a marked change in personality in that he was now relatively irresponsible and showed little respect for his fellows. Similar effects on the personality have been observed following frontal lobectomy in man, particularly if the operation is bilateral, and following the operation of prefrontal leucotomy which was introduced by Moniz in 1935 for the treatment of mental illness. In this operation, the frontal lobes are partially isolated by dividing the white matter connecting them with the thalamus. Effects of this operation extend from severe apathy to a mild flattening of emotional response with failure of concentration and lack of initiative. Memory and intellectual ability are little affected, but the higher faculties of judgment and sensitivity and the ability to appreciate the gravity of a situation, in terms of its future consequences, may be lost. These features account for the success of the operation in relieving intractable anxiety in chronic mental illness, but the side effects in terms of altered personality and social competence that sometimes ensue have limited its usefulness. Many attempts have therefore been made to modify the operation so that the patient can be relieved of stress without producing severe personality change. These have generally been aimed at producing restricted lesions in the inferior portions of the frontal lobe. The cingulate gyrus and the orbital part of the frontal lobe form part of the limbic system (see below). Operations on this part of the brain have been carried out to relieve severe obsessional disorders. The production of discrete stereotactic lesions in other parts of this system, such as the amygdala, is of interest in connection with the treatment of behaviour disorders associated with intractable epilepsy. The procedures at present employed in psychosurgery have been reviewed by Bond (1972).

Although the effects of lesions affecting one of the frontal lobes are less marked than with bilateral lesions, there is some evidence for specialization of function between the right and left frontal lobes in man. Thus, disease affecting either frontal lobe may affect performance in a variety of tests of intellectual function. Where the left side is affected, however, the overall deficit is greater and performance in tests depending on both verbal and non-verbal capacity is impaired. With lesions confined to the right frontal lobe there may be some impairment in non-verbal performance tests making use of visuo spatial material, but little or no deficit in verbal tests (Smith, 1966).

The Parietal Lobes

Sensation over the contralateral half of the body is represented in the postcentral gyrus of the parietal lobe of each hemisphere. The maps obtained by recording evoked potentials following sensory stimulation and by stimulation of the cortex are similar to those representing the motor area on the precentral gyrus. Damage to the postcentral area results in impairment, but not loss of sensation. The characteristic feature of cortical sensory impairment is that the subject loses the ability to recongize sensations which he can still perceive. Thus, it is possible to perceive an object touching the skin while failing to recognize its nature. The ability to distinguish the points of a divider touching the skin as two separate points may be impaired.

The posterior portions of the parietal lobe, and in particular those areas which border on the occipital and temporal lobes, are concerned with the recognition and organization of complex perceptions, especially those of vision and hearing. On the left cerebral hemisphere, the posterior parietal lobe is particularly concerned with language function, whereas the right parietal lobe is important for the perception of space and the body image. The posterior parietal lobe, however, is not solely concerned with perception. It is also concerned with the initiation and development of motor activity. Parietal lobe lesions thus also give rise to apraxia, a condition in which the subject is not paralysed but is unable to plan and execute specific actions. In general, the association areas of the parietal cortex are not accessible to direct experimentation. Our knowledge of the functions of this part of the brain has been largely derived from clinical and psychological testing of patients with localized intracranial lesions. The clinical study of the parietal lobe has been extensively reviewed by Critchley (1953).

The importance of the parietal cortex in the appreciation of pain is probably relatively small in comparison with subcortical structures. Pain is rarely a feature of disease affecting the parietal lobe and stimulation of the parietal cortex does not normally give rise to pain. In their detailed study of the effects of cortical stimulation on 163 patients, Penfield and Boldrey (1937) elicited a painful sensation only eleven times out of more than 800 responses and in no instance was the pain severe. However, there are well authenticated cases where sensory loss to pain has resulted from small injuries confined to the cortex (Marshall, 1951). In a few patients with intractable pain, it has been possible to reproduce the pain by stimulation of the postcentral gyrus and to relieve it by removal of the affected areas of cortex (Lewin and Philips, 1952). Pain has been recorded as part of the aura in a few patients with sensory epilepsy. There are a number of case reports of patients with cortical lesions who have spontaneous pain, similar to that of the thalamic syndrome. Head and Holmes (1911) considered that the thalamus was the centre where pain is experienced, but that the response to pain was nevertheless under some form of cortical control. The present evidence is difficult to evaluate, but seems consistant with the appreciation of pain depending on the interaction between cortical and subcortical structures.

The Temporal Lobes and the Limbic System

The temporal and occipital lobes contain the sensory cortex associated with hearing and with vision. This has been referred to in chapters 8 and 9. The association areas of the temporal cortex and the adjacent parts of the parietal lobe in the dominant hemisphere are of particular importance in relation to speech. The temporal lobes also appear to be necessary for registering and recall of experience. Those parts which form a portion of the limbic system may be concerned with emotional responses.

The cortex of the temporal lobe may give rise to epileptic discharges. Temporal lobe seizures may include, in addition to generalized convulsions, dreamlike states, episodes of automatic behaviour and peculiar feelings of familiarity, déjà vu. The implication drawn from this type of seizure, that the temporal lobe is concerned with emotional experience and particularly with memory, has been confirmed by stimulation studies carried out on the exposed cortex of patients undergoing surgery for the treatment of focal epilepsy (Penfield and Jasper, 1954). Stimulation of the convexity of the temporal lobe cortex has shown that this part of the brain is important, both in the interpretation of experience as it is occurring and in the recall of past experience. Penfield has found that stimulation of the first temporal gyrus of either the dominant or nondominant hemisphere will give rise to sudden feelings in relation to present auditory experience, whereas stimulation of a much more extensive area of the nondominant hemisphere will produce sudden interpretations of visual experience and sometimes the feeling of familiarity or déjà vu. In a small proportion of epileptic patients studied, it has been found that stimulation of the lateral surface of the temporal lobe, in particular the first temporal gyrus, can evoke hallucinations of experience that in some instances represent to the patient the reproduction of a past experience. The hallucination differs from memory in that it is more immediate and vivid. Sometimes if the parameters of stimulation are appropriate, the speed of the remembered events corresponds with the passage of time in a real experience. On the other hand, the patient may be aware that he is in the operating room and not actually undergoing the evoked experience (Penfield, 1966).

The infero medial portion of the temporal lobe includes the primitive olfactory cortex, or rhinencephalon, that together with the cingulate gyrus on the medial surface of the hemisphere and a group of subcortical nuclei including the amygdaloid complex, the septal tegion, certain thalamic and hypothalamic nuclei and the midbrain reticular formation comprises the so-called limbic system. This part of the brain is closely associated with that part of the cortex which is concerned with the sense of smell. Olfactory fibres enter the brain without passing through the thalamus and end in the olfactory tubercle close to the anterior perforated substance and in the uncus or pyriform area. It is probable that a few fibres also end in the medial nuclei of the amygdala. An important feature of this part of the brain is the hippocampus or Ammon's horn, that is a small structure composed of allocortex which lies close to the olfactory termination. The hippocampus is readily damaged by anoxia and a lesion in this situation may give rise to an epileptic discharge. It is connected to the hypothalamus by the fornix, which is a band of white matter that passes from the hippocampus to the mamillary bodies. These are connected by the mamillothalamic tract to the anterior nucleus of the thalamus, which itself is connected to the cingulate gyrus. Papez in 1937 postulated that this system which has connections between the hippocampus, hypothalamus, thalamus and cerebral cortex might be particularly important in connection with emotional responses. This hypothesis has stimulated a great deal of experimental work on the limbic system of the brain.

In the same year Klüver and Bucy described the effects of bilateral temporal lobectomy in monkeys. These included a change in behaviour so that the animals became relatively tame and no longer showed signs of anger or fear. At the same time they showed an abnormal tendency to examine objects by mouth where previously they would have used their hands. Although their visual acuity seemed to be unimpaired they no longer had the ability to recognize objects by the sense of sight. This feature, which they described as 'psychic blindness', was not present following unilateral temporal lobectomy. In a later study, they reported a marked increase in sexual activity that developed in the months following the operation (Klüver and Bucy, 1937; 1939). In 1955, Terzian and Dalle Ore described a patient who had undergone bilateral temporal lobectomy as treatment for psychomotor epilepsy associated with aggressive behaviour. Following the operation, he showed many of the features of the Klüver Bucy syndrome such as emotional apathy, abnormal sexual behaviour and insatiable appetite, but in addition there was a profound memory disturbance. In this patient, the operation included not only removal of the anterior temporal cortex on either side but also the amygdala and anterior hippocampus. In 1957 Scoville and Milner described the effects of operations which had been carried out in a series of psychotic patients to remove the mesial part of both temporal lobes sparing the temporal neocortex. After these operations, it was found that there was no defect of memory if the resection had been limited to the uncus and the amygdala, but a profound disturbance of memory followed removal of the hippocampus. There was one nonpsychotic patient in the series who had had intractable epilepsy. In this patient, following radical excision of the medial surface of both temporal lobes which included the anterior surface of the hippocampus, there was a severe defect of recent memory so that the patient could remember nothing for longer than a few minutes. There was also an extensive, but patchy, retrograde amnesia which gradually shrank. The inability to remember new things persisted, but in other respects there was no significant change in personality or in measured intelligence.

Unilateral temporal lobectomy has frequently been carried out with little impairment in memory. However, Penfield and Milner (1958) have described two cases in which unilateral lobectomy was followed by a defect in recent memory similar to that described above. One of these patients was later found at autopsy to have severe atrophy of the contralateral hippocampus. It would appear, therefore, that damage to the hippocampal regions has a grave effect on recent memory and on the process of memorizing. It is of interest that damage to the mamillary bodies, which may occur in Wernicke's encephalopathy as the result of thiamin deficiency, is also associated with a severe loss of recent memory, although here the memory deficit may also be associated with confabulation. The system of neuronal connections that joins the hippocampal regions with the mamillary bodies and the thalamus is therefore of cardinal importance in connection with the process of registering and consolidating memories.

SPEECH

In 1836, Marc Dax drew attention to the association between disturbance of speech and disease affecting the left side of the brain. This observation passed unnoticed until after 1861, when Broca demonstrated the brains of two patients with loss of speech before death, which in each case had a lesion affecting the inferior frontal convolution of the left frontal lobe. A full account of the history of these early observations on aphasia and the controversy they aroused has been given by Critchley (1970). Since that time it has come to be recognized that, at least in right-handed people, the dominant hemisphere for speech is the same as the dominant hemisphere in terms of motor control and handedness. However, although in right-handed subjects the left hemisphere is nearly always the one that is dominant for speech, the reverse situation does not necessarily occur in left-handed individuals. A large number of studies have now shown that in more than 50 per cent of left-handed subjects, language disturbances are more likely to occur in association with lesions affecting the left hemisphere (Humphrey and Zangwill, 1952). A few cases have also been described in which speech has been affected in a right-handed individual following disease of the right hemisphere. With left-handed subjects, cerebral dominance for speech appears to be less definitely established than in right-handed individuals and recovery from aphasia is sometimes more complete in patients who are left-handed. In children, cerebral dominance is not established until about the age of 4 years. Below that age, children with left hemisphere damage may escape serious disturbance of speech function. For several years after that, the right hemisphere retains the capacity to take over the function of the left as regards speech and gradual recovery from dysphasia may take place. On the other hand, aphasia is more likely to develop in children than in adults if the damage is to the right cerebral hemisphere (Goodglass and Quadfasal, 1954).

Of the methods which have been applied to the study of speech dominance, the first and most important has been the clinical method of studying the incidence of speech impairment in right and left-handed patients with clearly defined lesions affecting a single hemisphere. In this respect, the study of aphasia in patients who have sustained penetrating wounds of the brain has been particularly rewarding (Russell and Espir, 1961). Another method has been to observe the effects on speech of the injection of amylobarbitone into the right or left carotid artery, since injection into the dominant side may produce temporary aphasia and sometimes unconsciousness (Wada and Rasmussen, 1960; Serafetinides, Hoare and Driver, 1965). A third method has been to observe the effect on speech of unilateral electroconvulsive therapy. The study of the localization of the mechanisms of speech within the dominant hemisphere has been largely carried out by observing the clinical effects on language function of damage localized to particular situations in the hemisphere. Clinical studies have been supplemented by attempts to classify language functions and to explain disorders of speech in terms of what is known of the structure of language.

It is not possible to make a strict localization of language functions in relation to specific locations in the hemisphere, but careful study of cerebral lesions has shown that, in broad terms, certain general types of speech disturbance are associated with damage to particular regions of the brain. Thus, difficulties of verbal expression may be associated with lesions of the frontal lobe, in particular the third frontal convolution or Broca's area. Difficulties in understanding speech are predominantly associated with damage to the temporal lobe and the temporoparietal region. Lesions further back in the parietooccipital cortex may give rise to difficulties in reading and writing.

Penfield (1966) has pointed out that Wernicke's area on the first temporal gyrus is the major part of the brain in relation to speech, Broca's area and the supplementary motor area being of secondary importance. When an electric current is applied to any of these areas on the exposed brain, this may produce either vocalization or interference with speech, including complete arrest or merely hesitation and misuse of words. Damage to the temporal area may produce a very severe disturbance of speech in which the patient is not only unable to understand the spoken word, but expressive speech also suffers and he may talk jargon. Brain (1965) regarded this as a disorder of the central word schemes and this type of dysphasia is sometimes spoken of as central dysphasia. Geschwind (1965; 1970) has drawn attention to the clinical importance of the pathways connecting different cortical regions. Disconnection syndromes can affect many different functions including speech. One form of dysphasia that can arise in this way has been termed conduction aphasia. In this, there is no abnormality of either Wernicke's or of Broca's area, but the white matter joining the two is damaged. The condition resembles central aphasia but comprehension of speech is intact.

Hughlings Jackson (1931), in his analysis of speech disturbance, drew attention to the fact that in expressive aphasia the loss of propositional speech that occurs includes not only a failure to talk out loud, but also loss of internal speech, so that the subject is unable to put his thoughts into words. If speech disturbances are looked at in linguistic terms, expressive dysphasia with its loss of internal speech may be considered as a failure of a final encoding process (Jakobson, 1964). In the same way, receptive aphasia may be seen as a failure to decode the auditory perceptions which make up speech. Luria (1966) has interpreted this form of aphasia as a failure to identify properly the phonemic patterns of articulated speech.

LEARNING AND MEMORY

Perhaps the simplest form of learning is what is known as habituation, in which an organism becomes progressively less responsive to a stimulus that is repeated regularly. This can occur even in very simple forms of life where no nervous system has developed. At a more complex level, learning involves the facilitation of nervous pathways, so that stimuli may give rise to particular responses that have been established by the learning process.

An important experimental method that has been used to study learning and memory is that of conditioning which was developed by Pavlov (1927). In contrast to reflexes which are inborn and predictable, Pavlov described a set of acquired responses in which an unconditioned reflex becomes linked to a new stimulus to give rise to a conditioned reflex. A simple way to produce a conditioned reflex is to apply an indifferent stimulus in association with a stimulus that normally evokes a reflex response. If the two stimuli are applied in association a sufficient number of times, a stage is reached where the indifferent stimulus given alone will evoke the response. Pavlov's experiments were carried out on the dog. He used the flow of saliva evoked by food or acid in the mouth as the unconditioned response. If an indifferent stimulus, such as the sound of a metronome or a particular visual pattern were presented in association with food, the dog would eventually salivate after the indifferent stimulus even if no food were given.

In this experiment the timing of the two stimuli is important. Application of the indifferent stimulus should precede that of the unconditioned stimulus and both should occur close together. When a conditioned reflex is first established it is relatively non-specific in respect of the characteristics of the evoking stimulus but gradually the animal can be trained to distinguish between a conditioned stimulus which has been reinforced by repetition and similar stimuli which have not been reinforced. In this way, a dog can be trained to salivate after viewing a circle, but not an ellipse, and to differentiate between notes of different pitch where the interval separating them might be as little as an eighth of a tone. Pavlov used the expression nervous analysers to describe the mechanisms concerned in discrimination between different stimuli. He defined the analysers for particular sensations as including the peripheral receptors on the one hand, together with their afferent fibres and central connections. The process of differentiation is accomplished by combining one signal with the act of feeding and applying a different stimulus from time to time without this association. When a signal normally associated with food is given repeatedly, but not followed by food, the conditioned reflex is said to undergo extinction. Pavlov considered that both extinction and the process whereby the animal discriminates between two stimuli are due to a process of inhibition. This he termed internal inhibition, in contrast to external inhibit on that occurs when a conditioned reflex is blocked by the application of an extra distracting stimulus at the same time as the conditioning stimulus.

The conditioning processes which Pavlov described are known as classical conditioning. A number of procedures have since been developed whereby an animal can be trained to carry out certain tasks. In operant conditioning, the animal is given a reward such as a pellet of food that acts as reinforcement whenever it carries out a task such as pressing a bar in a Skinner box or finding its way through a maze. A modification of this is avoidance conditioning, where the animal learns to respond in a particular way to a sensory stimulus in order to avoid an electric shock. A sophisticated form of reinforcement is provided by the arrangement whereby an animal stimulates itself through chronically implanted electrodes to produce pleasurable or painful sensations, depending on the site of stimulation in the brain (Olds and Milner, 1954).

Pavlov considered that the cerebral cortex was particularly important in relation to conditioning, but it is now evident that many forms of conditioning can occur in the decorticate animal and also in forms of life with a relatively simple nervous system. Thus, earthworms conditioned by the association of light and an electrical stimulus can be trained to turn in a particular direction. A relatively highly developed invertebrate which has been extensively studied in connection with learning is the octopus, which can readily be conditioned in response both to food and to painful stimuli. In this animal, the sensory systems both for vision and for chemotactile sensation are well developed. It can be trained to discriminate both in respect of visual and tactile stimuli. It will readily attack any object which it associates with food and it can be trained not to attack a particular object if it is given an electric shock. If it is taught to associate a vertical rectangle with food and a horizontal rectangle with an electric shock, it can be trained to attack the one but not the other. It cannot distinguish oblique lines and it appears that the receptive fields of the retina cells are arranged in vertical and horizontal planes. The nervous system of the octopus is relatively uncomplicated. Young (1961, 1965 and 1966) has used it to develop a neuronal model for the memory system of the brain which is based on both its known anatomy and its mode of response to stimuli (Fig. 12.3). The optic lobes contain neurones with branched axons which have been called classifying cells. If these cells are capable of responding to more than one type of stimulus, they could initiate an appropriate response by acting on the appropriate effector cell through one of the branched axons. Which response takes place depends on the activity of memory cells that act to facilitate one of the branched axons, while the other is inhibited so that the appropriate response is evoked, depending on the memory of the previous stimulus. Young has called this system a mnemon and postulates that the brain can be conceived as a hierarchy of mnemons showing different grades of complexity.

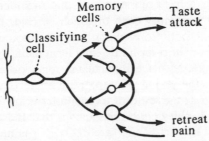

FIG. 12.3. The components of a single memory unit or mnemon. The classifying cell records the occurrence of a particular type of event. It has two outputs producing alternative possible motor actions. The system is biased to one of these, say 'attack'. Following this action signals indicating its results arrive and either reinforce what was done or produce the opposite action. Collaterals of the higher motor cells then activate the small cells, which produce inhibitory transmitter and close the unusual pathway. These may be called 'memory cells', because their synapses can be changed. Young, J. Z. (1965), *Proc. Roy. Soc. Ser. B.*, **163**, 285–320.

Although conditioning has provided much information in the study of learning and behaviour, the observation of group activity in animals has been useful in the study of adaptive learning and, in particular, the effect of learning on instinctive and inborn patterns of behaviour. Certain species of bird, such as the greylag goose, carry no innate capacity for the recognition of their own species and may develop a long lasting fixation on another species if they should see an individual of another species prior to contact with its own parent. This process of imprinting is of interest because it only occurs at particularly sensitive periods of development, is relatively permanent and can influence complex patterns of behaviour over long periods (Lorenz, 1937; 1969).

How memory traces are stored in the brain is unknown, but there is increasing evidence that the process may be related to changes in the protein structure of the cells that in turn may depend on changes which take place in the structure of RNA. Hyden (1961) has shown that if rats are exposed to rotatory stimuli there is a marked increase in the RNA content of the vestibular nuclei. The increase in the RNA content of the neurones is accompanied by a decrease in the RNA content of glial cells. Hyden has suggested that the glial cells may be intimately associated with the chemical processes involved in laying down the memory trace. Agranoff (1967) has shown that if goldfish are given an antibiotic which blocks protein synthesis, they can still learn to perform a simple task, but they lose the ability to consolidate a long term memory for the training procedure. Further evidence for the role of glial cells in memory storage comes from the observation that rats living in an enriched stimulating environment develop a thickened cerebral cortex with an increased density of neuroglia.

In clinical practice, it is usual to distinguish between short term and long term memory. On this basis it has been suggested that memory may be divided into primary and secondary memory each of which depends on a separate storage mechanism. It is evident, both from animal experiments and from clinical studies, that the consolidation of short term into long term memory can readily be interfered with by events taking place immediately or soon after the remembered stimulus. In this way, the period of retrograde amnesia which follows a head injury may be regarded as the result of trauma interfering with the consolidation of the memory trace. Lashley (1929) has shown that the ability to learn a task following the removal of part of the cerebral cortex is more dependent on the total mass of cortex removed than on which part of the brain is affected. Clinical studies, however, have shown that the hippocampal region is particularly important in the registering of memory, since loss of both hippocampal regions results in severe loss of short term memory although memories of the distant past persist.

Although memory is essential for mental processes, the faculty for forgetting is also important if thought is to be properly organized. The total capacity of the human memory is unknown and it is not understood to what extent it is possible to recall apparently forgotten material. The effect of electrical stimulation of the cortex in evoking past memories of past events in a few individuals as vividly as at the time they occurred is of interest in this respect, as is the existence of a few individuals who apparently have the capacity for total recall for past events in their lives (Luria, 1969).

THE ELECTRICAL ACTIVITY OF THE CORTEX

In 1875, Richard Caton was able to demonstrate continuous electrical activity from the surface of the brain of animals. These findings were confirmed by other workers and in particular by Prawdicz–Neminski (1925) who showed that potentials could be recorded through the intact skull of the dog. He was able to demonstrate two rhythms similar in frequency to the alpha and beta rhythms later described in man. In 1929, Berger showed that it was possible to record electrical potentials from the brain of the human subject. For this electrical activity, he introduced the name electroencephalogram. His earliest observations were made on patients who had skull defects resulting from neurosurgical operations. He followed these with studies on healthy subjects with intact skulls and later continued his observations on patients with epilepsy and other neurological disorders.

In 1934, Berger's observations were confirmed by Adrian and Matthews and since that time electroencephalography has developed into an important method for the study of cerebral activity in man. Since disease affecting the brain may affect the electrical potentials recorded from its surface, electrophysiological techniques have made important contributions to the clinical study of cerebral disease.

The Human Electroencephalogram

The potentials recorded from the human brain through the intact scalp are of low amplitude ranging from about 10 to a few hundred μV. They therefore require a high degree of amplification, so that recording apparatus may need to operate at a voltage gain of the order of 10^6. Since, however, they are of relatively low frequency they can be recorded after amplification by means of a pen recorder on moving paper.

Because it is important to localize the possible source of any electrical changes recorded, it is necessary to record simultaneously from different portions of the cranium. In practice this is done by using not less than eight amplifiers connected to a set of electrodes, which are placed over the skull according to a systematic pattern. Many different patterns of electrode placement have been devised, but one which has gained international acceptance is known as the 10–20 system (Jasper, 1958). In this arrangement 20 or more electrodes are placed on the skull according to measurements made from four landmarks. Appropriate switching arrangements make it possible to connect the recording amplifiers to the electrodes according to a number of different patterns or montages. EEG amplifiers have a balanced input and by convention, the leads to the two sides of each amplifier are referred to as black (grid 1) and white (grid 2) leads and the recording system is arranged so that the pen always gives an upward deflection when the black lead of the amplifier driving the pen is negative to the white.

In order to localize the possible source of an electrical disturbance, the recording system can be connected either as a unipolar or a bipolar montage. In the unipolar derivation, potentials are recorded between electrodes on the scalp, each of which is connected to one amplifier through its black lead and an indifferent or common reference electrode that may be attached to an ear lobe or other neutral point and to which all the white leads are connected. This method is not entirely satisfactory because no placement on the head is really indifferent. A modified method of unipolar recording is to use, instead of the indifferent electrode, what has been termed an average reference electrode. In this arrangement, the potentials are measured against a point that is connected to all the white leads in the same manner as the common reference electrode but, in addition, is connected to all the black leads through a set of equal resistors. By either unipolar method localization is made by comparison of the amplitude of the potential changes in the various channels. In bipolar recording, the potentials are recorded from pairs of electrodes that are placed on the scalp and to which the amplifiers are connected in series at common electrodes. With this arrangement, a focal disturbance near an electrode gives rise to a potential which is recorded out of phase by adjacent channels. A full account of the technical factors in EEG recording has been given by Cooper, Osselton and Shaw (1974).

The potentials recorded from the brain occupy a bandwidth of less than 60 Hz and the four principal wavebands commonly recorded are as follows:

(1) Alpha rhythm. This has a frequency of 8–13 Hz but most commonly occurs at a frequency of 9–10 Hz and the amplitude may reach 100 μV but is usually considerably less. In early infancy it cannot be detected by visual inspection of the record, although its presence can be demonstrated by frequency analysis. It may not become fully established until about the thirteenth year of life. It is recorded from the postcentral regions and is usually symmetrical, but especially in young people it may have a greater amplitude on the right side than the left. It is normally only present when the brain is idling and is blocked by visual attention. It is thus recorded when the eyes are closed. When the eyes are open, it disappears to leave only low voltage relatively fast activity (Fig. 12.4).

(2) Beta rhythm. This is a low voltage rhythm with a frequency which exceeds 13 Hz and the amplitude is seldom greater than 20 μV. It is recorded from the precentral part of the brain and appears to represent activity in the motor cortex. When recorded from the exposed cortex it can be blocked by voluntary movement (Jasper, 1949) but this blocking is less easy to demonstrate in the intact subject. In some subjects, a relatively high amplitude rhythm may be recorded from the central regionss at about half the frequency of beta rhythm. This is known as mu rhythm and it appears to be closely related to beta rhythm, perhaps as a harmonic, and is likewise blocked by movement of a contralateral limb (Fig. 12.5). During early sleep activity in the beta range of frequency is increased and may appear as short bursts or spindles of 14 Hz. Fast activity, similar in frequency to nautral beta rhythm, may also be recorded following intake of certain drugs such as barbiturates.

(3) Theta rhythm. This has a frequency which ranges from 4 to less than 8 Hz. It may form a substantial part of the background activity in children when it may be blocked by visual attention, but in the waking adult is scanty, generally with an amplitude of less than 20 μV.

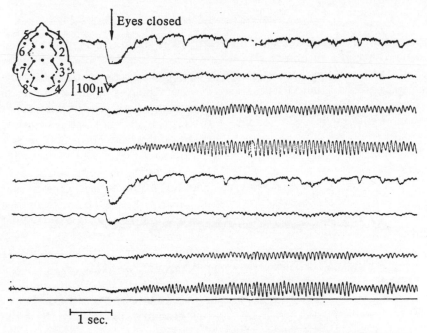

FIG. 12.4. EEG of healthy adult showing alpha rhythm present when eyes are closed. Time constant 0.3 sec.

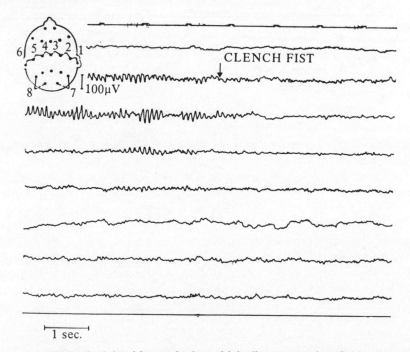

FIG. 12.5. EEG of adult with mu rhythm which disappears when fist is clenched. Artefact on channel 6. Time constant 0.3 sec.

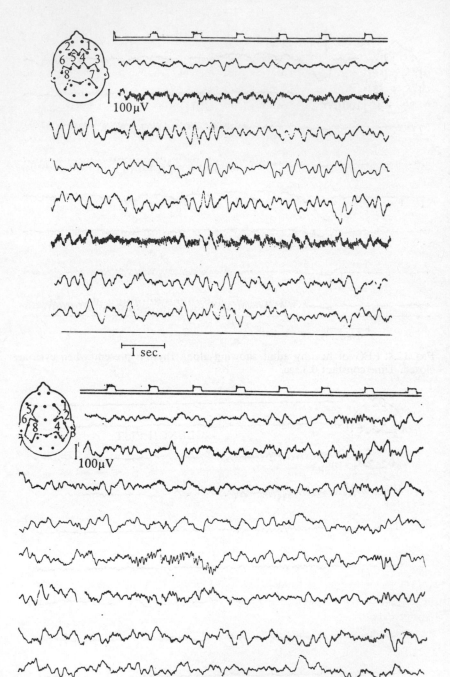

FIG. 12.6. (a) EEG of child aged 8 months awake but drowsy with eyes closed. Time constant 0.3 sec. (b) EEG of same child asleep; sleep spindles occur but are not synchronous as in adult.

(4) Delta rhythm. This includes all activity of less than 4 Hz. It is present as a normal rhythm in young children and may be the dominant rhythm in infants below the age of one year. In adults it is not normally seen when the subject is awake but is characteristically present in the deeper stages of sleep.

At birth and in the first month of life, the electroencephalogram shows little activity. Maturation is a gradual process, the adult rhythms not usually being fully established until between the ages of 13 and 18. During the first three months of life it consists of slow irregular activity which gradually gives way to rhythmical activity appearing over the occipital lobes. Alpha activity may begin to appear between the ages of 2 and 5, but at this time the record may be very complex with many different rhythms, the dominant frequency usually in the theta distribution. Below the age of 3 years, the alpha rhythm may be relatively unresponsive to eye opening. Before that age, theta activity will frequently respond to visual stimulation. Gradually, the slow activity becomes less evident as maturation develops, but in many individuals it may persist, particularly over the posterior temporal regions, until well after adult life is established (Figs. 12.6 and 12.7).

In their early studies of the EEG, Adrian and Matthews (1934) found that repetitive potentials could be recorded from the occipital region if the subject was exposed to a regularly flickering light. In general, flashes of light will evoke a response at flash frequencies of up to about 20/sec although a frequency of stimulation of around 10/sec is the most effective. Responses to flash can be recorded even in the newborn, but young infants will only respond to relatively slow rates of repetitive stimulation (Ellingson, 1960). The responses are characteristically positive with an amplitude which may reach about 40 μV (Fig. 12.8). In some individuals photic stimulation may give rise to paroxysmal discharges which occasionally can be associated with epileptic seizures. For that reason, photic stimulation has been widely employed as an activating procedure in clinical investigation.

A second activating procedure which is widely practised is that of hyperventilation. This gives rise to changes in the EEG that are secondary to the vasoconstriction of the cerebral vessels that follows lowering of the carbon dioxide tension in the blood. In children, this may produce a rapid change in the EEG which becomes dominated by symmetrical slow activity. In healthy adults, the changes are less striking, although slowing may take place in the presence of hypoglycaemia. In the presence of cerebral pathology, hyperventilation may be accompanied by paroxysmal discharges or by asymmetrical slow activity.

The Nature of Cortical Electrical Activity

In their early studies of the electroencephalogram, Adrian and Matthews considered that the 10 Hz rhythm, which is now known as the alpha rhythm, must represent synchronous activity of nerve cells in the occipital cortex. Since that

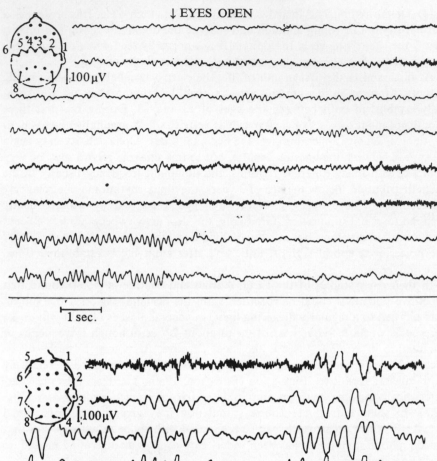

FIG. 12.7. (a) EEG of child aged 5 years. Time constant 0.3 sec. (b) EEG of same child after 1½mins hyperventilation. Time constant 0.3 sec.

time, the cortical origin of the different rhythms of the EEG has been generally recognized. It was originally considered that the potentials recorded from the brain must arise from the summated discharges of populations of neurones firing at approximately the same time. It is difficult however to explain the relatively slow changes of the cortical rhythms on the basis of discharging nerve cells since the duration of a single action potential is exceedingly brief in comparison with the duration of a surface potential. Evidence has gradually accumulated (see review by Purpura, 1959) that for the most part the slow potential changes

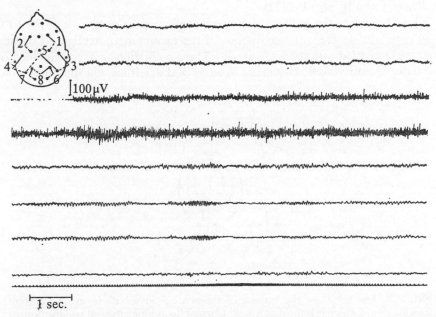

$100\,\mu\text{V}$

1 sec.

FIG. 12.8. Responses to photic stimulation; flash frequency on lowest line. Eyes closed. Photic responses most prominent channels 6 and 7. Time constant 0.3 sec.

on the cortex are not the result of discharging neurones but are due to changes in the postsynaptic potentials which occur in the soma and dendrites of cortical neurones. In this connection, the vertical arrangement of pyramidal cells in the cortex so that the cell bodies occupy the deeper layers and the dendrites, extend into and branch in the superficial layers is of particular interest.

The effect of an excitatory impulse arriving at a synapse connecting with a dendrite of a pyramidal cell is to depolarize the postsynaptic membrane so that the surface of the dendrite becomes negative. This will give rise to a flow of current from the positively charged soma to the dendrite. The vertically aligned pyramidal cell thus becomes a dipole with current flowing from the positive 'source' to a negative 'sink'. If a sufficient number of pyramidal cells are activated in the same way, a system of dipoles may be formed lying in parallel and at right angles to the surface, so that a negative potential may be recorded from the surface of the cortex. An inhibitory impulse acting on the soma to produce hyperpolarization would give rise to the same dipole configuration, but dipoles of opposite polarity would result either from depolarization of the nerve cell body or an inhibitory postsynaptic potential at the dendrite (Fig. 12.9). Assuming that cortical neurones can give rise to dipole arrangements of this kind, the potentials recorded by cortical and surface electrodes can be described according to the principles of volume conduction (Lorente de Nó, 1947; Woodbury, 1965; Hellerstein and Bickford, 1972).

A number of studies have now shown that the surface potentials of the EEG may correlate closely with oscillations of the membrane potentials of cortical neurones recorded with microelectrodes. These oscillations can be explained on the basis of postsynaptic potentials in soma and dendrites. On the other hand,

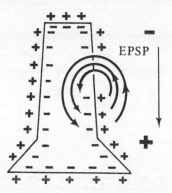

FIG. 12.9. The EPSP on the surface of the neurone gives rise to inward current flow the site of which is known as a sink. Current flows along the cell and the flow of current from positive source to negative sink is a dipole. Large potentials can arise when dipoles are situated in parallel. By convention the direction of the dipole is shown by an arrow pointing from sink to source.

correlation of the waveform of EEG sleep spindles in the anesthetized animal with spike discharges is variable and the slow potential changes persist even when spike discharges are suppressed by anesthesia. Long lasting depolarizations of cortical cells, however, are associated with the spike discharges that are recorded from the cortex during seizures induced by convulsant drugs such as metrazol (Li and Jasper, 1953; Jasper and Stefanis, 1965; Creutzfeldt, Watanabe and Lux, 1966).

If the potential changes in the cortical EEG are considered to be due to the slow build up and decay of postsynaptic potentials in cortical neurones, it is evident that the changes must take place in large populations of neurones at the same time. It is not, at present, certain how far the isolated cortex is capable of synchronous discharges in this manner (Kristiansen and Courtois, 1949; Burns, 1951) but the evidence suggests that in the intact brain the electrical changes recorded in the cortex are generated by impulses from subcortical centres.

Pacemaker Mechanisms

Although the site of origin of the cortical rhythms is unknown, the fact that the alpha and beta rhythms occur synchronously or nearly synchronously on each side suggests that the rhythms recorded on the two hemispheres may be derived from a common subcortical pacemaker. On the other hand, Adrian and Yamagiwa (1935) and Walsh (1958) have found evidence for two separate subcortical generators giving rise to the alpha rhythm on either side. Recently, it has been suggested that the alpha rhythm may be derived not from the cortex, but from the standing potential of the eye modulated by physiological tremor of the ocular muscles (Lippold, 1970). However, there is now a great deal of evidence to suggest that the nuclei in the thalamus and in the reticular formation are particularly important in the genesis of cortical rhythmical activity.

In 1941 Dempsey, Morison and Morison found that stimulation of the sciatic nerve in cats would give rise to an early primary response in the leg area of the sensory cortex and a late secondary response, which could be recorded over extensive regions of the cortex. The primary response was abolished by lesions involving the greater part of the thalamus, but the secondary response persisted unless the midline structures were damaged. Later, Morison and Dempsey (1942) found that stimulation of the lateral thalamic mass was followed by a localized surface positive potential on the sensory cortex but that stimulation of the medial thalamic area gave rise to a surface negative response, which could be detected over many cortical areas. They suggested that the primary responses arose from activation of the specific sensory thalamocortical projection system, whereas the secondary response was mediated through a non-specific thalamic system with diffuse connections. The secondary response, which they termed the recruiting response, differed in character according to the depth of anesthesia and the frequency of stimulation. In the deeply anesthetized animal, a single stimulus produced no response. However, slow rates of stimulation were followed by surface negative potentials, which increased progressively in amplitude. In lightly anesthetized animals, a single stimulus was followed by a train of potentials at a rate of 8–12 Hz that closely resembled the spontaneous activity recorded from the cortex during light anesthesia. If stimuli were given repetitively at a rate slower than 8–12 Hz evoked potentials occurred at this frequency which were similar, both in respect of frequency and in their tendency to wax and wane in amplitude, to spontaneous cortical activity (Dempsey and Morison, 1942). Exploration of the thalamus with depth electrodes has also shown that spontaneous bursts of rhythmical activity at 5–10 Hz can be recorded from a number of situations, in particular the non-specific nuclei in the intralaminar region (Morison, Finley and Lothrop, 1943). Many people have confirmed the presence of spontaneous rhythmical activity in the thalamus. It is evident that this can be recorded from many parts of the thalamus and not only from the non-specific nuclei and is present even when the thalamus is largely isolated from the cortex. Anderssen and Sears (1964) have suggested that this rhythmical activity may arise through a system of 'phasic recurrent inhibition'. In this way, a cycle may be initiated by a weak afferent stimulus exciting a relay cell. This acts through an inhibitory interneurone to inhibit a group of relay cells that later enter into a phase of post inhibitory exaltation in which they discharge synchronously and,

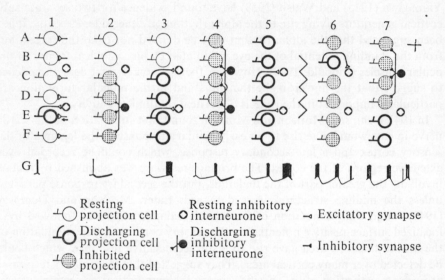

FIG. 12.10. Diagrammatic representation of the inhibitory phasing theory. Columns 1–5 represent stages in the development of a thalamic spindle and 6 and 7 two stages of the end. Anderssen, P. and Sears, T. A. (1964), *J. Physiol.* (*Lond.*), **173**, 459–480.

in the same manner, bring about inhibition of a still larger group of neurones that later discharge in unison. After a variable period, some cells drop out of the cycle which gradually comes to an end. In this way, a regular thalamocortical discharge can be set up that could initiate rhythmical activity in the cortex or alternatively act on and modulate a similar intrinsic mechanism already present in the cortex (Fig. 12.10).

The symmetrical distribution of the paroxysmal discharges in the EEG in certain kinds of epilepsy has led to interest in the midline structures of the thalamus as a possible source of an epileptic disturbance. Stimulation of certain parts of the intralaminar portion of the thalamus in cats can give rise to an 'arrest reaction' accompanied by a bilaterally synchronous spike and wave discharge, similar to that seen in petit mal epilepsy. Continued stimulation at sufficient intensity may give rise to convulsions (Hunter and Jasper, 1949). These and other observations have led to the view that petit mal, and other varieties of generalized epilepsy, arise from a primary subcortical disturbance in the thalamic region. Williams (1965) in a recent review considers that the integrity of the thalamus and the deep midline structures is necessary for the propagation of a generalized epileptic discharge but it is still uncertain whether these structures or an abnormal focus in the cortex or elsewhere is the primary source of this type of epileptic disturbance.

The Ascending Reticular System and Sleep

If the EEG is recorded when a subject is falling asleep, the earliest change to be observed is generally a reduction in the abundance of alpha rhythm and at the same time, slower waves in the theta range of frequency make their appearance. In light sleep, the amount of intermediate slow activity increases and bursts of activity at 12–14 Hz appear, which are known as sleep spindles. At this stage, a sensory stimulus, such as a sudden noise, may give rise to negative sharp waves which are recorded over the vertex or to a widespread complex slow wave discharge or K complex. As sleep deepens, the greater part of the record comes to consist of slow waves in the delta frequency at less than 3 Hz (Figs. 12.11, 12.12 and 12.13a and b).

In 1935, Bremer showed that if the fore-brain of a cat is isolated by dividing the midbrain between the colliculi, cerveau isolé, the animal remains in a state of sleep and the EEG is predominantly composed of large slow waves and spindle bursts. On the other hand, if the section is made at the level of the first cervical vertebra so that the brain is separated from the spinal cord, encèphalé isolé, the animal appears to be awake and the EEG shows the low voltage fast activity characteristic of wakefulness. At that time, afferent impulses in the classical sensory pathways were the only known influences ascending from the brain stem to the hemispheres. Bremer considered that the conduction of sensory impulses to the cortex was responsible for wakefulness and that loss of afferent stimuli led to sleep. Subsequent experiments by Moruzzi and Magoun (1949) showed that if electrodes were placed in the reticular core of the brain stem of an anesthetized animal, stimulation would abolish the synchronized discharges of the sleeping EEG and give rise to low voltage fast activity. The effects could be obtained by stimulation of the reticular formation in the medulla or in the tegmentum of the pons and midbrain, and in the subthalamus and dorsal hypothalamus. The excitable system appeared to comprise a series of reticular relays ascending to the basal diencephalon. Its threshold was low and it responded best to high frequencies of stimulation of up to 300 Hz.

K

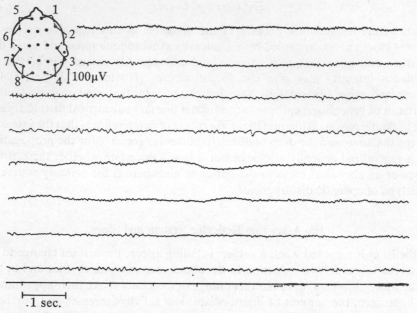

FIG. 12.11. EEG of drowsy adult with rolling eye movements. Time constant 0.3 sec.

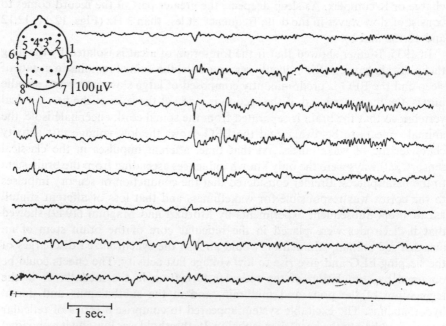

FIG. 12.12. EEG of sleeping adult with sleep spindles and vertex sharp waves. Time constant 0.3 sec.

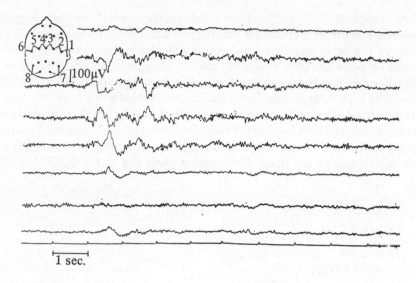

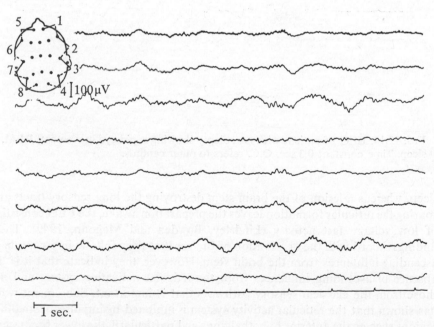

Fig. 12.13. (a) EEG of adult asleep showing K complex. Time constant 0.3 sec. (b) EEG of same subject more deeply asleep with widespread delta activity and traces of sleep spindles.

The encèphalé isolé preparation which remains awake in the absence of anesthesia is a useful preparation for studying the effects on the waking EEG of lesions of the brain stem that involve the reticular system. Elimination of the medulla or pons has little effect, but striking changes occur with lesions of the midbrain or diencephalon, so that the EEG activation pattern of fast activity is replaced by high voltage slow waves and recurrent spindle bursts similar to those seen in natural sleep and anesthesia. This effect has occurred particularly with tegmental lesions which involve the reticular formation and spare the brain stem afferent pathways. Thus, a lesion of the reticular activating system in the midbrain tegmentem or the basal diencephalon gives rise to the EEG changes of

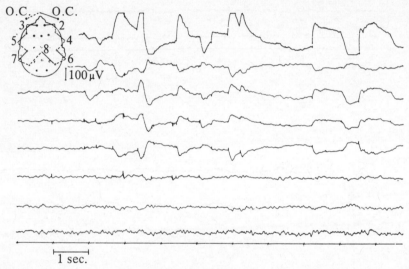

FIG. 12.14. EEG of patient with narcolepsy showing rapid eye movement, REM, sleep. Time constant 0.3 sec. O.C. refers to outer canthus.

sleep, whereas a lesion of the brain stem destroying the long sensory tracts and sparing the reticular formation leaves the preparation awake, the EEG consisting of low voltage fast activity (Lindsley, Bowden and Magoun, 1949). These findings accord with the observation of Bremer that sleep follows interruption of ascending influences from the brain stem. However, they indicate that it is the absence of ascending influences from the reticular activating system and not those from the classical sensory pathways that is important. Subsequent work has shown that the reticular activity system is inhibited by impulses from other regions such as the anterior hypothalamus and particularly the lower brain stem, so that sleep and waking evidently depend on the reciprocal action of different subcortical centres (Moruzzi, 1960).

If the EEG is recorded continuously during a night's sleep, it is seen that phases occur in which the slow waves of deep sleep are replaced by low voltage fast activity and the eyes show rapid conjugate movements. These phases may last up to about 20 min and do not usually appear until the subject has been asleep for an hour or longer. If he is wakened during this period he may report that he has been dreaming (Aserinski and Kleitman, 1955; Dement and Kleitman, 1957). During this rapid eye movement, REM, or paradoxal phase of sleep (Fig. 12.14), arousal may be more difficult than at other times. Electromyographic studies have shown that the muscles are in a state of virtually complete relaxation. In the cat, coagulation of the pons may prevent the development of paradoxical sleep and Jouvet (1965) considers that paradoxical sleep is brought about by action of the pontine reticular formation. The physiological significance of paradoxical sleep is unknown, but it clearly is important for the well being of the organism since if it is suppressed in an animal, by applying an arousing stimulus whenever it develops, subsequent sleep shows an increased percentage of REM sleep (Jouvet, 1965). A similar effect is observed in the human subject if drugs are administered, such as barbiturates or amphetamine, which suppress paradoxical sleep. If the drug is discontinued, after a period of time, the period of administration may be followed by a period that may extend into several weeks when the amount of paradoxical sleep is increased (Oswald, 1965). When a patient with narcolepsy falls asleep he passes directly into paradoxical sleep (Rechtschaffen *et al.*, 1963) and attacks of sleep paralysis may be due to awakening from this stage of sleep when the patient may find himself unable to move due to the profound hypotonia.

Cerebral Evoked Potentials

If a subject is exposed to a flickering light with the flicker occurring at frequency of up to about 30 Hz, rhythmical activity can be recorded from the occipital cortex at the frequency of the flicker or a harmonic of that frequency. This repetitive response to flickering light is of high enough amplitude to be recorded by standard EEG recording arrangements. This response to repetitive stimulation by a flickering light is an example of a specific evoked response in which a particular type of stimulus evokes a response in the part of the brain normally concerned in receiving the impulses relating to the type of sensation concerned. The K complex or the vertex sharp waves which occur in response to an arousal stimulus in light sleep are examples of non-specific responses that may occur in response to a variety of sensory stimuli. They are not confined to any particular situation in the cortex, although they are generally best obtained from the region of the vertex. Specific responses are of relatively short latency and can fairly readily be obtained from the skin overlying the striate and postcentral areas of cortex. They are less readily obtained from the auditory cortex and study of the non-specific vertex potential following auditory stimuli has proved helpful in the recognition of deafness, particularly in children.

The amplitude of cerebral evoked potentials recorded by means of scalp electrodes is of the order of a few μV and they are therefore difficult to distinguish from the background activity of the EEG. Dawson in 1947 was able to demonstrate cerebral responses to peripheral nerve stimulation by photographing superimposed sweeps on an oscilloscope. In 1960, Cobb and Dawson used an averaging device to study the characteristics of occipital responses to visual stimuli. At the present time, digital averaging computers are regularly used to record evoked potentials.

It is not yet possible to adequately evaluate the clinical place of evoked potential studies that at present can only provide information of a limited nature, some of it already accessible to less elaborate techniques. Visual evoked potentials (Fig. 12.15) may show asymmetries in the presence of cerebral tumours and may

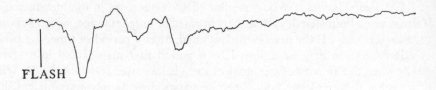

FLASH

10 μVolts

+100 msec.

Fig. 12.15. Average of 128 responses to light flash recorded between occipital and vertex electrodes from a healthy subject. There is considerable variation in the form of the visual evoked response dependent both on individual variation and recording technique.

be enhanced in some epileptic patients, particularly those who show photosensitivity. Somatosensory potentials may show a reduced amplitude and a prolonged latency in peripheral nerve lesions, and in spinal cord disease where the pathways conveying position and joint sense, but not those conveying pain and temperature sensation, are affected. In myoclonus epilepsy a proportion of patients have somatosensory potentials of abnormally high amplitude. The study of auditory evoked potentials following audiometric stimuli has proved of value in the study of deafness. It is particularly helpful with disturbed or handicapped children in whom it can be successfully carried out in sleep (Dawson, 1947b; Halliday and Wakefield, 1963; Halliday, 1967; Bergamini and Bergamesco, 1967; see review by Regan, 1972).

The Contingent Negative Variation

If a subject decides to carry out a voluntary movement, a negative potential with a duration of 1–2 sec can be recorded from the vertex immediately before the movement is carried out. This potential has been termed the 'Bereitschafts-potential' by Kornhuber and Deeke (1964 and 1965). This is probably similar to

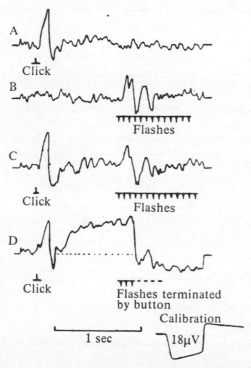

Fig. 12.16. Contingent negative variation. Average of response to 12 presenta-tions. A. Response in fronto vertical region to clicks. B. Flicker. C. Clicks followed by flicker. D. Clicks followed by flicker terminated by the subject pressing a button as instructed. The contingent negative variation appears following the conditional response and submerges the negative component of the imperative response. Grey Walter, W., Cooper, R., Aldridge, V. J., McCallum, W. C. and Winter, A. L. (1964). *Nature*, **203**, 380–384.

the contingent negative variation described by Walter and his colleagues (1964) in which a negative potential is recorded from the frontocentral region following a warning stimulus that the subject has learned will be succeeded by a stimulus which will involve the subject in carrying out an action or making a decision. In one experimental procedure, an audible click is followed after an interval of 1 sec by a series of flashes, which the subject is able to terminate by pressing a

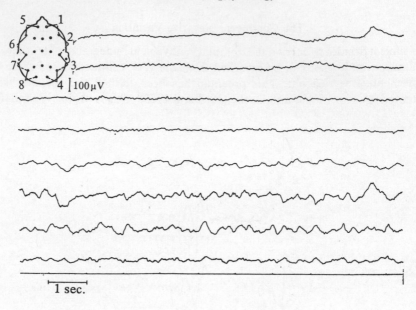

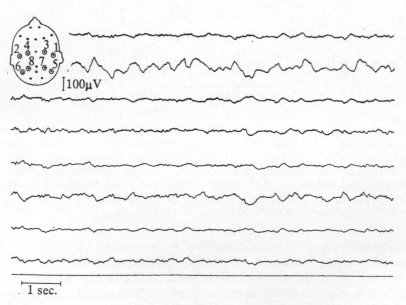

FIG. 12.17. (a) Left temporal lobe abscess, eyes closed. Bipolar recording. Time constant 0.3 sec. (b) Same patient. Average reference. Time constant 0.3 sec.

button. If this sequence of events is repeated a number of times, for example 12, and the potential changes recorded by means of an averaging device, the negative potential or expectancy (E) wave can be seen developing between the click stimulus and the flashes (Fig. 12.1b). There is considerable variation in the E wave between different subjects and in the same subject at different times, depending on the degree of motivation and the emotional state at the time the test is carried out. The contingent negative variation is of interest in the study of psychological disorders. There is evidence that the E wave may be sometimes difficult to obtain in criminal psychopaths, may show abnormal variability in patients with anxiety states and be abnormally persistent in patients with obsessional compulsive states (Walter, 1967).

The EEG in Cerebral Lesions

In 1936, Walter was successful in localizing cerebral tumours by means of the EEG. At about the same time Gibbs, Gibbs and Lennox (1937) studied the EEG changes which occur in association with epilepsy. A space occupying lesion may declare itself by giving rise to local slow activity in the EEG, since slow activity is the characteristic change that is seen overlying brain tissue in which the metabolism is disturbed (Figs. 12.17a and b). For this reason, a cerebral infarct may give rise to changes similar to those resulting from tumour and the issue may be clarified by serial records. If cerebral tissue is replaced by tumour tissue or by a porencephalic cyst, there may be an area of relative electrical silence. A subdural haematoma overlying part of the brain may lead to an apparent reduction in amplitude of the normal background activity on the affected side. A tumour may also exert its effect by causing a general rise in intracranial pressure that may be associated with disappearance of the normal background rhythms, which may be replaced by slow activity.

In epileptic subjects, a record taken between seizures may be normal, but many subjects may show paroxysmal spike discharges, which if they are focal, may provide information regarding the situation of the abnormal tissue that is giving rise to the epileptic discharge (Fig. 12.18). In petit mal, the 3/sec spike and wave discharge which occurs during a seizure is frequently present during interseizure records (Fig. 12.19). In many metabolic and degenerative disorders of the brain, the EEG is abnormal and single or serial records taken together with the clinical findings may contribute to reaching a correct diagnosis. In some circumstances, the EEG may be an exceedingly sensitive index to the acuteness of a disease process and in severe brain damage it may assist in evaluating the prognosis. When it is uncertain whether the brain is viable or not, the presence or absence of electrical activity in the EEG during a period of prolonged observation may be of critical importance. An important limitation of the EEG, on the other hand, is that even in conditions where the EEG is frequently helpful, normal records can be obtained even in the presence of significant

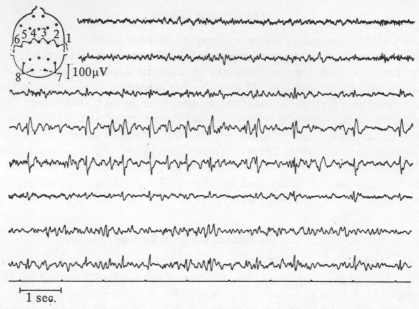

FIG. 12.18. Child age 7 years with cortical epilepsy to show left central focal discharge. Eyes closed. Time constant 0.3 sec.

↓ OPEN EYES

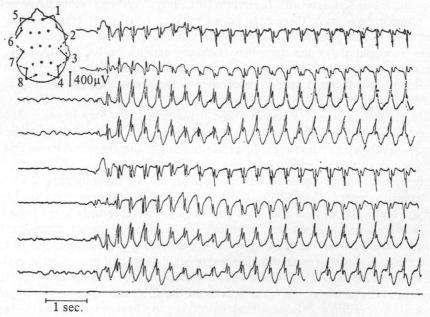

FIG. 12.19. 3/sec spike and wave discharge occurring in child with petit mal epilepsy after 2 mins hyperventilation. Spontaneous eye opening occurs during paroxysmal discharge. Time constant 0.3 sec.

pathology and a normal EEG does not in itself exclude cerebral disease. The clinical applications of electroencephalography have been reviewed at length by Hill and Driver, 1962, Hill and Parr, 1963, and Kiloh, McComas and Osselton, 1972).

REFERENCES

ADRIAN, E. D. and MATTHEWS, B. H. C. (1934). The Berger rhythm: potential changes from the occipital lobes in man. *Brain*, **57**, 355–385.

ADRIAN, E. D. and YAMAGIWA, K. (1935). The origin of the Berger rhythm. *Brain*, **58**, 323–351.

AGRANOFF, B. W. (1967). Memory and protein sysnthesis. *Scien. Am.* **216**, 115–122.

ANDERSSEN, P. and SEARS, T. A. (1964). The role of inhibition in the phasing of spontaneous thalamo cortical discharge. *J. Physiol. (Lond.)*, **173**, 459–480.

ASERINSKY, E. and KLEITMAN, N. (1955). Two types of ocular motility occurring in sleep. *J. Appl. Physiol.*, **8**, 1–10.

BERGAMINI, L. and BERGAMESCO, B. (1967). *Cortical Evoked Potentials in Man*. Springfield: Thomas.

BERGER, H. (1929). Das Elektrenkephalogram des Menschen. *Arch. Psychiat. Nervenkr.*, **87**, 527–570. Reprinted in *Electroenceph. clin. Neurophysiol.* (1969), suppl. 28. Ed. and translated by Gloor. P.

BOND, M. R. (1972). Psychosurgery. In: *Scientific Foundations of Neurology*. Ed. Critchley, MacD., O'Leary, J. and Jennett, B. London: Heinemann.

BRAIN, L. (1965). Speech Disorders. *Aphasia, Apraxia and Agnosia*. London: Butterworth.

BREMER, F. (1935). Cerveau 'isolé' et physiologie de sommeil *C.R. Soc. Biol. (Paris)* **118**, 1235–1242.

BURNS, D. D. (1951). Some properties of isolated cerebral cortex in the unanaesthetized cat. *J. Physiol. (Lond.)*, **112**, 156–175.

CATON, R. (1875). The electrical currents of the brain. *Brit. med. J.*, ii, 278.

COBB, W. A. and DAWSON, G. D. (1960). The latency and form in man of the occipital potentials evoked by bright flashes. *J. Physiol. (Lond.)*, **152**, 108–121.

COOPER, R., OSSELTON, J. W. and SHAW, J. C. (1974). *EEG Technology*. 2nd Edn. London: Butterworths.

CREUTZFELDT, O. D., WATANABE, S. and LUX, H. D. (1966). Relations between EEG phenomena and potentials of single cortical cells. I. Evoked responses after thalamic and epicortical stimulation. II. Spontaneous and convulsant activity. *Electroenceph. clin. Neurophysiol.* (1966), **I**, 1–18; **II**, 19–37.

CRITCHLEY, M. (1953). *The Parietal Lobes*. New York: Hafner Publishing Co.

CRITCHLEY, M. (1970). The Origins of Aphasiology. In: *Aphasiology* (Chap. 6). London: Edward Arnold.

DAWSON, G. D. (1947a). Cerebral responses to electrical stimulation of peripheral nerve in man. *J. Neurol. Neurosurg. Psychiat.*, **10**, 134–140.

DAWSON, G. D. (1947b). Investigations on a patient subject to myoclonic seizures after sensory stimulation. *J. Neurol. Neurosurg. Psychiat.*, **10**, 141–162.

DEMENT, W. and KLEITMAN, N. (1957). Cyclic variations in EEG during sleep and their relation to eye movements, body motility and dreaming. *Electroenceph. clin. Neurophysiol.*, **9**, 673–690.

DEMPSEY, E. W., MORISON, R. S. and MORISON, B. R. (1941). Some afferent diencephalic pathways related to cortical potentials in the cat. *Amer. J. Physiol.*, **131**, 718–731.

DEMPSEY, E. W. and MORISON, R. S. (1942). The production of rhythmically recurrent cortical potentials after localized thalmic stimulation. *Amer. J. Physiol.*, **135**, 293–300.

DIMOND, S. (1972). *The Double Brain.* Edinburgh: Livingstone.

ELLINGSON, R. J. (1960). Cortical electrical responses to visual stimulation in the human infant. *Electroenceph. clin. Neurophysiol.*, **12**, 663–677.

FERRIER, D. (1876). *The Functions of the Brain.* London: Smith, Elder and Co.

GAZZANIGA, M. S. and SPERRY, R. W. (1967). Language after section of the cerebral commisures. *Brain*, **90**, 131–148.

GESCHWIND, N. (1965). Disconnexion syndromes in animals and man. Part I, *Brain*, **88**, 237–294. Part II, *Brain*, **88**, 585–644.

GESCHWIND, N. (1970). The clinical syndromes of the cortical connections. In: *Modern Trends in Neurology.* No. 5. Ed. Williams, D. London: Butterworths.

GIBBS, F. A., GIBBS, E. L. and LENNOX, W. G. (1937). Epilepsy: a paroxysmal cerebral dysrhythmia. *Brain*, **60**, 377–388.

GOODGLASS, H. and QUADFASEL, F. A. (1954). Language laterality in left-handed aphasics. *Brain*, **77**, 521–548.

HALLIDAY, A. M. (1967). Changes in the form of cerebral evoked responses in man associated with various lesions of the nervous system. *Electroenceph. clin. Neurophysiol.*, suppl., **25**, 178–192.

HALLIDAY, A. M. and WAKEFIELD, G. S. (1963). Cerebral evoked responses in patients with dissociated sensory loss. *J. Neurol. Neurosurg. Psychiat.*, **26**, 211–219.

HEAD, H. and HOLMES, G. (1911). Sensory disturbances from cerebral lesions. *Brain*, **34**, 102–254.

HÉCAEN, H. (1962). Clinical symptomatology in right and left hemispheric lesions. In: *Interhemispheric Relations and Cerebral Dominance.* Ed. Mountcastle, V. B. Baltimore: Johns Hopkins Press.

HELLERSTEIN, D. and BICKFORD, R. (1972). Electrical activity of the brain. In: *Scientific Foundations of Neurology.* Ed. Critchley, MacD., O'Leary, J. and Jennett B. London: Heinemann.

HILL, D. and DRIVER, M. V. (1962). Electroencephalography. In: *Recent Advances in Neurology and Neuropsychiatry.* Ed. Lord Brain, 7th Edn. London: Churchill.

HILL, D. and PARR, G. (1963). *Electroencephalography.* London: Macdonald. 2nd Edn.

HUMPHREY, M. E. and ZANGWILL, O. L. (1952). Dysphasia in left-handed patients with unilateral brain lesions. *J. Neurol. Neurosurg. Psychiat.*, **15**, 184–193.

HUNTER, J. and JASPER, H. H. (1949). Effects of thalamic stimulation in unanaesthetized animals. *Electroenceph. clin. Neurophysiol.*, **1**, 305–324.

HYDEN, H. (1961). Biochemical aspects of brain activity. In: *Man and Civilization: Control of the Mind.* Ed. Farger, S. and Wilson R. New York: McGraw-Hill.

JACKSON, J. H. (1931). *Selected Writings.* Ed. Taylor, J. 2 Vols. London: Hodder and Stoughton.

JACOBSEN, C. F. (1936). The functions of the frontal association areas in monkeys. *Comp. Psychol. Monog.*, **13**, 3–60.

JAKOBSON, R. (1964). Towards a linguistic typology of asphasic impairments. In: *Disorders of Language.* Ed. de Reuck, A. V. S. and O'Connor, M. Ciba Foundation Symposium. Boston: Little, Brown and Co.

JASPER, H. H. (1949). Electrocorticograms in man. *Electroenceph. clin. Neurophysiol.*, **2**, 16–29.

JASPER, H. H. (1958). Report of the committee on methods of clinical examination in electroencephalography. *Electroenceph. clin. Neurophysiol.*, **10**, 370.

JASPER, H. H. and STEFANIS, C. (1965). Intracellular oscillatory rhythms in pyramidal tract neurones in the cat. *Electroenceph. clin. Neurophysiol.*, **18**, 541–553.

JOUVET, M. (1968). Paradoxical sleep—a study of its nature and mechanisms. In: Sleep Mechanisms. *Progress in Brain Research*, **18**, Ed. Akert, Balley and Schadé. Amsterdam: Elsevier. 20–57.

KILOH, L. G., McCOMAS, A. J. and OSSELTON, J. W. (1972). *Clinical Electroencephalography*. 3rd Edn. London: Butterworths.

KLÜVER, H. and BUCY, P. C. (1937). Psychic blindness and other symptoms following bilateral temporal lobectomy in rhesus monkeys. *Amer. J. Physiol.*, **119**, 352–353.

KLÜVER, H. and BUCY, P. C. (1939). Preliminary analysis of functions of the temporal lobes in monkeys. *Arch. Neurol. Psychiat. (Chicago)*, **42**, 979–1000.

KORNHUBER, H. H. and DEECKE, L. (1964). Hirnpotentialänderungen beim Menschen vor und nach Willkürbewegungen, chargestellt mit Magnet band speicherung und Rückwärtsanalyse. *Pflügers Archiv.*, **281**, 52.

KORNHUBER, H. H. and DEECKE, L. (1965). Hirnpotentialänderungen bei Willkurbewegungen und passiven Bewegungen des Menschen: Bereitschaftspotential und reafferente Potentiale. *Pflügers Archiv.*, **284**, 1–17.

KRISTIANSEN, K. and COURTOIS, G. (1949). Rhythmic electrical activity from isolated cerebral cortex. *Electroenceph. clin. Neurophysiol.*, **1**, 265–272.

LASHLEY, K. S. (1929). *Brain Mechanisms and Intelligence*. Chicago: Chicago University Press. Republished 1964, New York: Hafner.

LEWIN, W. and PHILIPS, C. G. (1952). Observations on partial removal of the postcentral gyrus for pain. *J. Neurol. Neurosurg. Psychiat.*, **15**, 143–147.

LI, C.-L. and JASPER, H. (1953). Microelectrode studies of the electrical activity of the cerebral cortex in the cat. *J. Physiol. (Lond.)*, **121**, 117–140.

LINDSLEY, D. B., BOWDEN, J. W. and MAGOUN, H. W. (1949). Effect upon the EEG of acute injury to the brain stem activating system. *Electroenceph. clin. Neurophysiol*, **1**, 475–486.

LIPPOLD, O. C. J. (1970). Origin of the alpha ryhthm. *Nature*, **226**, 616–618.

LORENTE DE NÓ, R. (1947). *Studies from the Rockefeller Institute for Medical Research*, **132** (2) Chap. 16, pp. 384–477.

LORENZ, K. Z. (1935). Companions as factors in the bird's environment reprinted in *Studies in Animal and Human Behaviour*, Vol. 1. London: Methven, 1970.

LORENZ, K. Z. (1969). Innate Bases of Learning. In: *On the Biology of Learning*. Ed. Pribram, K. H. New York: Harcourt, Brace and World Inc.

LURIA, A. R. (1966). *Higher Cortical Functions in Man*. London: Tavistock Publications.

LURIA, A. R. (1969). *The Mind of a Mnemonist*. London: Jonathan Cape.

LURIA, A. R. (1973). *The Working Brain*. London: Penguin Books.

MARSHALL, J. (1951). Sensory disturbances in cortical wounds with special reference to pain. *J. Neurol. Neurosurg. Psychiat.*, **14**, 187–204.

MILNER, B. (1962). Laterality effects in Audition. In: *Interhemispheric Relations and Cerebral Dominance*. Ed. Mountcastle, V. B. Baltimore: Johns Hopkins Press.

MORISON, R. S. and DEMPSEY, E. W. (1942). A study of thalamo cortical relations. *Amer. J. Physiol.*, **135**, 281–292.

MORISON, R. S., FINLEY, K. H. and LOTHROP, G. N. (1943). Spontaneous electrical activity of the thalamus and other forebrain structures. *J. Neurophysiol.*, **6**, 243–254.

MORUZZI, G. (1960). Synchronizing influences of the brain stem and the inhibitory mechanisms underlying the production of sleep by sensory stimulation. *Electroenceph. clin. Neurophysiol.*, **13**, 231–256.

MORUZZI, G. and MAGOUN, H. W. (1949). Brain stem reticular formation and activation of the EEG. *Electroenceph. clin. Neurophysiol.*, **1**, 455–473.

OLDS, J. and MILNER, P. (1954). Positive reinforcement produced by electrical stimulation of septal area and other regions of rat brain. *J. comp. and physiol. psychol.*, **47**, 419–427.

OSWALD, I. (1965). Some psychophysiological features of human sleep. In: *Progress in Brain Research*, **18**, Sleep Mechanisms. Ed. Akert, Bally and Schadé, Amsterdam: Elsevier. 160–169.

PAPEZ, J. W. (1937). A proposed mechanism of emotion. *Arch. Neurol. Psychiat. (Chicago)*, **38**, 725–743.

PAVLOV, I. P. (1927). *Conditioned Reflexes*. An investigation of the physiological activity of the cerebral cortex. New York: Dover Publications Inc. 1960 (republication of translation first published in 1927 by Oxford University Press). Translated and edited by Anrep, G. V.

PENFIELD, W. (1966). Speech, perception and the uncommitted cortex. In: *Brain and Conscious Experience*. Ed. Eccles, J. C. Berlin: Springer-Verlag.

PENFIELD, W. and BOLDREY, E. (1937). Somatic motor and sensory representation in the cerebral cortex of man as studied by electrical stimulation. *Brain*, **60**, 389–443.

PENFIELD, W. and JASPER, H. (1954). *Epilepsy and the Functional Anatomy of the Human Brain*. London: Churchill.

PENFIELD, W. and MILNER, B. (1958). Memory deficit produced by bilateral lesions in the hippocampal zone. *Arch. Neurol. Psychiat. (Chicago)*, **79**, 475–497.

PIERCY, M. (1967). Studies of the neurological basis of intellectual function. In: *Modern Trends in Neurology*. 4. Ed. Williams, D. London: Butterworths.

PRAWDICZ-NEMINSKI, W. W. (1925). Zur Kenntnis der elektrischen und der Innervations vorgänge in den funktionellen Elementen und Geweben des tierischen Organismus. Elektrocerebrogramm der Säugetieri. *Pflügers Archiv. Physiologie.*, **209**, 362–382.

PRIBRAM, K. H. (1966). A neurophysiological approach to the analysis of the neuro-behavioural deficit that follows frontal lesions in primates. *Proceedings of the Eighteenth International Congress of Psychology*. Moscow, 1966. Reprinted in *Brain and Behaviour*. 3. Memory Mechanisms. Ed. Pribram. K. H. Harmondsworth: Penguin Books Ltd.

PURPURA, D. P. (1959). Nature of electrocortical potentials and synaptic organizations in cerebral and cerebellar cortex. *Int. Rev. Neurobiol.*, **1**, 47–163.

RAMÓN Y CAJAL, S. (1894). La fine structure des centres nerveux. Croonian lecture, March 8, 1894. *Proc. roy. Soc.*, **55**, 444–468.

RECHTSCHAFFEN, A., WOLPERT, E. A., DEMENT, W. C., MITCHELL, S. A. and FISHER, C. (1963). Nocturnal sleep of narcoleptics. *Electroenceph. clin. Neurophysiol.*, **15**, 599–609.

REGAN, D. (1972). *Evoked Potentials in Psychology, Sensory Physiology and Clinical Medicine*. London: Chapman and Hall.

RUSSELL, W. R. and ESPIR, M. L. E. (1961). *Traumatic Aphasia*. London: Oxford University Press.

SCOVILLE, W. B. and MILNER, B. (1957). Loss of recent memory after bilateral hippocampal lesions. *J. Neurol. Neurosurg. Psychiat.*, **20**, 11–21.

SERAFETINIDES, E. A., HOARE, R. D. and DRIVER, M. V. (1965). Intracarotid sodium amylobarbitone and cerebral dominance for speech and consciousness. *Brain*, **88**, 107–130.

SMITH, A. (1966). Intellectual functions in patients with lateralized frontal tumours. *J. Neurol. Neurosurg. Psychiat.*, **29**, 52–59.

SPERRY, R. W. (1964). The great cerebral commisure. *Scien. Am.* **210**, 42–52.

TERZIAN, H. and DALLE ORE, G. (1955). Syndrome of Klüver and Bucy reproduced in man by bilateral removal of the temporal lobes. *Neurology (Minneap.)*, **5**, 373–380.

WADA, J. and RASMUSSEN, T. (1960). Intracarotid injection of sodium amytal for the lateralization of cerebral speech dominance. *J. Neurosurg.*, **17**, 266–282.

WALSH, E. G. (1958). Anatomy of alpha rhythm generators studied by multiple channel cross correlation. *Electroenceph. clin. Neurophysiol.*, **10**, 121–129.

WALTER, W. G. (1967). Electrical signs of association, expectancy and decision in the human brain. *Electroenceph clin. Neurophysiol.*, supple., **25**, 258–263.

WALTER, W. G., COOPER, R., ALDRIDGE, V. J., McCALLUM, W. C. and WINTER, A. L. (1964). Contingent negative variation: an electric sign of sensori-motor association and expectancy in the human brain. *Nature*, **203**, 380–384.

WILLIAMS, D. (1965). The thalamus and epilepsy. *Brain*, **88**, 539–556.

WOODBURY, J. W. (1965). Potentials in a Volume Conductor. In: *Physiology and Biophysics*. Ed. Ruch, T. C. and Patton, H. D. Philadelphia: Saunders.

YOUNG, J. Z. (1961). Learning and discrimination in the octopus. *Biol. Rev.*, 36, 32–96.

YOUNG, J. Z. (1965). Croonian Lecture. The organization of a memory system. *Proc. Roy. Soc. Ser. B.*, **163**, 285–320.

YOUNG, J. Z. (1966). *The Memory System of the Brain*. London: Oxford University Press.

INDEX